DESIGN
the Dream

A Veterinarian's Preconstruction Primer

DESIGN
the Dream

A Veterinarian's Preconstruction Primer

Thomas E. Catanzaro, DVM, MHA, FACHE

Insights by veterinary-specific architects

Daniel D. Chapel, AIA
Tony L. Cochrane, AIA
Lawrence A. Gates, AIA
Paul Gladysz, AIA, CSI
Mark R. Hafen, AIA, NCARB
Sam Salahi, AIA
Mark J. Schmidt, AIA
Wayne Usiak, AIA

Working appendices by veterinary-specific consultants

Steve Amsberry, DVM
Robert W. Deegan, DVM
Thom A. Haig, DVM

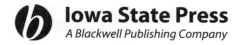

Iowa State Press
A Blackwell Publishing Company

Thomas E. Catanzaro, DVM, MHA, FACHE, Diplomate, American College of Healthcare Executives, received his DVM from Colorado State University and his master's in healthcare administration from Baylor University. Dr. Catanzaro was the first veterinarian to receive board certification with the American College of Healthcare Executives. Dr. Catanzaro has the largest veterinary-exclusive, diplomate-led veterinary consulting team in the United States. He is the author of the *Building the Veterinary Practice* series and eight veterinary practice management books, most published by Iowa State Press.

© 2003 Iowa State Press
A Blackwell Publishing Company
All rights reserved

Iowa State Press
2121 State Avenue, Ames, Iowa 50014

Orders: 1-800-862-6657
Office: 1-515-292-0140
Fax: 1-515-292-3348
Web site: www.iowastatepress.com

Authorization to photocopy items for internal or personal use, or the internal or personal use of specific clients, is granted by Iowa State Press, provided that the base fee of $.10 per copy is paid directly to the Copyright Clearance Center, 222 Rosewood Drive, Danvers, MA 01923. For those organizations that have been granted a photocopy license by CCC, a separate system of payments has been arranged. The fee code for users of the Transactional Reporting Service is 0-8138-2922-4/2003 $.10.

♾ Printed on acid-free paper in the United States of America

First edition, 2003

Library of Congress Cataloging-in-Publication Data

Design the dream: a veterinarian's preconstruction primer / [edited by]
Thomas E. Catanzaro; insights by veterinary-specific architects, Daniel D.
Chapel . . . [et al.]; working appendices by veterinary-specific
consultants, Steve Amsberry . . . [et al.].—1st ed.
    p. cm.
Includes bibliographical references.
   ISBN 0-8138-2922-4 (alk. paper)
   1. Veterinary hospitals—Designs and plans. I. Catanzaro, Thomas E.
   SF604.7.D47 2003
   725'.592—dc21
                           2003001004

The last digit is the print number: 9 8 7 6 5 4 3 2 1

Contents

Preface

THIS REFERENCE was conceived and developed as a prearchitect primer text. Many of the veterinary-specific architects were gracious enough to provide insightful chapters discussing the pros and cons of the critical path planning considerations involved in the decision and commitment for veterinary practice remodel, upgrade, and/or new construction. The practical application appendices were developed to offer insights by the consulting team of Veterinary Practice Consultants®, who have visited over 2,500 hospitals in the past decade. The American Animal Hospital Association (AAHA) *Design Starter Kit for Veterinary Hospitals,* third edition, is still the landmark prearchitect design reference, but *Design the Dream* is intended to provide the narratives and planning perspectives to expand and clarify the AAHA set of design planning ideas. As the principal author of this reference, I was committed to bringing the industry leaders together and sharing their perspectives in a single prearchitect text, to ensure each potential veterinary practice could access the needed resources before investing future earnings.

As an evolutionary perspective, I was trained in architecture before medical administration and was a healthcare administrator before becoming a veterinarian. Over a decade after veterinary school graduation, I was also trained as a facility planner as part of my Baylor University healthcare administration master's degree program and must pass boards (oral and written) every five years to stay certified. The veterinary-specific consultants are beneficial to a practice's perspective by keeping the "form follows function" approach in the forefront. End-of-chapter summaries add the consultant's perspective to the architect's advice, allowing the reader to have a balanced approach to the prearchitect process. The bibliography lists all texts cited in this book along with other useful references.

The authors are the best of the best. They care enough to share their knowledge in a public domain text that can be used by their less-knowledgeable regional and local competitors. This sharing starts the joining process that is critical for bringing colleagues together again. It helps the veterinarian understand a complex subject that is seldom taught, never explained, and usually approached only once in a career. I sincerely appreciate the contributions of these authors and hope that each reader visits them in some veterinary exhibit hall and says thank you for sharing.

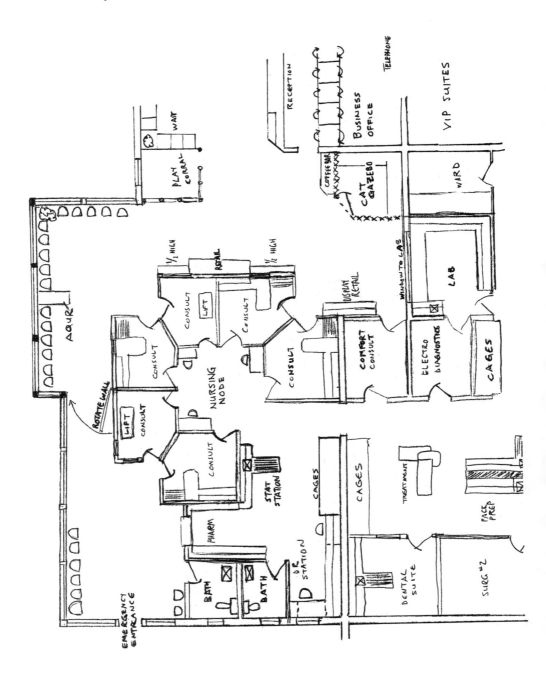

Introduction: Even in Veterinary Practices, Form Follows Function

The doctor can bury his mistakes but an architect can only advise his client to plant vines.

Frank Lloyd Wright

IT HAS BEEN a revelation to me, as a practice consultant who has visited over 1,500 veterinary hospitals in the past decade, to see how practices try to adapt to a facility that no longer fits their style or the expectations of clients. The concept of practice consultants, accountants, interior design specialists, and architects working as a team to tailor a facility to a specific practice philosophy and practice style has come of age; to do less is to ignore the future potential of a practice and limit the associated growth of liquidity.

Use all the methods analytical,
Bring every detail into play;
Planning just to please the critical
Can cause the team to lose their way.

The practice *must* control the architectural engagement, from the description of needs, to the wish list, to the practice habits. For instance, some practitioners prefer center islands for working on animals, some want peninsulas, and now with Occupational Safety and Health Administration (OSHA) and smaller staff members, most want lift tables in treatment as well as in the consultation rooms. In production practices, the chute system must have a squeeze and head catch. Are there physical limitations that must be considered in your practice? These limitations might include

- open architecture—client through-view in selected areas
- visibility of cages/run patients from the treatment room

- boutique and pet resort ambiance
- reduction of hallways and single-use circulation spaces (expensive)
- nasal oxygen, IV pump space, cardiac monitoring access, etc.
- surgery suite and isolation units visible from treatment
- imaging space capable of X-ray, ultrasound, endoscope, and ECG procedures
- nursing nodes for high-density scheduling support
- computer technology, CRT/LCD hardware, software integration points
- medical record legal sufficiency and access
- staff and client amenities
- security at parking and access, prescreening before admission to facility, alarms, etc.

Build a team of advisors who will give you what you need and want, and beware of symmetry demands by anyone, especially the architect who wants the outside to look good *before* determining the inside function!

> **Zoned Systems and Schedules**
> In *Zoned Systems & Schedules for Multi-Doctor Practices*, the modern methods of staff utilization and the new delivery methods are discussed (available from www.v-p-c.com). It is assumed that anyone reading this text has assessed high-density scheduling for their practice concurrent with the use of veterinary extenders to leverage the primary provider's time and control facility operations.

Prebuilding concerns are more than the capital available and the quality of the blueprints. The environment (catchment area) must have a quantitative set of forecasts developed to predict the pet ownership trends, the purchasing trends of the community, the zoning parameters and subsequent site selection to capitalize on household locations, and transition planning (getting away from the old facility and old habits). A traditional site model formula for most general companion animal practice situations is often

$(1 \times \text{access}) + (3 \times \text{visibility}) + (5 \times \text{population}) + \text{practice constants} =$ site quality

while the formula for an urgent care (emergency) practice or specialty practice should describe reality, such as

# of referring full-time equivalent (FTE) doctors + cost of occupancy
+ practice constants = site quality

If your practice has been dealing with the "big boys," the consolidators of this industry, you have heard about "EBITDA" (net earnings before interest, taxes, depreciation, amortization, and owner goodies). Gross and growth are the keys to practice resale value with the consolidators. The success target is 16–20 percent of gross income, and the practice value is

$\text{EBITDA} \times 5 = \text{practice value}$

The first bottom-line question: Will the front door swing as often as needed because of what we are doing for the community? Veterinary companion animal practices have become more complex and facilities need to address the trends of the future, to include

- need for sixty million dollars of community income per FTE doctor in catchment area
- need for a population of 4,000 per FTE doctor in catchment area
- need for a pet population of 1,500–2,000 per FTE doctor in catchment area
- number of owners (if more than one, governance structures are needed)
- building and land ownership
- equipment limited liability company (LLC)/corporate structure
- administrative leadership versus chief of professional services leadership (healthcare)
- production per square foot of existing facility prior to construction
- staff man-hours per transaction (1.3 is usually effective staff utilization)
- doctor man-hours per transaction (0.33 is usually very effective)
- Less-expensive office space "upstairs" or use of basement for temperature control
- gross income production required to exceed building and land cost within three years in new facility

The addendum to the bottom-line question: Will the front door swing as often as needed because of what we are doing for the other practices in the community? Veterinary urgent care (emergency) practices have become more complex and facilities need to address the trends of the future, to include

- need for twenty-three to twenty-six referring veterinarians in a stand-alone emergency facility
- reduced general practice referral rate when colocated with daytime specialists
- need for a population of over 100,000 in the primary catchment area
- reduced population criteria when colocated with daytime specialists
- twenty-four-hour (24/7) critical-care services without disruption of other specialists
- multiworkstation treatment area with closely available stat lab capabilities
- Internet access for literature review services to referring practices
- training space for adjunctive benefits for referring practices
- shift access/parking security, including video monitors and alarm services
- telephone referral support, including automatic forwarding for referring practices
- security of dispensing pharmacy and safety in consultation rooms
- doctor and nursing stations within the facility flow instead of office isolation
- boardroom for shareholders to set policy and precedent

Whether planning a new general practice, a merged practice complex, an urgent care (emergency) facility, or just making a few minor adjustments, the long-range plan of the practice must be clearly identified. Realistic goals must be established for a balanced cash flow that matches the wants and needs of the staff, veterinarian(s), and ownership. This simple concept is where most practice owners find indecision the rule; they don't know where they want to be in five to ten years, much less what kind of facility or practice they want to get them to that point. There are four reasons for this indecision:

1. Every veterinarian is a product of accumulated practice bias, from those who taught us in veterinary school to those who have hired us in our quest for independence. Some of this bias has caused practice methods that will require specific facility arrangements to remain functionally effective, while other bias reduces the effectiveness of an emergency hospital.
2. The perfect facility for all veterinarians has never been found; while open architecture has great benefits for healthcare delivery, it has reduced client comfort aspects associated with it (e.g., noise control). The alternatives depend on patient needs, client expectations, staff development, and state-of-the-art techniques that can be incorporated into a specific practice philosophy.
3. There are very few doctors who can afford to build a true "total service" veterinary facility in today's economy, and very few localities that can support such a facility. Cobalt therapy, CAT scans, nuclear magnetic resonance imaging (NMRI), and similar emerging diagnostic and treatment capabilities have not developed the client demand and payment capability to support the services.
4. Building a larger, more complex, expanded service facility, by definition, is something the practitioner has *never* done; this void of knowledge would make anyone hesitant to step off boldly into the unknown.

The role of governance is a major concern in facility planning when there is more than one owner or one fiscal entity involved. In these multileader cases, a governance board structure is required for best results. While the board must approve the plans, review the budget projections, and physically sign for the expenditure commitment(s), the actual operators need to be the hospital administrator and project coordinator (governance concerns and administrator utilization are discussed in detail in *Veterinary Management in Transition: Preparing for the Twenty-First Century*).

Don't Kill Your Dream—Just Execute It!

Feasibility studies must include an assessment of staff capabilities as well as demographic considerations. Budgets and practice philosophies for a new "joint enterprise" seldom are compatible in the initial planning steps, especially with governance boards comprised of shareholders who have never been urgent care (emergency) veterinarians or true landlords, nor trained as board members. The preliminary design begins by addressing space utilization—exclusive versus primary versus shared access—and often addresses what you want versus what you can afford. Many architects use hallways and walls to define space, rather than require board credentialing of the clinical participants; the latter allows a tighter and more cost-effective emergency/specialty practice facility.

Potential uses must be realistically evaluated. Income centers and joint tenants must be assessed to determine profit potentials compared to space allocations. Economy of scale considerations often mean looking at facility-owned equipment in joint-use space rather than service-controlled equipment in exclusive-use space. Concurrently, in the central hospital, affiliation, or joint-use veterinary model, neighborhood outpatient veterinary facilities need to be seen as daytime space users and colleagues rather than access competitors.

Unlike building your first mom-and-pop practice facility, larger complexes actually show that the selection of a contractor can be mediated by hiring a knowledgeable healthcare facility contract manager, and the quality of previous construction efforts by each contractor must be evaluated before hiring the low bidder. Tying contractor payments to percent completion often causes time and quality to conflict, but it is the recommended technique if you have an adequate quality assurance system in place.

In renovations and expansions of existing facilities, sequencing of construction is critical to ensure practice liquidity is maintained. Remodeling is not just done during the slow time for the practice. Effective sequencing requires a team effort by the owner and architect to ensure cost-effective construction, which is why veterinarians have such a problem. Very few architects understand the demands and needs of a veterinary healthcare emergency facility; human healthcare facility standards are too high and residential standards are too low, which is why veterinary-specific architects have emerged as a benefit to this profession. The transition planning must provide a template for change, to include

- developing an actual flow plan of clients and patients as well as staff
- review of equipment requirements compared to practice capabilities of the future
- planning the premove demands of healthcare delivery and housekeeping
- evaluating the marketing requirements and community information plan
- revision of the practice literature/image, from business cards to client handouts
- training programs for the staff, with a realistic schedule for completion
- psychological issues associated with change management and human acceptance
- move management control factors, clear responsibilities, and accountabilities
- installation and start-up operations, within assigned troubleshooting authority
- postoccupancy problem solving when the facility fails to operate as expected

When I wrote the AAHA *Design Starter Kit for Veterinary Hospitals,* third edition, I stated clearly that practices needed to conduct a staff orientation to the design intent—a walk-through of the drawings with the staff, explaining how to read the plans and discussing the design intent of each area. I forgot to tell veterinarians to listen to their team, to promote discussion of alternatives by the people who will actually use the areas. Maybe that is why the top level of most all cage banks is high-quality stainless steel storage areas, or why there is never enough storage space for all the supplies the veterinarian wants to have on hand. Maybe that is why a doctor's lounge is planned before the staff break area, or why there is no place for staff to eat or take a quick break and have a cup of coffee. This may be the reason some reception areas are sequestered behind an island counter, where receptionists are unable to assist the senior citizen (a population that is growing five times faster than any other demographic group), or why there are inadequate patient movement aides (e.g., scissor gurney, stretchers, etc.) close to the front door for hit by car (HBC) emergencies, or even inadequate Internet communication or computer capabilities within the operational areas.

So the Integration of Many Occurs

The goal of this book is to inform the practice manager/administrator, board member, facility planning team, and veterinarian of the process, pitfalls, and terminology of veterinary facility programming and design. The process of planning, building, or renovating is highly technical and, to the uninitiated, often fraught with problems. This book is intended to explain the programming and design of veterinary healthcare facilities in sufficient detail to establish a common language and understanding between architects and engineers on the one hand and veterinarians and practice managers/administrators on the other. The process of creating a new building, or altering an existing one, is described from conception to construction initiation.

Initially, the need for thorough planning by and for the facility is considered. The plans and programs of a veterinary-specific facility set the facility's future and are the key to its survival and growth in a demanding marketplace. Long-range building concepts, including the incorporation of current structures, the mechanical energy plant, and site potential and phasing, establish the future of the physical facility for the next twenty years. Careful planning by veterinarians, managers/administrators, and outside consultants can assure not only the financial viability of the practice but also its survival vis-à-vis regulatory agencies. For these reasons, the first topics addressed in this book are the need for planning and the different levels of planning.

This complex process requires the integration of a wide variety of professionals into a planning team. Members of the practice staff and technical experts need to work together to create the new programs, a new facility flow, and an actual structure to support them. The issues of who should be on the planning team, what such a team does, when it is needed, and how it operates are considered. The various types of consultants needed for facility programming and design are described, as are their skills and expertise. Technical planning and design services include architects and engineers (civil, structural, mechanical, and electrical) plus value management services, equipment specialists, and construction management. The bidding process is defined and appropriate construction management discussed. In addition, pricing design is presented and its value to the institution considered.

Initial planning considerations are then presented: What general physical plan is being considered; how the current physical plant is to be incorporated; what the space requirements, cost constraints, time schedules, and codes and standards that must be included are.

These efforts are then brought together in overall facility design development. Issues that cross facility zone lines are included. Traffic, movement of patients and materials, communication flow, parking, site, and needs for adjacent space must all be incorporated into systems and processes that are designed to integrate them.

Construction of the facility requires the development of working drawings and specifications based on programming and design. The legal relationships among the client, architect, and general contractor are defined. The actual construction, including changes and inspections, is the final step in the production of the building and varies with each municipality, so it is covered only in planning consideration terms in this text.

Throughout the process, the practice team must consider the larger community it serves (including the trends of the community as seen by city and county planners, long-term master plans and plots, plus street expansions, parks, and man-made geographic barriers planned for the future) and should take the time to solicit public support for the expansion or construction efforts. Good public relations are invaluable. Groundbreaking and opening ceremonies are an excellent opportunity to reach the public. A council of clients is usually available from existing clients and could be developed from homeowner groups when it is a new practice in a new area (see *Building the Successful Veterinary Practice: Volume 3: Innovation and Creativity* for the details on a council of clients).

Planning any facility for animal needs must focus on the population to be served. The patients, the species and their characteristics, and the past professional experiences in previous veterinary facilities should be described and included in the design if the habits are essential to ease of use; bringing bad habits into new construction can cause dysfunctional plans (e.g., excessive hallways in specialty hospitals due to academic veterinary teaching hospital [VTH] experiences of specialists). In a healing institution, aesthetic as well as physical and emotional needs of the staff and providers are important to the eventual patient outcome; the layout of public areas greatly affects patient, client, and family impressions of value and competence.

The details of operational programming for zone needs are considered next. Utilization and planning ratios determine the site and flow of each zone, based on federal guidelines and the author's architectural and consulting experience. These requirements include not only floor space but also relationships within the practice zone and with other zones. In addition, zones vary in their need for equipment, spatial efficiency, and patient or staff amenities.

Interior design defines furnishing, finishes, and general appearance of the building's interior. It is especially important in public and patient areas because there it affects the person's facility. This often requires a layout and color specialist who is not in the practice. The interior design should have a five-year accent change plan included. Thoughtful interior design can also increase staff efficiency and satisfaction.

The process of creating a new facility, or a new section of a facility, is long and complex. The many steps and resources available are described here in sufficient detail to enable those not trained in architecture or construction to understand and use the programming and design process to produce the most appropriate facility for their specific needs.

The First Rule of Architecture

Whether evaluating the interior or exterior of a facility, *form must follow function*. Many architects require a symmetry of exterior design, regardless of the interior needs; sometimes this is demanded by community zoning regulations, but more often it is only an architectural bias. Some architects require a treatment room island although the practitioner prefers a peninsula; most have never even assessed an urgent care, emergency, or specialty practice for appropriate patient flow. There are some architects who have seen the veterinary facility plans of the 1970s that separate reception of cats from dogs and large examination room systems with small treatment areas and minimal cages; they feel that is best for a veterinary practice. Worse, they design a special use veterinary practice with minimal consideration of the emerging lessons learned for out-of-hours, expanded daytime services, and/or joint usage by specialists. As with computer systems, whenever the seller (architect or contractor) states that *"the practice flow only has to change a little,"* it should send a red flag up warning the buyer that the seller is not capable of tailoring a product to fit the practice's need. These discussions are needed, but after the design or construction facts are laid out and the costs are understood, the practice function must be able to dictate the form. For this reason, the "Insights and Perspectives" following this introduction are from someone at an average practice instead of from an architect as in the other chapters; this perception is why we decided we needed to write this text.

Some simple statements that may help to evaluate design concepts:

Good architecture lets nature in. (Mario Pei)
Clients want a warm and inviting reception, in space as well as staff.
The client areas are an opportunity to market by presentation alone.
Form follows function. (Frank Lloyd Wright)
Without competing price quotes, you will always pay too much.
When someone charges you by a percentage of construction costs, why should they help conserve your spending?!

And one final thought on veterinary architecture, design, facility form, function, equipment, and material concerns:

It's not cheaper things that we want to possess,
But expensive things that cost a lot less.

Insights and Perspectives

Building a New Facility—The Dream Becoming a Reality
A typical practice manager

I recall when I first became involved in building the new veterinary facility, it was exciting, almost like a childhood adventure. We planned and talked for hours about how we were going to build it, what it would look like, the equipment, how it would flow, and the various areas that we would incorporate. It would be unlike any other hospital! At the same time I noticed a slight feeling of intimidation, as I had never been in charge of helping to actually build a new hospital. I was very aware of the enormous cost and the consequences my lack of experience might bring. The purpose of this article is not to defame the individuals who were a part of our experience, but rather to show the hurdles I encountered moving through this process. I hope others may learn from my experience and be better equipped to identify problems as they begin to arise, rather than finding themselves amid confusion and frustration, costing thousands of dollars . . . and trying to figure out what to do.

We started with veterinary-specific architects and had some learning curve experiences. One architect out east made it very clear that he did not respect a woman's thoughts and played the "big man" in design. The veterinary-specific architects closer to us were nice but would not do a design-build veterinary facility (they talked about a conflict of interest and a lack of checks and balances), but they were more than happy to advise us on the contractor selection and provide periodic on-site oversight. We wanted more. We sought out a veterinary practice consultant who seemed to have some design and construction experience (he wrote the AAHA *Design Starter Kit,* and we used the second and third editions during our planning).

When I came into the project, it had already been in process for three years by the practice owner (we were building a new facility in the vicinity of our existing, overcrowded, old but trustworthy, little clinic). I started by going through the political issues such as zoning, city annexation, and neighborhood meetings. When we had the very first design-build phase by a nonveterinary architectural firm, we still had Tom Cat as our consultant, and asked him to come in and help design the flow of the floor plan in detail. We had what we felt was a nice design for the hospital and a basic layout for the boarding facility. At this point we were looking at a total of 24,000 sq. ft. and approximately a $2.6 million budget. We were very happy with the progress at this point, but the company informed us that they normally work on much larger projects and would not be able to go any further with our project as it was too small.

We made arrangements with another nonveterinary architect and design-builder and began the process all over, negotiating contracts, going through the initial design phase, and laying out the floor plans. In the beginning it seemed fine. We had several meetings where we went over in detail what we wanted, what we felt our standards were, ideas pertaining to the flow of the floor plan, the quality that we were anticipating, a description of the two-story boarding facility, and the general appearance of the building. We then began to notice that there seemed to be confusion regarding the quality level of the facility and the specific materials that we would use. We requested that they visit a few other hospitals in the area that we felt represented the quality we were looking for. They had never built a veterinary hospital before or dealt with a boarding facility, let alone a two-story boarding facility. As we began discussing gutters, various floor drains, and the slopes necessary for proper drainage, there seemed to be a great deal of confusion. Again we suggested they come out and look at our existing facility. We gave several other recommendations, drew pictures and diagrams, and explained in detail. Again . . . we went to the next meeting, and it was as if they did not comprehend a word we said; at this point we began to feel frustrated. We tried once again to explain what we wanted, and again recommended that they visit our boarding facility and others to form a concept of how to design and build this aspect of the project.

We began to express a feeling of concern among ourselves and tried to figure out how we could help them to understand what we were looking for. Again . . . the next meeting that we had with the structural engineers, plumbers, and electricians, we went into detail about the boarding facility. The architect was drawing pictures for the builder and explaining it in a variety of ways. The structural engineers were discussing the different possibilities for how it might be done. We thought, all right! They finally got it. They understand. We relaxed, felt a surge of enthusiasm, and anxiously awaited our next meeting to see the drawings.

It was during our next meeting that we would be going over the pro forma for the first time. When we first revised the pricing structure, our working budget was now up to four million, according to the design-build architect firm. This was a bit of a shock. Again we sent the bid to Tom Cat, who reviewed the projected construction numbers and went back to the design-build architect firm with his estimate of $2.26 million, rounded up to $2.5 million for contingency planning. The design-build architect firm immediately (within twenty-four hours) said they were overly conservative and it really should have been bid at $2.5 million (concurrently, the architecture portion of the design bid went from $400,000 to $226,000, on itemized bidding). We tried to remain open-minded as we went into the next phase, thinking that we would be getting the materials that we had specifically requested. But as we began reviewing it, this was not the case. They told us that we couldn't build it within our budget without using cheaper materials. When we got to the boarding facility, we were absolutely shocked to discover they had designed and priced out a one-story facility and the floor drains were completely wrong. When we questioned this, the project manager acted as if he didn't even know we were talking about a two-story facility. We were beside ourselves! I felt as though I was in a nightmare; I could not believe what I was hearing and seeing! After we became visibly upset, he also told us that we couldn't build a two-story boarding facility because it wasn't structurally sound. We left this meeting in total dismay, wondering what we were going to do.

We decided to call and discuss how we felt with the architect the next day. We requested a meeting to talk about it. At first he expressed his feelings of dissatisfaction with the project manager and said that he too was stunned by his attitude and the comments he had made, although he was defensive and appeared very frustrated by the fact that we were upset. We then called the owner of the firm and requested a meeting. After talking with him in detail about our experience with his company, he appeared concerned and said that he wanted to check it out and get back with us. We agreed.

He called a couple of days later and set up a meeting. When we attended the meeting, he stated that he was standing by his project manager and would be keeping him on the job. The architect became visibly upset and shook his head, but was silent. We stated that while we appreciated their position, we would not be working with them. We left the meeting in dismay, again wondering what we would do.

To further complicate matters, our bank representative was not responding to repeated calls; we found out he had left the company. We were assigned a new representative, who came out to introduce himself and appeared to be ready to move forward with us. Two weeks later we learned he had also left the company. We were assigned a third rep. A few weeks into this relationship, he began asking us for paperwork we had given to the company some time ago. We inquired as to whether or not he had our files and was aware of our situation. He reluctantly informed us that they had lost all of our paperwork during the personnel transfers, so we had to resubmit all our financial information. They then informed us that they would not be able to offer us the same deal we had with the previous representative. Again, we became very weary. What did this mean? We were already into a half-million-dollar loan only to find out they could not guarantee us financing?

We then decided to use a design-builder who specialized in veterinary hospitals. We had picked up information from a conference we had attended and decided to give them a call. This company seemed very interested in the project and agreed to fly out and talk with us. We expressed our reservations about the previous builders, of their not being concerned or giving any kind of priority to our project. I expressed to the principals that I did not have experience in coordinating a building project and would need their help in keeping me informed of anything that was necessary for me to take care of. I was concerned by their out-of–state location, but they assured me that it would not be a problem. They would fly in regularly for meetings, and if anything was required of me, they would inform me and give me explicit instructions. We felt that they were competent and would be concerned about doing a good job, as they were trying to build their reputation in the veterinary field. Once again . . . we started the process over.

We began the design phase using the initial footprint previously developed and expanding on it. As we went through the design phase, they started with an initial "water hazard and tree obstacle course" design that would win awards and drown any kids, cats, or small dogs, but after a few reviews and exchanges (including using our consultant as leverage with them), we had a plan and all seemed well. They seemed to have good ideas, and we finally came up with what we felt was a good design. We set the budget at our previous "high level" of $3.4 million, and appeared to be in that arena. At this point a liaison was introduced as taking over our project, and I was informed that all communication would go through him. We then began the process of submitting paperwork to the city for approval. At this point it became apparent to me that it was going to be my responsibility to coordinate the architect and contractors, set the deadlines, put together all the plans, and actually go down and do the submittals. After the city responded, I would fax all the comments to the various contractors and send copies of the redlines to our liaison. It also became apparent at this point that our liaison was somewhat confused, as every time I would ask him questions he wasn't sure. He would state that he would get back with me, which, ultimately, he seldom did. We started having problems with the plans we were submitting—they had a lot of minor, repeated mistakes. Some of these mistakes had to do with simply not communicating with the other contractors making submittals and coordinating their blueprints. We also began noticing that some of their costs seemed to be off and their projections did not represent large portions of hidden costs, specifically in the site costs and landscaping. I began questioning our liaison about these, and he didn't even know enough about the project or the pricing to respond to my questions. He kept saying he would have to find out, but would never call me back. When I asked about it again, he would say he forgot and would have to find out, again.

The bank continued to request a variety of information documents; every time we gave them something, they would request more. Then they wanted projections; we gave them projections. Then they wanted three-year projections. Then they decided they wanted them done professionally. Then they wanted a revised business plan. Then they wanted current financial information . . . then . . . and it went on and on!

The contractors began telling me that our liaison was not communicating with them and wanted me to ask him questions. I began frequent phone calls to tell our liaison that he needed to talk to people. He needed to provide them with information and site plans and agree upon a schedule to help meet the deadlines. It began to get frustrating at this point, as we were never meeting with the architects to review or discuss concerns with the project. Multiple direct phone calls to the architects went unanswered, and in some cases, appeared to be ignored on purpose. Everything was done by phone, fax, or FedEx, with no flights as promised. There was no feeling of concern or urgency on their part and we received virtually no response after repeated inquiries.

Then our liaison began arguing over the deadlines for the technical review submittals, stating that he needed more time. We again called the principals to express our concerns with this liaison and the poor quality of work we were receiving from their firm. They became argumentative and defensive, stating that it was not their job to coordinate the project. During our last technical review, the liaison wanted to set deadlines back two weeks, even though he had already had four weeks to work on making any corrections necessary. I told him we needed to keep moving, and he agreed. He asked me if this was considered our second technical review because he wasn't sure what he needed to submit. It almost didn't make sense. Then as we approached the deadline, he was having a lot of trouble with very simple issues; I told him whom to call to get the answers. He then missed his deadline for FedExing the prints to me, so I told him to e-mail them and we would plot them ourselves. He did this, and we plotted and put the plans together ourselves and submitted them, only to have them once again rejected for the same reasons they were previously denied.

During my conversation with the city planner, she stated that she would not be willing to work with this liaison in the future as she was on the phone with him constantly, and he seemed as though he didn't know what was going on. She felt he was wasting her time. I then called the principals to tell them of my experience and to request someone else be put on the project. They told me they would discuss it and get back with me. A week or so later, I received a letter in the mail stating they had reorganized the project, and that the liaison would be heading it up and they had complete confidence in his ability to handle the job. I couldn't believe it! A letter! Not even so much as a phone call? I felt almost scared at this point. This was our whole life, our livelihood. This was a very big deal to us and they were dismissing it as though it were insignificant. I had lost my trust in them. I wondered, if this is what we are experiencing at this point, what's it going to be like when they actually start to build it? What will we go through then?

I expressed concern that they were not giving our project any priority and had fallen behind on the schedule. I then requested that they send me copies of all the work that they had done up to that point so I could evaluate where they were on the project. It took them several days to get copies of their work to me. I felt as though they were scrambling to put things together during this time.

After careful consideration, we decided to terminate our contract. I drew up and sent them a letter stating our intentions. We were already $140,000 into the project with them, and were looking at the possibility of having to start over. Naturally, they began to demand payment for what they felt we owed them. During this process they claimed that we had no rights to any of the work that we had paid for, and that they owned full copyright. We could not use any of it without their permission. $140,000 wasted! At this point, we felt discouraged and drained of energy. We had no enthusiasm left for what was once our dream! We felt like quitting! It didn't seem worth it anymore; the emotional letdown was almost heartbreaking.

We then picked up and once again moved forward. We went back to the first company we started with, which by this time had a new department that worked on smaller jobs, and they resumed our dream. It was during this time that we discovered our last architects had seriously underbid the project by $1.4 million and had hidden over $700,000 in costs. If we had continued working with them and used their pro forma to obtain our bank loan we would have never been able to finish the project. So, as these things usually go, it was a blessing in disguise.

As we continued the process with our original design-build company, we went in with our knowledge far advanced from our previous encounters of the bizarre kind; all appeared to be going well. Throughout the design phase and all of the city submittals, I haven't had to take action. We have regular meetings and they keep us abreast of what's going on and provide us with information we need to make decisions. Now, however, we are looking at financing. The original design-build firm's bid was $3.4 million, talked down to $2.5 million, but was now up to $4.6 million. We had to do some serious rethinking to bring it back into the $3.4 million ballpark. Now the bank has denied financing, and we are going through the stages of applying at multiple banks, submitting endless paperwork, and divulging personal information to massive institutions.

But . . . what the heck . . . what you learn is you have to play it like a game! If things don't work out, you pull back, regroup, think it through, form a new strategy, and try a different approach. While I admit I do not have nearly the excitement and enthusiasm I started with, I do have a strange sense of calm and feel as though I am truly in control, not of them or what they do, but of how I choose to interact!

I don't ever want to be the type of person who criticizes or tears people down to make a point, although it needs to be made. I believe people create their own karma and live on the reputation they build by their actions and the kind of integrity with which they live their life. While I cannot change who they are or how they choose to do business, I fully control how *I* conduct myself and how *I* choose to do business. The real challenge is that no matter how positive you are, if surrounded by negative people they will bring you down to their level. Our perception of life . . . like happiness . . . is a choice, not a defined set of circumstances.

We are continuing, and though this has certainly been a long, arduous learning experience, we *will* build our new hospital!

Ms. L.G., design school of hard knocks graduate

Tom Cat's "Form Follows Function" Review Issues

- Every fifteen minutes of planning saves over an hour of implementation time.
- On-site urgent care services are only needed from seven to eleven in a general practice—and you can always charge extra for urgent care.
- Nothing replaces client service!
- Transition into a new facility starts a year before the move—get professional planning help for this task.
- A new outside practice image usually brings in 15 percent new business.
- Plumbing and heating, ventilation, and air-conditioning (HVAC) will be over 30 percent of the construction budget—ensure a reputable subcontractor.
- Caring providers are confident patient advocates—two "yes" options.
- Three consultation rooms per outpatient doctor allows greater access and higher productivity—a doctor station behind each three-room group helps.
- High-tech planning requires high-touch delivery.
- Staff leveraging requires a practice culture based on continuous quality improvement and recurring training programs—plan the space to allow this.
- Hospital zoning is required to use larger facilities effectively.
- Companion animal veterinary facility demographic profiles parallel dry cleaners, stand-alone drug stores, and day care centers—car counts are virtually worthless in suburban and urban environments.
- Cats usually do not like dogs, but separate doors are not required.
- Personal liquidity of the owner will decrease from the first moment of planning to at least two years after occupancy—just plan on this fact of life and tighten your personal spending belt.
- Connected cat condos allow cross sell of empty units during slower times.
- Very important pet (VIP) suites start at six feet by eight feet, are usually eight feet by eight feet with half doors, and include high-touch care (frequent walks)—you can charge significantly for this service too (more than forty dollars per night per animal).
- Male practitioners seldom select the appropriate colors for a facility.
- Form follows function. Design the facility without walls before drawing the first line—know what you need and how it needs to work for you!
- Use a veterinary-specific consultant to "align" architects who do not listen.
- When the first floor plan is sketched, put onion skin paper over it and give each staff member a different colored pencil to trace their daily travels—look for congestion points and walking spaces, as well as access to storage areas.

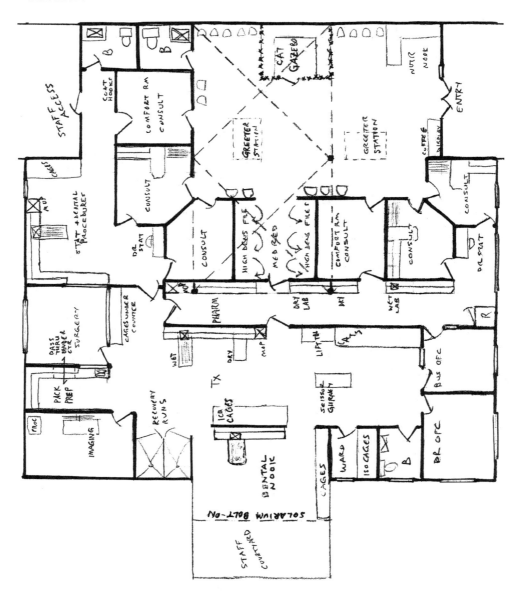

Retro-fit laboratory ~4,800 sq. ft.

Contributors

Architects

Daniel D. Chapel, AIA
  Chapel Associates Architects,
    Inc.
  8201 Cantrell Rd., Suite 360
  Little Rock, AR 72227-2453
  501-225-5900
Tony L. Cochrane, AIA
  Gates Hafen Cochrane
    Architects, PC
  735 Walnut St.
  Boulder, CO 80302
  303-444-4413
  www.GHCArch.com
Lawrence A. Gates
  Gates Hafen Cochrane
    Architects, PC
  735 Walnut St.
  Boulder, CO 80302
  303-444-4413
  www.GHCArch.com
Paul Gladysz, AIA, CSI
  BDA Architecture
  9016 Washington St. NE
  Albuquerque, NM 87113
  505-858-0180
  www.BDAArc.com

Mark R. Hafen, AIA, NCARB
  Gates Hafen Cochrane
    Architects, PC
  735 Walnut St.
  Boulder, CO 80302
  303-444-4413
  www.GHCArch.com
Sam Salahi, AIA
  Architectural Planning and
    Service Limited
  1080 Cherrywood
  West Chicago, IL 60185
  630-876-5357
  S.Salahi@worldnet.att.net
Mark J. Schmidt, AIA
  Knapp Schmidt Architects
  2809 Fish Hatchery Road #201
  Madison, WI 53713-5020
  608-271-0140
  MJSarchitect@aol.com
Wayne Usiak, AIA, NCARB
  BDA Architecture
  9016 Washington St. NE
  Albuquerque, NM 87113
  505-858-0180
  www.BDAArc.com

Veterinary Practice Consultants® Authors

Steve Amsberry, DVM
Thomas E. Catanzaro, DVM, MHA, FACHE
Robert W. Deegan, DVM
Thom A. Haig, DVM
Catanzaro & Associates, Inc.
   18301 West Colfax Ave. Bldg. R-101
   Golden, CO 80401
   303-277-9800
   www.v-p-c.com

DESIGN
the Dream

A Veterinarian's Preconstruction Primer

Planning Needs

1

HEALTHCARE administrators and facility planners have become the key to community human health programs and facilities in the United States. Regional planning and federal controls have supplanted the local physicians and hospital boards as primary forces in determining a community's healthcare program. In veterinary medicine we have a lot of latitude, so much, in fact, that the checks and balances are seldom in place to prevent poor planning, overspending, or contracting disasters. The veterinarian has always been the operating manager of his or her facility, but now, because of sophisticated facilities; multiple doctor ownership; and in some cases public and private financing, control of proprietary interest, major insurance controls, and reduced utilization of facilities, the veterinarian has been thrust into an expanded leadership role. In most multiple-owner, multiple-doctor, and multiple-practice entity facilities, a trained hospital administrator is needed, first as the project manager for the planning and construction, then during the transition into the new facility, and continuing as the practice administrator and implementation agent for the board (see *Veterinary Management in Transition: Preparing for the Twenty-First Century*, chapter 2, for the details on governance issues).

The veterinary profession has become more complex in the past couple of decades, with a scarce labor force to match. The healthcare administrator has a correspondingly complex management role in any practice: Every area of social need, including housing, welfare, ecology, defense, and education, is addressed in the new veterinary medical healthcare programs. Although we deal here with design and preconstruction concerns of veterinary facilities, it must be noted that a strong management and leadership team is essential to the daily functioning of a facility and must be included in expansion plans.

The process of creating a new or expanded facility begins with a plan based on the practice's history, current situation, and future projections. Each practice fills definite needs in its community, from ambulatory services to highly specialized practices. These animal health needs, along with the community's ability to pay for them, must be specified before the practice owner or governing board can commit planning and construction monies for an appropriate facility. The plan must consider all aspects of the practice's role:

1. Community plan: How does the practice fit into the broad community and county program of meeting veterinary service needs? What are potential special interest areas for the providers of the practice? What are the public health requirements? Are there bioterrorism concerns?

2. Service area (aka catchment area): Who are the people served by the practice? Where do they work and live? What are their animal healthcare needs? What is the dual income level of the families, requiring special availability/ access?

3. Patient needs: What are the present family animal health considerations (zoonotic sentinels of disease)? How many visits per year per animal is the expectation set by the practice in the client's mind? What services are needed in the community catchment area? What should be the day admission rate when the consultation room is *not* abused by doctors? What are the emerging future needs?

4. Medical staff: What prompts a doctor to join the staff? Is the hospital AAHA certified? What reasons do clients have to refer a patient to a doctor of this facility? Where do the practice's doctors live? What will be the urgent care demands on the veterinarians and staff?

5. Practice staff: What major benefits and needs are available to attract and retain a proper number of skilled staff? To attract and hold nurses/technicians? To attract and evolve the client relations staff, and maybe even telephone receptionists? To provide a nurturing environment to pet resort, boutique, and animal caretaker staff?

6. Organization: How does the chain of command and internal makeup of the organization affect the fulfillment of client, patient, and staff needs? What are the historical workload demands within each zone of the practice? The projected costs of the future workload demands within each zone of the practice?

7. Physical plant: What is the current size, location, and cost of the existing facility? What is its probable future use of the facility? If it is a new facility in a new location, what are the full time equivalent (FTE) demands of the catchment area? What will differentiate this practice facility in the client's mind? Is there room for expansion later, and do the new renovation/construction plans make provision for future expansion(s)?

8. Financial feasibility: Can the client payments and other practice funds cover new construction or renovation costs? Does the practice need to continue operating during the renovation? If operations must continue, must the facility have phased construction in the renovation plans? If it is an existing practice, has the building and land been exteriorized into a separate legal entity owned by an expanded family group? Has the equipment been exteriorized into a separate legal entity owned by an expanded family group? Has the construction loan "request for term sheet" to financial institutions included review of credit card rates, money market sweep accounts, contingency line of credit, self-collateralizing equipment line of credit, all separate from the base construction loan?

A variety of planning studies can be executed to aid the practice ownership. A long-range plan and facility master plan are often necessary in order for local and county regulatory agencies to grant overall approval of any specific program or space addition. The long-range plan defines the practice's role and future program goals and defines the market. The facility master plan translates the role and goals into a defined physical space plan.

The other types of studies described are unique to specific needs in further refining or implementing a long-range plan. The practice-specific plan is an integrated planning effort of current and potential veterinary practices in a community, to help define patient count needs per FTE doctor impacting the catchment area.

Long-Range Plan

The long-range or master plan covers the following areas:

- demographic study of catchment area
- study and definition of community veterinary care needs and available services
- analysis of veterinary professional staff
- organizational plan of the practice—current and proposed
- size and physical concept of current plan and future expansion plans
- environmental impact and landscape architecture proposed
- financial feasibility

This type of study defines the present service area or market, the socioeconomic characteristics, inventory of other practices in the area, present scope of problems, utilization, volume, present organization, fiscal condition, building and site limitations, and medical staff analysis. These conditions are projected into the future and form the basis for a plan. The plan, which usually covers between five and ten years, defines the practice's goals for the future. The financial portion of this plan is conceptual; it estimates what can be done. Although this plan is often referred to as the master plan or long-range plan, it amounts to a projection of goals, not specific plans for development.

Facility Master Plan

The facility master plan covers the following areas:

- site analysis
- evaluation of the existing facility utilization
- projection of new/expanded facility needs
- profile of program and service utilization present and future
- development of options in veterinary healthcare delivery
- recommended development scheme and an alternative
- energy plan based on an engineering study

– construction budget
– construction schedule

The master plan combines program goals with site and facility needs in order to plan for several phases of construction, with a long-term facility plan of about twenty years. The facility master plan presents solutions to limitations caused by growth of programs and beds or by facility condition and age. This plan should take into account

– the environmental character of the site and facility
– transportation access and parking
– topography
– soil conditions
– building datum levels
– zoning considerations and variances needed
– building age and potential
– availability and restrictions of utilities
– energy usage and condition
– functional relationships
– space assignment
– staffing characteristics
– budget considerations

Such a plan provides a guide to all remodeling and future construction; it will be the document submitted to the planning and community regulatory agencies.

The planning staff of the practice can set up a committee that, together with consultants, will frame a statement of the practice's role and goals. Such a statement should cover the following areas:

1. Practice planning roles
   mission focus
   primary goals and objectives
   inpatient holding needs and type of runs/cages
   inpatient scope of service plans
   outpatient services and consultation room programs
   ancillary services being considered
   personnel (veterinarians and staff)
   potential growth targets
   workloads, activity ratios, and space requirements
2. Review of previous plan
   master site plan
   parking and transportation access needs
   land acquisition
   affiliated, merger, or owned satellite facilities
   building potential
3. County and local regulations
   conformance to the AAHA standards (whether a member or not)

practice-specific plan review by the regulatory agencies
any joint plans with nearby practices
4. Financial feasibility
    debt and borrowing potential
    income production capabilities
    building program potential

The facility master plan is a very effective tool for all physical planning and renovation. It indicates the most cost-effective way of constructing space for short-term needs. When a particular space decision is made, the practice can see immediately what effect it will have on other zones and programs. As goals and programs change, the master plan can be adjusted. It also predicts the need for cages, runs, replacement equipment, or service base adjustments, responding to caseload projections. The master plan aids in community planning because it establishes the individual practice's target markets and operational goals.

Practice-Specific Plan

The practice-specific plan determines

– market share of the planning catchment area, defined as pets per FTE veterinarian, community income of catchment area population per FTE veterinarian, and specific potential client profiles for predicting access rates
– projected utilization based upon outpatient visits, inpatient admissions, and scope of services projected (also included are community outreach and teaching needs)
– projected impact of ancillary services (e.g., a pet resort or full-service grooming operation averages approximately 23 percent guest referrals for veterinary care)
– site and building potential and limitations

The practice-specific plan is usually developed by a veterinary-specific consultant. It is designed to integrate the individual practice's plans with those of other practice pressures impacting the catchment area. The number of patients per veterinarian in the United States ranges from 900 to 1,800 pets per veterinarian. This ratio cannot be standardized because different practices have different needs; client access varies, scope of service varies, fees vary, and return rate expectations vary. Even the weather plays a role in seasonal demands on a practice! The practice must understand what possible impact these factors can have on its plans and be prepared to make voluntary healthcare delivery adjustments.

One of the first practice-specific plans was developed by PSI for practices using its software. PSI built a computer-based model to extract data from a practice's database, in service and sales factors by practice, comparing it by type of practice and comparing it to other similar practices around the county.

This exciting model was used to develop the Practices of Excellence in the mid-1990s. In the new millennium, NCECI developed the Exam Room software for use by AAHA and AVMA members; it adjusts for differences in type of practice and size of practice, and the model provided the range of numbers for similar practices. Part of the plan was directed at practice potential, in order to allow practices to understand where they stood on the range of limitations and potential. As veterinary practice consultants, we are able to develop rating methods for specific practices and assess the functional aspects of their standards of care and scope of services, offering alternatives, developing their staff, and assessing the potential of their building(s) and site potentials and limitations. The potential of each practice can be developed and tracked when supported by a veterinary-specific consultant, which lends to projections presented to financial institutions as well as the improvement of liquidity *before* the construction phase. Each year the practice-specific budget is adjusted to veterinary healthcare delivery preferences in the specific community and picks up changes due to primary, secondary, and tertiary movement of patients to alternative community practices.

Operational Planning

Operational planning determines current and projected space needs within a facility and is necessary for productivity assessments; it is the written program for an architectural project. It also takes a look at service utilization and program concepts based upon current and projected inpatient and outpatient markets. Past and present ratios of procedures per doctor or per patient are studied, projected, and compared with national averages (average is only the worst of the best—or the best of the worst—so it should not be a practice goal). Where national numbers may suggest a ratio of ten to twenty laboratory tests per doctor per day, a practice with high-density scheduling and a trained staff for follow-up, as well as an automated clinical laboratory, may actually perform up to fifty tests per doctor per day. Staff limitations or demands as veterinary extenders when invoicing can also affect these numbers dramatically. Operational planning studies establish a zone-by-zone description of needed space ratios outlining the consultation room demand and use, number and type of surgeries, scope of imaging services, concurrent treatment room services, laboratory capabilities, and ancillary services.

In the early 1980s, AAHA tried to formulate a typical companion animal practice layout in terms of staff mix, patient care concepts, and standards of care. Client preference and practice services varied too greatly for such standardization. Any size practice may serve best in a given situation, and no typical layout can adjust to all needs. Doctor or owner bias, patient mix by services or by illness, type of utilities required, client and/or community demographics, staff availability and training levels, and various communications concepts can completely change a design. Each zone planning team needs to refer to the *AAHA Standards for Veterinary Hospitals* to determine the state of the art for basic operational data as their planning guidelines. Again, whether your practice is a member or not, this is a set of guidelines established by a board of veterinarians and therefore an industry standard. This information, in descriptive form, makes up the operational program.

Both veterinary-specific consultants and informed consulting architects can offer operational planning services; the planning can also be performed in-house if members of the staff have a diversified practice background and are well informed of the standards and regulatory requirements of the profession and community.

Functional Planning

The consulting architect should *not* dictate room-by-room square footage, while the veterinary-specific healthcare consultant should mentor a practice leadership through the options to be considered based on the practice's needs. Operational planning comes first and defines *major* needs (often we see this as bubble diagrams, but very few practitioners are happy with only the conceptual appearance). The operational plan is then developed into a functional plan, which lists every room and suggests net sizes for most rooms as well as total zone size and facility footprint (where it occupies the space on the dirt).

The key to functional planning is not just a room list but understanding that travel and adjacencies will affect operational costs for the life of the facility. The initial cost of the building is insignificant compared to the cost of running and staffing it over twenty years, sometimes eighteen to twenty times the initial cost. Therefore, no one can set the exact room sizes until concepts of space engineering and travel patterns are developed. For instance, in healthcare facility planning, an elevator (lift) is considered zero distance between floors, yet in veterinary medicine, since we are not used to elevators and multifloor facilities, we seldom consider the benefits of subsurface space or second-floor clinical space. We actually like to plan for MRI, CAT scan, and radioisotope imaging to be subsurface to save shielding requirements, while we like to place the surgery suites on the second floor to allow larger natural light windows to be used. In one specialty facility where we did space utilization among six specialty practices, we used these up and down concepts to spread 28,000 sq. ft. across three floors (one was subsurface from the front, but has a hillside back truck ramp for major equipment access), and only eight linear feet of pure single-use hallway.

The architect usually develops cost limits per gross square footage based upon construction cost goals and veterinary program needs. The exact functions will change size depending upon support or column needs, mechanical shafts, exit requirements, code standards, and space design. The essential control of functional planning is gross space and number of corners in the footprint (the more corners, the more cost—see appendix C). Individual zone functions are best listed by physical position such as number of client access and waiting, desk/reception positions (location of personal workspace often based upon number of staff in a zone and utilization plan), cabinet and counter needs, patient flow, and patient-staff-client separation and movement.

An approved functional plan is required to set construction cost, to allow the architect to proceed with the design of the building, and to assure the owner of a balanced planning approach, as well as to provide the practice manager/administrator an approved document in case of in-house staff changes.

Materials Management Study

The cost savings of automated materials-management systems are based upon a life-cycle analysis of manual labor versus labor time saved. A study on this issue should be contained in the long-range plan or facility master plan for combined specialty practices under one roof, but is seldom needed for general practice settings.

The detailed design of a materials-handling system is a composite of trips, times, and amounts that could be automated through a physical structure. This process must be included in the design contract and should be performed by an independent veterinary-specific consultant working with the architect or by the veterinary-specific consultant or architect working with various manufacturers. Since many manufacturers offer consulting contracts on a fee basis as part of the design effort, ensure there is a *full-disclosure* clause in the architect's contract or veterinary-specific consultant letter of engagement to ensure this person is not being paid twice for the same effort. You also want to ensure that he or she is working for you instead of someone else who can profit from the advice.

Staffing Study

Personnel costs are a fact of life in this labor-intensive profession. A good study of staffing can allow the practice to plan the most appropriate staffing patterns for its needs. High-density scheduling, consultation room access, treatment room workstations, nursing time, patient mix, scope of services projected, and management habits are very important in computing cost of care per procedure (or for a zone space). Various communications and paper-handling systems can affect staffing pattern and work site locations. Each method should be studied and its state of the art investigated. Progressive management and productivity can be overstated, but staff cost greatly affects all budgets and should be given due attention. Staff planning requires a combination of the skills and knowledge of practice administration, and a knowledgeable veterinary practice consultant can start the transition process in your existing facility to ensure there is a smooth transition to the new facility. Since the rule of $A^2 = G^2$ must be applied (if you **A**lways do what you have **A**lways done, you are going to **G**et what you have always **G**otten), this is seldom something that can be performed in-house.

Equipment Planning

The planning and design of fixed equipment (that is, equipment built in to a hospital facility) is the architect's responsibility. Moveable equipment (that is, equipment replaced, moved from existing locations, or simply portable equipment) is not typically the architect's responsibility but it could be added to his work and to his fee. Most reputable architects recommend an veterinary-specific consultant for this service. The consultant would program, list, and specify moveable items in each room during the design stage. Working closely with the architect or project manager of the practice, the consultant would challenge the space needed for each item of equipment requested by the staff and look at compromises for the equipment as well as location in the respective zone for traffic-flow enhancements. This allows for full coordination of the required mechanical and electrical services, counter or floor space, and proper functioning at the bench or table level.

The equipment consultant deals with technical medical equipment. In contrast, the interior designer deals with furniture and accessories, which is best handled by another community expert. In most established practices, moveable medical equipment accounts for 10 to 15 percent of the construction cost.

Typical equipment planning includes

- familiarization with the practice methods
- operational analysis of the equipment needs
- definition of storage spaces and material flow networks
- interviews with the staff and doctors
- analysis of existing capital expense resources
- preliminary lists of equipment
- equipment maintenance needs and POCs for workbooks
- revised list of equipment
- layout of moveable equipment
- ensuring the project manager has all technical specifications
- advising the project manager on bidding, procurement, and placement

Financial Feasibility Study

Major accounting firms make financial feasibility studies their business. Experts in the veterinary field know financing mechanisms and their application to a specific project. Because of the fact that a legal responsibility is assumed in the financial market, the best consultant often saves the most in time and cost. More awareness and sophistication is needed by individual veterinary practices in this critical area. The future of even the best-developed planning hinges on the cost picture. An aggressive and accurate financial plan is required for every project from the outset. This study determines the practice's debt capacity to fund a project and recommends the methods to enhance searching the funding mechanisms available at the current and projected money market.

Fiscal considerations include

- working from a position of the buyer—a power position—no begging!
- a general working floor plan for fiscal proposal discussions
- projected building costs, equipment costs, and contingency costs (+ 10 percent)
- a list of three small and three large financial institutions for interview
- on-site practice interviews of the financial institutions
- potential requirement for D&B (Dun & Bradstreet) or Environmental Phase 1
- needs for demographic assessments or forecasts
- for established practices, no personal guarantees required
- transferability of the debt in case of sale or partnership realignment
- clarity in the pro forma costs (building, equipment, contingency)
- clarity in what to request in the term sheet submissions
- ensure each knows a full package will be supplied to all financial institutions based on what the individual institutions requested, so first bid can be the best bid by each institution in their term sheet
- establish a deadline for term sheet submission
- ensure the financial institution addresses known estimates for:
  building loan amount and interest, as well as payment plan
  equipment secured line of credit (LOC) (self-collateralizing)
  contingency funds (LOC for two months' operating expenses)
- if the financial institution wishes to be the depository for the practice, ensure:
  sweep account costs for deposits
  money market interest rates for each sweep
  credit card processing costs
  banking and checking costs
  other banking benefits to practice and staff

Eyes Wide Open Factors—Tom Cat's Consultant's Perspective
- If you plan to renovate for under $100 a square foot, you will probably be scrimping on materials and equipment.
- If you plan to build new for $120 a square foot, you are probably related to the contractor or live in an overbuilt community with extra contractor crews and subcontractors sitting idle.
- If you are planning new veterinary facility construction at $150 per square foot and already own the land, with utilities already run to the property, you are working in the correct playing field for the new millennium.
- The second floor, when used for offices, is often about 50 percent of the first floor construction costs, while the basement is often about 30 percent.
- Most architects charge by a percentage of the final construction cost, rather than by time, so many of them love to add on the nice-to-have extras; concurrently, their commission goes upward.
- Many architects love hallways, allowing for over 20 percent of the total floor plan to be circulating space. It does not have to be this much.

- HVAC/plumbing will be at least 25–30 percent of the construction cost—but do not scrimp on the hospital zones and drainages needed to control odors, noise, and fresh air circulation.
- A flat roof saves about three dollars per square foot during initial construction, but seldom has the curb appeal or moisture protection of a pitched roof.
- Outside zoning requirements can add up to 45 percent cost overrun due to parking, beautification requirements, curb cuts, and street access; ensure your contractor and architect fully explain the zoning requirements for external spaces.
- Many funding sources are available, and some come with a major consequence called interest rates. Everything is negotiable (which we often do as agents for our clients), including interest rates over commercial prime, money market sweep accounts, credit card rates, interest for equipment lines of credit, personal guarantees, and even whether the note will be resold or not.

Insights and Perspectives

Eyes Wide Open, Eyes Wide Shut—Riding the Emotional Roller Coaster
Wayne Usiak, AIA, NCARB

It wasn't so long ago that you drove by what looked like a nice site for a veterinary hospital, perhaps every day on the way to work. On your day off, you decided to finally call a realtor to inquire about it. After some preliminary fact-finding, you arranged to purchase the site over the next few years. Finally paid off three years later, you approached an architect friend at a dinner party where he sketched an idea on a cocktail napkin. You had a client who was a general contractor, and the three of you got together and within six months built a simple, economical new veterinary hospital.

Unless you're from Mayberry, those days are gone. This was all before strict zoning, Yellow Page advertising, the S & L disaster, spay-neuter clinics, the Americans with Disabilities Act, environmental awareness, animal humane hospitals, neighborhood associations, architectural review committees, and complex building code regulations. It's a new world!

Whatever the reason you decide to embark on building a veterinary facility, I can assure you that you are in for an emotional ride. There are highs and lows, long looping high g-force turns, and twisting drops to make your stomach leave your body. Some of them are even fun! Certainly the result is almost always worth the ticket price, and failures of the well-prepared are few and far between. But still, everyone gets the ride.

Strategize—Your First Step

Real success will only be achieved when a balance is achieved between your personal and professional life. A successful business that leaves your personal life in ruins is no success. You must develop separate but codependent plans as your strategy to success—your business plan and your building plan. Your business plan will develop your professional goals based on your personal situation. Once this is completed, you can develop your building plan—the three-dimensional structure that will allow you to go forward to achieve the business plan.

The Business Plan

Your business plan will be founded in two parts. The first part, based on MBA modeling, is important but not the subject of my focus. The MBA model would include market definitions, demographic analysis, competitor analysis, marketing plans, cash flow projections, financing needs and options, and pro forma financial statements.

The business plan that is the focus of my discussion includes five quite different components:

1. Comfort zone
2. Financial requirements
3. Professional goals
4. Personal goals
5. Exit strategy

Each of these areas, when developed and outlined, will allow you to develop a project meeting your long-term life goals and achieve the aforementioned balance.

Comfort Zone

Your comfort zone will be defined by your practice mission statement. Is there a professional milestone you wish to reach by your career's end? Is there a type or style of practice you want to develop? Philosophically, what type of practice do you want? The more concisely and completely you can define your philosophy and goals, the more you will be able to structure your practice to achieve them.

It appears clear that four practice types are emerging as the dominant prototypes for twenty-first-century veterinary medicine. Your own practice may be a subset of one of these, but will more than likely fall within one of the categories.

1. Multidoctor general practice: Containing three to twenty DVMs, this practice forms the backbone of today's medically focused, successful veterinary practice. A key ownership consideration in this type of practice involves commitment to professional hospital management with practice growth.
2. Pet care centers: Offering a broad spectrum of medical and nonmedical whole-life caregivers and products, these practices are also referred to as mega-practices and one-stop shops. Key to their philosophy is the client coming to the practice for all pet care needs from adoption and medical care to food and ancillary retail products as well as training, boarding, grooming, etc.

3. Boutique practice: Typically one- to three-doctor practice specializing in pet wellness in a focused area. Feline practice is the simplest model, but neighborhood doctor general practice, holistic practice, and other microspecialty practices fit this prototype.
4. Specialist/referral practices: These practices usually rely on one of the three prototypes above for client referrals. Usually staffed by board certified DVMs in various medical specialties, they can be individual discipline specialists or offer a full spectrum of specialist doctors. Twenty-four hour critical care/emergency care practices have a synergistic relationship with specialist practice and often are combined for gained efficiency.

Financial Requirements

Your financial requirements will, to a large part, be determined by the debt service your practice can support. These will include land, professional fees, finance costs and fees, building costs, equipment and furnishings, moving/relocation, and operational/personnel costs. The first six can be readily projected, but the last item will most likely be a SWAG, based largely on how fast projected business increases occur.

Professional Goals

We have all heard the expression "be careful what you ask for"; often what we ask is more than we bargained for. In defining your professional goals, you must determine what kind of veterinarian you want to be—clinician, practice manager, mentor, or part-time of each. Often, choosing the latter is the simplest answer, but remember the cliché "jack of all trades, master of none." Understand the reasons you have been successful thus far, and don't lose that competitive edge. Then understand what it will take to achieve the next level, and provide for trust, skill level, and support structure within your practice. Growth can cause you to become what you never envisioned, or worse yet, what you never wanted to become. When my own firm grew from five to twelve, I found my architect time diminishing and my management time increasing. I learned words like human resources, staff turnover, and practice management. I wanted to design veterinary hospitals but I was doing less and less of that! Yet if we were to continue in our practice as industry leaders, we needed to continue to offer the services of our on-staff specialists, and that meant twelve to fifteen employees. I needed a partner to share and divide the practice management duties if I was to continue active project involvement, which I felt was a key to our past success.

Your personal goals statement will allocate your time in developing life balance between your personal and business lives. When your practice was young, the two were probably indelibly intertwined, often the definition of nepotism. Everyone was focused on getting the business off the ground. Once the business becomes self-sufficient, a separation needs to take place between business and personal lives to gain equilibrium. Your personal time investment cannot be at the expense of family. You must determine the time allocation the practice receives and then use good management techniques to keep within your target.

Inevitably, increases in time allocations to the business will be at the expense of personal life issues. This may be fine occasionally but, if occurring too often, will lead to a compounding effect and can cause you to lose sight of your original goals with suddenly disastrous results.

Exit Strategy

Perhaps the most important plan to have in mind as you begin to plan a building project is your exit plan. Looking down the road ten, fifteen, twenty, or twenty-five years can be a daunting task, especially when looking out over just one year is so difficult. Still, someday you will leave the practice, and how the real estate plays into your plan is a critical component of your exit strategy. You may just want a small two-exam-room building, a single-table treatment room and surgery, and a maximum of five employees to reach your state of professional equilibrium. The question is, at get-out time, will that same dream be shared by another veterinarian or be an economically viable business model in the future? Will you have a marketable product? You can have both by planning ahead. Purchasing or optioning enough site to allow a future owner to double or triple that building under their tenure can ensure that you have built flexibility into your exit plan.

Bricks and mortar will continue to be a key component of veterinary service delivery. This gives the veterinarian two exit strategy income streams—the practice and the building. They can and should be considered separately in the exit equation. You may sell the practice but continue as landlord until the new owner can afford to finance the real estate. This monthly income stream, while keeping the entire principal value in your portfolio, can enhance your retirement income. In some cases, the real estate may appreciate beyond the value of what a veterinary practice can afford, and the new practice owner may have to relocate while you reap the benefits of a high-performance real estate investment. I'm not suggesting you can plan on any of this, but maintain flexibility to accommodate several options, and don't think that *your* goals will end the dream.

Use Your Resources

Developing your business plan isn't a lone endeavor. You should consult a variety of resources to gain a comprehensive understanding of the consequences of each decision. A practice management consultant can provide a valuable sounding board and impartial party for your ideas. While your strong emotions about a certain decision may cloud your clear thinking, a consultant is free of that involvement and tends to be more results-oriented. He or she has probably seen someone in your situation before and can provide you the benefit of that past experience. Your accountant knows your financial capabilities and understands your total financial statement, not just your business performance. He or she knows you personally, your risk profile, and your family situation, and certainly understands your total financial picture and your ability to bear debt structure.

Don't forget to include your family. Fathers, mothers, spouses, and even children may be invited to participate, at least at the opinion level. Each of them will certainly add perspective to each component of your business plan. Your architect, site engineer, attorney, and realtor can assist with other specific decisions as well. Architects can offer construction cost information and construction schedule durations. Veterinary specialist architects can assist in these as well as exit strategy options and will be more specific regarding finance issues and specific building needs. Realtors can assist in their knowledge of zoning and comparable site costs.

The Building Plan

You're now quite confident you know your business goals, the model, what you can afford, and how it all fits your family life. So now you want to build! Except, you're a veterinarian. Now the problem here is that most veterinarians I know are fairly competent at a pretty wide variety of skills. You have to be. In your first practice, business was built on a shoestring. When the exam rooms needed painting, you worked in the evening and painted them. When you bought a new cage bank, you installed it. When you finally could afford real cabinets and a wet sink in treatment, you put those in too. So it's pretty tough to tell you *not* to do something. So instead I'll tell you what *to do*. You read between the lines. Your job is to be a leader, the conductor. You don't have to play the instruments. Your first job is to know everyone else's job and to understand all the jobs needed to complete the project.

This begins with the municipal development review process. It typically begins with a zoning review, followed by a site plan and/or architectural review, culminating in the plan check for a building permit. In these reviews government agencies tell landowners what they can build on their parcel, how large it can be, how tall it can be, how much parking it will have, how much and what type of landscape is allowed, how trash is to be picked up, and how rainwater is to be diverted. Additionally, they decide if the building style is acceptable to them and ask the neighbors for their approval. Some towns have refined the bureaucracy to a fine science, requiring six reviews by twenty-four agencies with any rejection putting you back to the end of the line to start again. Naturally, with each review there is a fee. The key for the conductor is to understand the process, the time frame, and the submittal requirements. Architects, engineers, landscape architects, attorneys, and realtors should provide the content. You provide the assembly, delivery, and—naturally—the fee.

Another interesting project component involves utilities. It is not enough that they are there, though that's the first question. Sanitary sewer, storm sewer, domestic water, fire protection, gas, electric, and telephone should all be verified. Once the needed utilities are confirmed, inquiry should be made as to size adequacy and tap fees. Fees in the tens of thousands of dollars are not unheard of for utility expansion charges, a nice way of back charging for line installation costs. Often if a municipality or developer has provided inadequate fire hydrants in an area, you must pay to install additional hydrants in order to meet the fire code. Your architect and engineer are valuable assets here in projecting potential utility usage and respective service sizes needed. In addition to the reviews and fees mentioned above, we have completed projects in revenue-creative towns featuring fees for energy, microfiche, city beautification, child care, traffic mitigation, creek impact, reinspection (whether you get one or not), aerial mapping and encroachment. All we wanted to do was build a veterinary hospital! Believe me, these add up. On this particular 15,000 sq. ft. hospital/boarding facility the fees were $157,000!

Your Architect's Job

As the project designer, your architect will provide a needs analysis, quantify the space requirements, establish quality standards, conceptualize the building design, coordinate their engineer team, and finally develop the architectural and engineering systems into documents to secure a building permit. The architect will assist you in selecting a contractor and then endeavor to act in your behalf to prevent defects and deficiencies in the construction. Your job is to be available to answer questions, provide requested data, and review and comment on presented designs in timely fashion. And pay.

Your Engineering Team

Several engineering disciplines may be required over the course of your project. Mechanical, electrical, and structural engineers are almost always necessary and usually provided by the architect within his fee. Civil engineering is required for site hydrology (storm water), utilities services, roads and parking, and site structures (retaining walls, catch basins, manholes, etc.). The civil engineer is typically selected, directed, and compensated by the owner with coordination by the architect. Environmental consultants may be required depending on site and municipality specific circumstances. Phase one environmental surveys document prior usage and potential sources of contamination.

Geotechnical engineers provide soils analysis and design guidelines for foundations and pavements. Their fees are almost saved later by allowing more efficient structural designs. Structural engineers working without the benefit of a soils analysis will design for a worst-case scenario resulting in more expensive footings, foundations, and earthwork preparations. Geotechnical fees are cheap insurance against foundation failures or exorbitant structural overdesign.

Two types of surveys are needed. A boundary survey will document property lines, corners, and overall size. A topographical survey indicates land contours, roads, other improvements, utilities, and large vegetation. A survey is one of the first things needed for preliminary planning and design.

Finally, the landscape architect, not technically an engineer, provides landscape design and layout, plant selection, and irrigation. Often using a landscape plan is a preliminary site design requirement of municipalities.

Your Financial Team

Financing has become the highest-stress part of project development. Typically, veterinarians approach their local banker, with whom they have a stellar record. The banker, typically a branch manager or vice president, assures them that "a 6,000 sq. ft. new office will be no problem, just bring in the plans and we will arrange the financing." The veterinarian takes his word, retains an architect, and tells him or her, "I have financing in place." The architect completes a building design and the owner takes the construction drawings to the bank and duplicate sets to the contractor. The contractor prepares an estimate, while the banks have their appraiser complete an appraisal. Now the fun begins. The contractor estimates everything noted on the plans—every faucet, air conditioner, exhaust fan, cabinet, and finish. He gets actual prices from specialty subcontractors in each trade. The appraiser prepares a more general estimate, based on average buildings recently constructed within their database. Guess how many are state-of-the-art, twenty-first-century veterinary hospital, investment-quality buildings? Right. None. So, the appraiser's estimated value of the building is significantly lower than both the architect's and the contractor's. Unfortunately, the bank lends money based on the appraiser's figure. The branch manager takes the loan request and the appraisal in front of the loan committee (he failed to mention he needed to do this when he told you "no problem") who promptly deny the loan request based on the undervalued appraisal. The bank tells the veterinarian to build a smaller building, get rid of the expensive exhaust fans, put in cheap flooring, or let my house builder build you a hospital. All too often, in the end the veterinarian must make up the difference between the appraised cost and real cost with a bridge loan or second mortgage on his home to keep the building he knows he needs to succeed (and have something worth selling.) Recently, specialist lenders in the marketplace specializing in veterinary hospital loans have streamlined the process with higher loan-to-value ratios and improved appraisals. They attend most of the national veterinary trade shows or advertise in national veterinary publications. Still, it is difficult for the veterinarian to abandon his local bank, even when they so often leave the veterinarian stranded.

Be a Boy Scout—Be Prepared

The two most valuable commodities we never seem to have enough of remain consistent in all life's endeavors—money and time. They remain so in the veterinary building project.

Even in today's 24/7/365, fax, FedEx, or e-mail it to me now society, a building project is a time-consuming affair. As with all investment-based endeavors, time is money. So the dilemma is to get it as fast as possible. The time-line for your project contains the following major line items and durations (see table 1.1). The time-lines listed for the design function (programming, schematic design, and construction documents) are what our firm finds average for a veterinary-experienced designer. About twice this amount should be budgeted for designers unfamiliar with veterinary terminology or function.

An average duration and chronological location for each major task is provided. Financing, preliminary governmental approval, and building permitting are, unsurprisingly, the most unpredictable and usually create the greatest

Table 1.1 Typical Project Schedule

PHASE	Month 1	Month 2	Month 3	Month 4	Month 5	Month 6	Month 7	Month 8	Month 9	Month 10	Month 11	Month 12	Month 13	Month 14	Month 15	Month 16
Programming	A															
Schematic design		A	A													
Construction documents				A	A	A										
Appraisal							O									
Financing	O	O		O		O		O						O		
Permitting							O/A/C	O/A/C								
Construction									C	C	C	C	C	C / C+	C+	C+

Notes:
Primarily architect tasks = A
Primarily owner/bank tasks = O
Owner/architect/contractor Tasks = O/A/C
Primarily contractor tasks (up to 5,000 sq. ft.) = C
Primarily contractor tasks (5,000 sq. ft.–30,000 sq. ft.) = C+; add 1 mo/4,000 sq. ft. for 4 mo

20

delays. Once again research of your specific site, bank requirements, and municipal review procedures will allow you to develop more project-specific time-lines. Table 1.1 lists no time duration for zoning processing or site plan review, as these may not be necessary on all projects, and when required, vary greatly. Research your municipality requirements and add their stated time durations to this schedule cumulatively.

The first three activity lines of the project schedule are programming, schematic design, and construction documents. These functions are primarily architect-driven. The needs analysis and assessment (programming) phase should take about thirty days. Following an acceptable space summary, the schematic design will commence and take an average of sixty days. Once approved, the architect will complete the construction documents for permit and bidding use. Three months should be allowed to complete construction documents for projects up to 8,000 sq. ft. Each 4,000 sq. ft. over this will require an additional thirty days.

Following construction document completion, those documents will be given to your bank for appraisal and your selected contractor(s) for pricing. These activities take three to eight weeks. This should not be the first time you have made inquires regarding financing. Four different early interaction times are shown for financing. At the project outset, you should contact a financing consultant to determine your acceptable debt load to assist in establishing a project budget. You would also be well advised to consult with a practice management consultant to project revenues from the new facility and any new or expanded service offerings. At the completion of schematic design, you should return to discuss changes from the original plan. Perhaps the building size has increased, or additional equipment can be foreseen. Will this change the financing picture? The third time is to submit for an appraisal and the fourth to institute the construction financing.

Permitting can begin as soon as the construction documents are completed. We find the average to be sixty days, though we have seen six months in bureaucrat-rich municipalities.

Finally, once a permit is issued and a contract for construction is agreed to, construction can begin. Construction averages five to six months for projects up to 5,000 sq. ft. Not much reduction is found for smaller projects, though tenant improvements in shopping centers can be completed quicker. Add one month for each 4,000 sq. ft. additional to 25,000 sq. ft. This gives us a total project duration from programming to occupancy of fourteen to twenty months.

Developing a comprehensive total project budget is paramount to success (see table 1.2). It is truly amazing how many people put their hands in your pockets before it's all finished. It's okay to forget a few minor charges or costs here and there, particularly if you have a contingency set aside, but like the government on a small scale, a few thousand here and there too many times and pretty soon you're talking real money—and real problems. In attempting to develop a rule of thumb for a total project budget, site costs need to be deleted from this equation. They are too variable and location sensitive. This leaves professional fees, financing costs, building construction costs, permitting and approval costs, furnishing and equipment, and occupancy/relocation/operations costs. Table 1.2 is a form I have developed listing all these costs. Based on past experience and these line items, total project budgets range from 1.25 to 1.5 times the building construction cost. A quick rule of thumb I have is to figure your building construction cost (realistically) and add a third. Remember that site costs have been excluded from the equation and must be added to the total project budget for a true gross total. I have prepared categories with line items for an average project example in table 1.2. You may discover costs unique to your municipality or situation that need to be added to this form, but it is as comprehensive an average representation as I have been able to prepare. Once again, use your resources (realtor, architect, engineer, practice management consultant, etc.) to develop realistic entries for each line item. Address each line item, even if it is zero. Finally, maintain a contingency of 3 to 5 percent of the total cost, not construction cost. Things *will* go wrong. You never know when or where they may come from, but errors and omissions are to be expected on such a complex endeavor. A fund needs to be established to address them. Three to 5 percent is an average based on an experienced, professional team. If you choose to take on certain responsibilities yourself, or use nonveterinary-project-experienced team members, expect this number to increase, and budget for it. Hopefully, the savings will cover the difference.

The transition to project closeout, occupancy, and initial operations will be a reflection of the preparation and experience of previous project phases. If chaos has ruled during design and construction, this trend will continue, making this transition eventful, in an unfun way. However, if you've been the prepared conductor, with a methodical approach, this transition is the realization of the dream you've harbored since veterinary school. We liken it to the first new car experience times ten. After a recently completed project by a veterinarian who was a model conductor, we were touring the complete hospital. I asked if he ever walked in and was overwhelmed by the whole thing, and needed to remind himself, "I did this and it's all mine."

He smiled, and told me, "Every day."

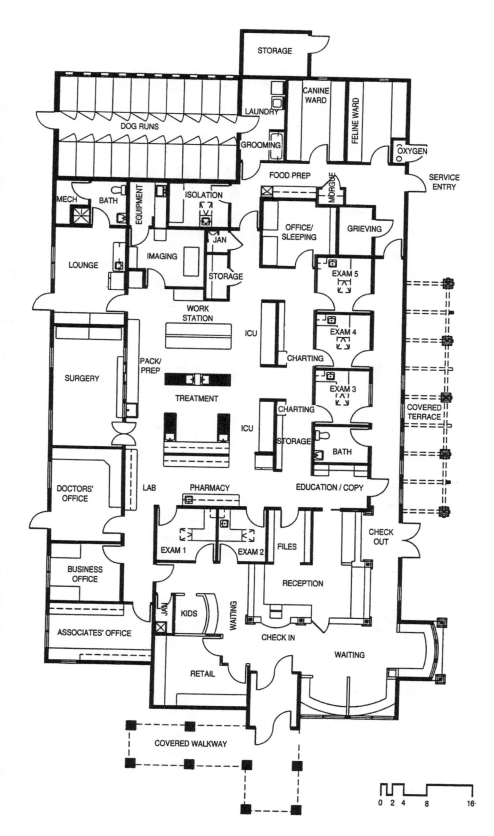

STORAGE

CANINE WARD

LAUNDRY

FELINE WARD

GROOMING

OXYGEN

SERVICE ENTRY

DOG RUNS

FOOD PREP

MORGUE

MECH

BATH

EQUIPMENT

ISOLATION

OFFICE/ SLEEPING

GRIEVING

JAN

LOUNGE

IMAGING

STORAGE

EXAM 5

WORK STATION

ICU

EXAM 4

CHARTING

SURGERY

PACK/ PREP

EXAM 3

TREATMENT

CHARTING

COVERED TERRACE

ICU

STORAGE

BATH

DOCTORS' OFFICE

LAB

PHARMACY

EDUCATION / COPY

EXAM 1

EXAM 2

FILES

CHECK OUT

BUSINESS OFFICE

RECEPTION

ASSOCIATES' OFFICE

JAN

KIDS

WAITING

CHECK IN

RETAIL

WAITING

COVERED WALKWAY

0 2 4   8   16·

23

Table 1.2 Average Project Cost Form

Site costs: _____
1. Land purchases   _____
2. Attorney fees   _____
3. Title insurance   _____
4. Closing costs   _____
5. Boundary survey   _____
6. Architect/consultant fees   _____
7. Environment fees   _____

Financing costs: _____
1. Appraisal   _____
2. Construction loan interest   _____
3. Construction loan fees   _____
4. Perm loan fee (bank)   _____
5. Perm loan fee (SBA or other)   _____

Professional fees: _____
1. Architects/engineers (bldg. design)   _____
2. Surveyor (topographical)   _____
3. Geotechnical (soils borings)   _____
4. Hydrology/drainage (civil)   _____
5. Interior design   _____
6. Landscape architect   _____
7. Regulatory agencies submittals   _____
   * Zoning (prof fees & gov proc)   _____
   * Design review board (pf & gp)   _____
   * Planning (pf & gp)   _____
   * Code enforcement—plan ck (gp)   _____
8. Special consultations (Utility, Envir.)   _____

Construction costs: _____
1. General contractor/subcontractor   _____
2. Utility construction   _____
3. Site improvements (walls, features)   _____
4. Water, sewer, gas, impact, fees   _____
5. Transformers, elect. reqmts., fees   _____
6. Traffic engineering costs   _____
7. Sign   _____
8. Builder's risk, other insurance   _____

Occupancy and equipment costs: _____
1. Moving/relocation   _____
2. Advertising/mailing/promotional   _____
3. 6 month operations increases   _____
4. Printing   _____
5. Furnishings (desks, tables, chairs)   _____
6. Stainless steel equipt. (cages/runs)   _____
7. Hospital equipt. (tables/lights, etc.)   _____
8. Special equipt. (X-ray, etc.)   _____
9. Telephones, computers, etc.   _____
Subtotal: _____
Contingency costs: (3–5% subtotal)   _____
Total budget cost: _____ _____

2

The Design Team

IN MOST MUNICIPALITIES, it has become impossible for the practice owner or hospital administrator to deal with the local government bureaucracy without expert advice. Consultants or architects can be hired for special studies on every aspect of the facility construction or expansion, from engineer reports, to setting up a more effective hospital flow, to coping with multiple codes.

Team-based planning is an excellent concept, and a local design and planning team can be highly beneficial to the goals of the practice ownership. The role each expert plays in his or her area of expertise, the value of that special knowledge to the project, and the impact on the total project costs should be evaluated so that each project is strong and unique. The practice's professional and administration staff are responsible for the needs of the people they serve, staff and clients alike. The degree to which needs are met is a function of the experience, innovative ideas, organizational paradigms, and age mix of these groups of people. The veterinary-specific consultant draws on the expertise of people in every area of the profession and combines this expertise with his own to come up with a plan for implementing the practice's plan. The architect's recommendations usually focus on the total operational past of the experience and wishes of the practice owner(s), regardless of the future of the practice in the community. There must be provisions for the demographic assessment of the catchment (service) area market, the financial future of the practice with old versus new delivery formats, any projected staff changes in function or specialties, multiowner/multipractice bylaw makeup, capital expense equipment sharing plan, and veterinary healthcare delivery programs projection; this is seldom within the scope of the architect or contractor.

The veterinary-specific consultant acts in many capacities, but the most important function is to provide an independent professional opinion. The final plan must be based on an unbiased look at the total operation. Therefore, the veterinary-specific consultant is usually retained to develop new operational and functional programs as well as to mentor the ownership in long-range planning.

The roles of the veterinary-specific consultant and consulting architect in design and construction are that of programmers of effectiveness. Once the practice's role in the community has been established, the operational and functional plans must be established. They should be based on the facility and staff utilization projections and compared to national experiences (see chapter 1). The veterinary-specific consultant relates the needs and requests of the practice manager, staff, and zone coordinators to innovations and operations that they may not be aware of due to limited past experiences.

Veterinary-specific consultants are now nationally listed/organized (see www.AVPMCA.org) but many do not work on individual facility construction. Looking at the past publications of any veterinary-specific consultant will often tell you where the consultant believes his or her expertise lies; most only publish in areas where they have expertise and a comfort zone. Fees are not regulated, and the cost of the on-site portion will vary depending on the scope of services. The size of an independent veterinary-specific consulting firm's staff can vary from one person to twenty. Many major consulting corporations and accounting firms are also acting as healthcare consultants, but few have veterinary-specific departments.

Consulting fees used to be based on a percentage of construction costs; services can include operational staff roles and healthcare delivery program planning, staff analysis and training, fixed equipment recommendations, materials-handling concepts, zone and systems operation and staffing, and functional programming. Because of the increased sophistication in each of these subjects and the practice of bidding professional fees as a lump sum or price, the fee is now usually based upon projected number of hours and duration of the project. On any specific consulting project, beware of consulting support systems that are based on only costs or only increases in profits. The consultant does not usually control these unless they just address the fee schedule or construction costs. Neither is centered on client access nor even the practice ownership's desires for effective operations in a new facility.

Practice managers/administrators and/or project managers may need multiple consulting and building design services at every stage of planning. Because of the amount of traditional ownership control and review in veterinary projects, this is seldom accepted as essential in today's veterinary facility planning market. With the new—and very sophisticated—competition for every client, alternatives in patient services, and the cost of new construction, the practice itself must now get others involved in the planning. Full-time veterinary-specific consultants, veterinary-specific architects, healthcare facility planners, professional engineers, and market planners have become common as veterinary-specific resources. Many national and state veterinary associations have listed architects, engineers, and planners as veterinary-specific, but the fact is that these are not screened individuals and they are not endorsed, but often are a fee-for-listing association income resource. The Association of Veterinary Practice Management Consultants and Advisors (AVPMCA) organization (see www.AVPMCA.org) has a code of ethics and a membership review capability, but again, is not an expertise review agency. The organization is just listing its members and has in its bylaws provisions for removing membership privileges if there is a proven ethics violation of significant magnitude. Ongoing professional veterinary-specific management contracts are also a current trend in many practices, especially when preparing for a new facility and as they adapt to the new expansion and delivery modalities.

Practices must depend on outside consultants for feasibility and construction studies. Further, few practices have developed a recurring need for their own architectural and engineering people, so each project is a new search for expert resources that can be trusted, whether it be accounting support, plans for new buildings, major renovations, or even changes in operational effectiveness. Many of these are also highly developed specialties in today's veterinary market, and are needed only a few times in a facility's history, so a trusted veterinary-specific consultant is often used as the linchpin for checks and balances within the design team.

Sorting out what consulting is needed and how much of it can be done in-house is a difficult task. The various consulting and architecture services described in this text are only the major ones available to the trained project manager/hospital administrator (being placed by the VPC Brokerage, www.v-p-c.com). There is, however, an expert consultant for any subject one can think of, which is the "good news" and "bad news" all in one concise statement.

Architects

It is well established that everyone believes that he or she can be an architect, but that a professional must be hired to assume the liabilities!

The architect is most often seen as the leader of the design team. As such, he or she must listen and evaluate the needs and desires of all parties in the practice and consulting team. The architect must formulate shapes, sizes, and materials that will meet the dreams of the practice ownership as well as the function and flow of the staff, the client, and, most important, the patient.

The practice normally selects its architect through an interview procedure or by commissioning an architect who has performed satisfactory work for a friend in the past. Schedules that define reasonable fees for certain classifications of project type and volume are published in this book, and construction estimates are provided in the appendices as well as in the chapters. The architectural costs should include all basic design and blueprint services plus total engineering costs.

Architects usually earn their bachelor of architecture degrees in a five-year university curriculum. Their training is based on a combination of mathematics and art. Besides standard liberal arts course work, the architecture student concentrates on a design sequence that outlines the theory, history, and detail of architectural design and concept. Because of his or her training in art and engineering, the architect emerges as a social designer, able to deal with the needs of animals, vegetables, and human beings. There are many specialties that architects can pursue, veterinary medicine being just one. The selected architect may be a specialist, but the design tasks include everything from animal runs to office space.

Most veterinary-specific architects' offices range from one or two to ten or twenty employees. Some veterinary-specific firms now include in-house design-build elements and may employ additional construction managers and engineers. Major veterinary-specific firms often contain interior design resources, act as equipment consultants, and offer construction management assistance.

The following four types of architectural firms are involved with healthcare:

1. Engineering architect: These firms are usually managed by engineers and offer a full scope of services. They compete at a high level and produce excellent functional buildings with an emphasis on systems management and technical detail.
2. Design-build architect: The design-build firm takes a project from design to finished construction, carrying out most of the engineering in-house. The fees of such firms seem lower but are equal when compared to the combined design, engineering, and general contracting.
3. Local architect: The size of a firm does not indicate its quality; the actual team from a large firm working on a major facility may only number eight to ten architects and an equal number of engineers. Local firms vary in size and earn 10-80 percent of their commission in healthcare facility design. Engineering may be done in-house or by a contracted consultant. The practice of joint venturing with a nationally recognized veterinary-specific architectural firm is also common because the "local" firm may have experience in zoning and local regulatory issues but not much experience in veterinary-specific projects.
4. Veterinary-specific design architects: The veterinary-specific design firms are usually national and international and have an established home base but travel to the site as needed. They offer veterinary-specific healthcare design expertise that includes master planning, layout, equipment, and programming for projects ranging from university medical center planning, to shelters, to primary care companion animal centers, to production animal chute systems, to specialty practices in mega-facilities. In many cases, they offer veterinary-specific facility design review services through national veterinary associations or independently to practices and local architects, in order to share their expertise at reduced costs to the practice owners.

Although architects must take a national registration examination, each state has its own licensing requirements . The architect and engineer must have this state license because of the effect that design has on public safety. Incorporation is allowed in the architectural profession, but it does not limit the liability of the individual architect. Each firm carries error and omission liability insurance to protect it in case of legal action. Error and omission is defined in each separate action, but it can be summed up as follows: *"If an item is left out of the construction for any reason, then the owner has never paid for it and it should be added at his expense. If an item is installed in the construction correctly as specified and does not physically work, then the architect or engineer has erred."* There are, as might be expected, many variations on this rule.

Another commonly misunderstood legal aspect of the contract should be mentioned. If the owner specifies a top dollar amount to be spent in construction, the architect is permitted to determine what materials, equipment, component systems, and types of construction are to be included and may adjust the scope of the project to bring it within that limit. This means that the architect must advise against and possibly refuse any unreasonable cost items or disproportionate program elements. This is very difficult for an architect to do because the emphasis in the project is always on what will benefit the owner.

The architect, then, has a very complex role, acting as judge, artist, businessman, lawyer, accountant, and patient.

Selecting the Architect

The interview process is difficult and tiring. The list may start with four national and three local firms and be shortened to a selected few. The practice's selection committee may sit through four presentations a night, hearing equally good demonstrations of expertise. We have interviewed architectural firms as a practice's consulting arm and as a consultant for specific design planning projects, so we know the process can be grueling.

The following areas may help narrow the choice:

- Find out which member of the architectural firm will handle the job and evaluate his or her responses. You will be working closely with this person for over a year, and this is the key to a secure selection.
- Study the proposed team and its organization's appearance. Ask about the engineer's experience and request a reference of complete work.
- Check the firm's references.
- Explain your needs and the goals of your project, such as design excellence, mechanical systems, and functional concerns, and ask questions as to how these can be best met for your practice.
- Relate the fee quoted to the larger cost of construction and efficient operation of the practice. Do not pick the lowest fee just because it is low. Once a fee is verbalized, it greatly influences a committee. However, this fee amounts to only 6-8 percent of the total amount you will spend for construction; money is not saved if the building operation does not work. Consider that each year and a half of operations will often cost as much as the initial construction. It is important to trust in your selection.

Engineers

By definition, engineers apply the physical laws of science for the benefit of mankind. The scope of engineering work is enlarged by the scientist's increasing understanding of our physical world.

Civil Engineers

Historically, engineers who worked on nonmilitary projects became known as civil engineers. Three main divisions of civil engineering exist today:

1. Transportation, whether by land (including railroads, highways, and rapid transit), water (including canals, port and harbor improvements, and improvements to navigation such as lighthouses), or air (airports)
2. Structures, including buildings and bridges
3. Sanitation, including the collection, treatment, and distribution of potable water as well as the collection, treatment, and disposal of wastewater such as storm water and polluted water

Civil engineers contribute their talents to veterinary hospital construction in three areas:

1. Site planning
2. Structural design
3. Construction

Site planning is the art and science of arranging the uses of land. The site planner designates these uses in detail by selecting and analyzing a site, forming a land-use plan, organizing vehicular and pedestrian traffic, developing a visual form and materials concept, readjusting the existing landform by design grading, providing proper drainage, and, finally, developing the construction details necessary to carry out the project. Although he or she may determine the overall uses of a site, this is not always the case. The site planner, does, however, arrange to accommodate the activities the client has specified; this is especially important for haul-in mixed animal practices, so ensure that your desires are stated up front in each planning meeting. These components must relate to each other, to the site, and to structures and activities on adjacent sites, as the site—whether it is large or small—must be viewed as part of the total environment. Site planning is done professionally by landscape and other architects, planners, and engineers.

Structural design of buildings involves determining how the entire building and its parts are to resist the loads to which they will be subjected and communicating this information to the builder. In long-term building flexibility, single-span construction, or post-and-beam construction, is preferable over supporting wall construction, so ensure the structural design takes this factor into account.

Civil engineers are leaders in the construction industry. The construction contractor's work will probably be under the control of a civil engineer employed by the contractor. (*Note:* Because this book deals primarily with the preconstruction concerns of veterinary-specific facilities, I will not elaborate on the civil engineer's construction role.)

Civil engineers have earned bachelor of science degrees in civil engineering and may have earned advanced degrees in one of its specialties. Engineers who design facilities to be used by the public are required to be registered by the state in which they practice. Requirements for registration vary but typically include the bachelor's degree or equivalent experience (generally four or five years of design responsibility) and successful completion of a written examination. The engineer responsible for the preparation of drawings describing construction requirements must place his or her seal of registration on the drawings. Registered engineers are referred to as "professional engineers" and use the initials "P.E." after their names.

How is the civil engineer's work done, and how can he or she help the owner, practice manager, hospital administrator, or project manager optimize the facility being designed? Regardless of who allocates the available space for buildings, access roads, parking, and open space, the location and design of features outside the building is vital to their function. The role of the civil engineer in the site-planning process is frequently to define precisely the location of all new features and to design new roads, parking, and water and drainage utilities. The owner/practice manager/hospital administrator should provide information from the master plan with regard to allocation of site uses and economic constraints. The architect is usually called upon to provide plans showing existing site improvements, property boundary description, topographic survey, and any other special surveys dictated by a particular site.

In developing the site plans, the engineer applies good practice to the requirements of the practice, architect, municipality jurisdiction, private utilities, and other engineering disciplines. He or she will want to balance the earthwork so there will be no need to haul earth to or from the site and to design drainage so that normal flows are self-cleaning. The materials the engineer specifies will be compatible with those already in use to minimize maintenance. His or her solutions will be aimed at long-run economy, considering first cost, maintenance costs, and operating costs.

Frequently, the budget for new construction will not allow the higher first costs that design for long-run economy dictates. In this event, it is incumbent upon the engineer to present alternatives and their relative costs so an intelligent decision can be made. For example, paving is a significant part of site development cost that is often compromised. Anticipated traffic loading, soil, and weather conditions may indicate the need for a total pavement thickness of ten inches, but only eight inches can be purchased with the money available for construction. The engineer may advise a mixed animal practice that maintenance costs will be significantly higher with eight-inch pavement, and that two inches of pavement will be required after several years' use anyway. Thus, the cost of paving could be much higher if only eight inches are originally constructed.

The engineer's work is not completed once the construction contractor is selected. The engineer must then represent the owner and architect to see that the work required by the contract is furnished both in quantity and quality. Independent testing laboratories are required to run various on-site tests of the work to evaluate its quality. Sometimes the engineer may carry out these tests, but usually the contractor is required to furnish them. The contractor may obtain them on a least-cost basis. Although this arrangement may be satisfactory, it is usually preferable for testing to be done by an independent laboratory, paid directly by the practice, in order to avoid possible conflicts of interest.

Structural Engineers

The structural engineer's role is that of providing the optimum support for the building. On any large, multidiscipline, specialty practice construction project, several structural engineers and draftsmen may work under the direction of the structural engineer primarily responsible for the work. Coordinating structural work with the architect and other engineers is absolutely essential in hospital projects. The structural engineer, like any other professional, must stay informed on the latest technology in order to render the best service to clients.

How does the structural engineer work? With increasing frequency, engineers are turning to computers for help. A mathematical model of a proposed building can be described to a computer, various loading conditions can be applied, and the computer will indicate changes that need to be made. The speed of the computer allows for a greater number of preliminary investigations. For all the advantages of computers, however, the structural engineer must still decide on the structural system to be used.

The engineer employs a scientific approach. First, all structural systems that meet the major requirements of the project are considered. The question of full spans versus weight-bearing systems will probably be resolved at this point. Assuming that a frame system is indicated, the structural engineer, with the architect, then determines the column pattern that will suit the architectural requirements. Using this pattern, studies are made, with or without computer assistance, to suggest the most economical framing schemes utilizing structural steel and reinforced concrete. Preliminary plans are drawn up for these schemes so that costs can be determined. The most economical one is then selected. It is in this preliminary stage of design that the structural engineer can effect the most savings.

The supporting capability of the soil on which the building will rest is a principal factor in determining the structural system to be used and the cost of the foundation. The structural engineer will advise that a soils engineer be engaged to conduct a boring and testing program and recommend the most suitable type of foundation. A skillful soils engineer may save thousands of dollars in unnecessary foundation cost.

Once the structural system has been selected, the engineer designs the building in detail, working from the top down. The design of structures is something of a chicken-and-egg problem. Given the same loading, the size and method of attachment of members in a frame has a significant effect on the load each individual member carries. Conversely, the size and method of attachment of an individual in a frame is a function of its individual loading. Consequently, framing members are sized (based on assumed loading), the method of attachment is determined, and the frame is analyzed to check the assumed loading. Changes are made when necessary. This trial-and-error approach is simplified greatly by accurate judgment in the selection of original member sizes and attachments.

All of the structural engineer's judgment, design, and analysis are of little value until they are communicated by drawings and specifications. Clear, neat, and complete drawings and specifications have a beneficial effect on the cost of construction by lowering the risks of construction contractor error.

Being certain that the owner gets the quantity and quality in construction that he or she pays for is the reason for inspections and testing during construction. Daily inspection of most projects is desirable. It may also be available from the construction manager, the project manager working for the owner of the practice, an independent inspector hired by the owner, or the architect or engineer. In any case, both the architect and the engineer need to be on the job to review construction with the contractor and inspectors to make certain that the requirements of the contract are being met, to provide interpretation of their plans and specifications when required, and to provide direction when changed conditions are encountered or when the owner desires changes not included in the contract. Never allow any change to occur without specific advice of the architect or engineer.

Mechanical and Electrical Engineers

The task of the mechanical engineer is to study the conservation of energy and apply it in the most efficient and economical way. The plumbing engineer is responsible for the processed water and the liquid waste of the entire structure. The electrical power designer must be aware of the public utility supply and rates so that an economical power distribution and emergency supply is obtained. A lighting designer is a key member of the engineering staff because he or she enhances all spaces through lighting and affects the mood and correct optical levels of the entire hospital staff. Let us review some of the problems that face mechanical engineers as the basic structure is being designed.

A building or space is a thermal container. Within any veterinary facility, a heating, ventilation, and air-conditioned environment for human and animal comfort is to be maintained, regardless of the season or climate. Thermal considerations in the construction of a building shell include

- efficiency of modern HVAC unit(s)
- thin panel versus massive wall
- insulation and glass wall shading
- partial versus total glazing
- three-zone HVAC (client, staff treatment, animal areas)
- radiant heating, double glazing, and other life-span economies
- roof construction (pitched roofs are only about three dollars a square foot more than flat roofs, look more user friendly to clients, and leak far less)

All of these constitute the outdoor design conditions. These factors, along with the internal space load of lights, motors, people, animals, and special heat-producing equipment (such as sterilizers, drying cages, computers, or staff lounge equipment) are required to calculate the air-conditioning load. It must be emphasized that an estimate of the actual cooling-heating load is essential before an air-conditioning system and equipment are selected. Knowledge of advances in the technology of solar space conditioning, recycled waste, total energy generation, and alternative fuels is the responsibility of the modern engineer. Because 30 percent of the cost of most veterinary buildings is spent on plumbing and HVAC system construction, it is vital to apply life-cycle analysis and value management to the engineering concept.

Each practice presents a unique problem. There is no universal solution to the selection of an HVAC system, even after the problem is defined, the physical circumstances evaluated, and the actual load of heating and cooling requirements established. The engineer must have an appreciation of the structure, its thermal capacity behavior, and the capabilities of the contemplated system. He or she must fully understand the interaction of the space with external and internal thermal loads and select a system that will effectively cancel these loads (including positive pressure surgery, negative pressure isolation, separate thermostat requirements, animal area minimal exchange requirements [e.g., greater than ten total exchanges per hour], and dumping of "conditioned air" rearward), without compromising the needed sound and smell barriers of a veterinary facility. It should be mutually agreed by all concerned that the equipment installed, the control of the system, and the building must be integrated to be successful.

After having established the requirements for blending the air-conditioning system into the basic structure, the architect-engineer team must consider the thermal load. They must devise a structure that is architecturally and acoustically acceptable and pleasing and that incorporates all possible forethought to minimize the air-conditioning load. Orienting the building with regard to sunlight and shade is essential. Heat gained from the sun through 150 sq. ft. of unshaded glass facing west is 12,000 Btu (requiring one ton of cooling) compared to 1,200 Btu (requiring 0.10 ton of cooling) for 150 sq. ft. of unshaded glass facing north. The total thermal load has a bearing on the space required for air-conditioning equipment and for transmission and distribution of the heating-cooling medium.

Systems Building

The objective of systems building is to lower cost by standardizing mechanical, electrical, and structural systems in a way that reduces on-site labor costs. Such systems are particularly effective where a large number of repetitive spaces are needed, for example, in wards, pet resorts, and boutiques. The integration of mechanical, electrical, and structural systems requires the involvement of the manufacturer in design. These integrated systems become building blocks. A variety of sizes of buildings can be constructed simply by changing the number and arrangement of the blocks. Systems building might be applied to the repetitive portions of a hospital, such as the office space and wards in a larger facility, but the present state of the art makes them less practical for most other areas of the hospital.

The professional mechanical and electrical engineer is trained, during his or her formal education, in many types of engineering studies, from space to undersea design. A young engineer will specialize in a field and after gradua-

tion will develop his or her expertise in a specified discipline. HVAC systems engineering involves both a mechanical and electrical specialty and can be further broken down into the following areas:
- heating, ventilation, and air-conditioning
- plumbing and process piping
- energy application
- control monitoring systems, including security systems
- communications, including AV, computer, Internet, and telephonic needs
- electric power distribution, including explosion proof where needed
- electric lighting design, aesthetic as well as functional

Setting Fees and Bidding

The basic percentage fee is based on the total construction cost of a project; it is higher if the project is smaller, because major services are the same for any size project. Over the past years, percentage fees have not risen along with the cost of living index because they are adjusted by a percentage applied to an escalating construction cost index. A fixed fee, or per diem fee, is also common to the profession, and is usually based on an hourly rate of $75-$175, depending on the status of the individual working on the project.

By the early 1990s, many states had begun bidding architects' and engineers' fees as a lump sum price. This price is based on a set of plans, or scope, that defines square footage, and on a construction cost estimate. The architect calculates the number of hours necessary to complete the project and multiplies that number by a direct cost loading factor, an overhead (general and administrative cost) loading factor and a profit factor to obtain his or her lump sum price. Travel and related expenses may be directly reimbursable or included in the cost. This type of bidding initially violated the professional ethics of architects, but it is now widely used by private industry.

Competition has driven architectural and engineering fees down over the past few years by about 10-15 percent. The total fee seems enormous, but, if broken down by the duration of the project and by services included, the architect's profits are found to be similar to those of any other professional. Included in the architect's lump sum fee are the following:

- exterior elevations for submission to zoning
- multiple working design drawings and elevations
- construction documents, including specifications for doors and windows
- negotiations for zoning variances required with municipality
- mechanical and electrical engineering
- structural engineering
- civil engineering and landscape design
- travel and printing cost

The American Institute of Architects' (AIA) standard contract has been tried and tested over many years, and it defines well the basic services of an architect.

The two methods of obtaining a construction price are competitive bidding and negotiated bids. In competitive bidding the owner advertises for general construction prices (including mechanical, electrical, site, and architectural) or separate major work (general, mechanical, and electrical). Competitive bids are received, and often the lowest bid is awarded the contract if the subcontractor's expertise can be verified based on the architect's drawings (it is easy for a disreputable contractor to low bid a project when change orders are used to pump up the prices after receiving the bid). In the negotiated (or cost-plus-materials) bid, a single contractor is selected. He works to a budget, charging for his time, overhead, profit, and materials.

Construction Management—Project Management

Construction management of human hospital projects began in the 1960s. Now, almost all projects include a construction manager for saving time. The ideas that originated in construction for developers were applied to hospital projects. For example, the practice of fast-tracking was first applied to speculative projects, such as apartment construction, in order to avoid price escalation. Fast-tracking involves beginning the foundation construction before the final building design is finished. It forced architects and engineers to complete their design and drawings before the total calculations and thoughts processes were concluded. Architects felt threatened because someone else now controlled their schedules and the process of design. Mechanical engineers could not accept design from the first floor up in order to offer advanced packages that might be built and bought sooner. The intended purpose of construction management had to be cleared up because negative attitudes were being formed among the construction manager, the architect, and the engineer. Clearly, these attitudes did not benefit the practice/hospital ownership. Through experience and sometimes difficult contract trauma, most of the problems have been resolved, and the initial concept of saving money now approaches reality.

Therefore, the newest member of the veterinary design team is now the project manager. His or her role is to see that all other members of the design team are satisfied with their products in the structure, use, cost, and schedule when compared to the owner's requested functional plan. Generally, few members of the team are satisfied. Too often clients who have done their own project management are heard to say, "Well, it is not really what I expected or what I wanted," or they blame the contractor or architect for cost overruns caused by small modifications asked for *after* the bid is established.

This condition of dissatisfaction is slowly changing with the help of project management and the project manager. The project manager creates circumstances during the design phase that result in a hospital that satisfies all members of the design team. He or she works methodically and continually to be sure that the knowledge and views of each member are heard and used even as the design is in process. The project manager sees the practice owner as a learner who, as time passes, increases his or her understanding of what is wanted versus what is really needed to open for business at completion. The project manager ensures that these views are clarified and brought to the design team's attention in ways that the design team members can respond to within the limits of schedule and budget. The design team members are also learning that their latest and best notions can be used by the practice only if the practice team can understand the value of their ideas for the new facility or the functional use of the new facility.

How can one ensure that all information is communicated quickly, absorbed readily, and acted upon? By hiring a dedicated project manager for all major veterinary construction projects. He or she ensures early continuing clarification of values, purposes, wants, and actions. The project manager performs the following functions:

- understanding the practice owner's expectations
- understanding the constraints on the practice budget
- understanding the expectations and limitations of the architect, engineer, and contractor(s)
- helping the design team communicate their expectations and needs to one another
- helping the architect and engineer make changes and stay within schedule and budget
- monitoring and reporting issues that seem likely to delay design or cause dissatisfaction among members of the design team
- preparing and conducting special problem-solving sessions to clarify values and objectives, improve design, maintain or lower cost, maintain or shorten schedule, improve life-cycle costs, and improve energy design and costs
- employing the methods and procedures of all problem-solving systems, including value engineering, practice core value clarification, design-to-cost, Kepner-Tregoe, Pert diagrams of work flow, and modified Delphi techniques for consensus

All of the project manager activities are intended to bring about the best possible value in design excellence, cost, and schedule. Project management methodologies may be divided into seven areas:

1. Practice team knowledge development
2. Information collection and interpretation
3. Problem identification
4. Alternative creation
5. Alternative selection
6. Implementation to the satisfaction of the design team
7. Transition planning from old facility to new

Team knowledge development allows the project manager to insert reality into the system to determine wants versus needs. All decisions have consequences, and in facility planning, most decisions carry a cost, either to the practice or to the design team member. The project manager walks a fine line in minimizing undue expenses to the practice while ensuring proper and timely remuneration for the expertise provided by the consultant(s), architect(s), and engineer(s).

Information collection and interpretation methods include Delphi forecasting, descriptive surveys, interviews (both to teach and to learn), programmed group exchanges (value verification and clarification), and review of scope, criteria, drawings, and specifications. The aspirations of the practice owner and design team are compared to expectations, and the understandings of each design team member are presented to ensure that all members of the team keep the purposes and objectives of the others before them.

In identifying problems, the project manager uses the above methods as well as cost models, energy models, and checklists to highlight at the earliest stages those areas that can be handled before they become major problems in design excellence, cost, or schedule.

Special techniques are used to compare such things as square feet of usable space per procedure zone, percentage of interstitial space actually used for mechanical-electrical functions, floor to ceiling heights, structural design of similar structures in similar conditions, and patient transportation distances and time. Special procedures are also used to ease adaptation to new ideas from the practice and from the architect and engineer. All things are reviewed from the standpoint that they can be done if . . . rather than from the standpoint that they cannot be done because . . . The project manager is the facilitator of an effectively operating veterinary practice when occupancy finally occurs.

Those methodologies that are drawn from value engineering need special mention. Value engineering is a set of concepts and methods used to adjust designs to acquire the best total value. Using definition and analysis of function, value engineering is aimed at achieving the lowest total cost commensurate with design excellence. Specific methods include function analysis, brainstorming sessions, matrix comparisons, and analysis of life-cycle costs.

The project manager employs all of these methods and ensures that the work is thorough, successful, and in line with the wishes of the design team and practice ownership. He or she paves the way for the design team by facilitating cooperation and understanding and by identifying potential areas of delay, design problems, and cost improvements. The project manager acts upon all of the above as approved by the design team and practice owner(s).

For example, suppose a veterinary facility design is budgeted for $1.2 million because "increased capacity" was a goal. The design team reports six months later that it will cost over $0.4 million more to build it as designed. The project manager should have verified the "increased capacity" need initially by looking at consultation room use, appointment fill rates, and existing facility utilization, then worked with the practice team to ensure the new functions, as seen by the veterinary-specific consultant, could be implemented and utilized to increase productivity. If the "increased capacity" was *not* needed, the initial design plan should have been sent back for redesign. If the "increased capacity" was needed, and the design team of mixed disciplines—including the architect and veterinary-specific consultant—concurred, presented a design within budget, and no "change orders" were authorized, then the cost overrun must be brought back to the design team as inappropriate fee assessments by contract. This overrun followed the architectural review and contract award phases and therefore cannot be approved as an afterthought. The project manager finds ways of bringing the cost in line with the budget and needed functions without reducing the scope of the hospital.

The project manager is a technical expert and as such is subordinate to the design team and practice owner. He or she is a manager, problem-solving leader, counselor, coordinator, and monitor. It is the project manager's job to make sure that all members of the design team and practice are pleased with the result of their labors.

The advantages of including a construction manager (or project manager) early in the design phase can be great. For example, the construction/project manager is familiar with

- current building systems that are available at a competitive price
- current labor and industrial prices, enabling him or her to ensure proper estimates
- subcontracting trades that can advise on detail
- specification review
- cost consulting and scheduling
- value engineering
- studies of life-cycle cost
- energy cost and conservation
- project time-line management
- inspections for owner and preinspections for municipality requirements
- insurance programming
- permit coordination and tracking actions
- samples and testing
- design and specification coordination

This knowledge, if applied in the design phase, can lead to cost improvements, time savings, and fewer change orders. The expected contingencies now budgeted and used should be reducible. Most construction/project managers only produce the general condition items in the construction of a project, manage the subcontracts and overall project schedule, and do not directly build any of the project with their own labor forces. Seldom are they general contractors, so they could not perform construction even if the ownership requested. Some veterinary-specific architect-engineer firms offer construction management services. The design-build firm incorporates construction management as an automatic step in its process.

The project/construction manager's responsibilities in the concept and pre-construction phase of design include

- reviewing project cost model and budget
- reviewing preliminary project master schedule

- conducting a site visit
- reviewing concept phase with architect and engineer and agreeing upon it
- updating master schedule and cost model
- ensuring the preliminary construction schedule, including staging, is understood
- finding alternative capital expense systems and evaluating cost
- analyzing HVAC and lighting/electrical systems requested
- recommending package documents for possible fast-track construction
- reviewing specification development and construction details
- identifying long-lead items and phasing concerns for subcontractors

The bidding and construction phase requires the project/construction manager to prepare the bid list, release bid packages to selected bidders, receive bids, review bids, and recommend an award of work. He or she manages general conditions on the site, including start-up and overall supervision, and supplies voluntary alternatives submitted by the bidding contractors. The project/construction manager receives the contractor's proposed manufacturers and provides recommendations on them to the practice owner, architect, and engineer. Based on data provided by the contractor, the project manager, architect, and engineer assess substitutions and recommend changes to the practice owner. Based on the client's reactions, the project manager advises the contractors of approvals and rejections of submitted manufacturers.

While this is a preconstruction planning text, the project manager has substantial duties during the construction phases, which should be mentioned here for a better understanding of the practice value of this key person:

- Shop drawings and equipment cuts from the subcontractors are sent to the project manager for review and approval. The project manager will return unacceptable drawings and cuts to the contractors.
- Contractor-approved shop drawings are sent to the architect and engineer for approval.
- Toward the end of construction, the project manager is responsible for working with the design team for drafting the certificate of substantial completion. This process includes

  a punch list of incomplete work prepared in conjunction with architects and engineers

  after completion of the punch list by the contractor, a conference with practice owner and architect-engineer firm to confirm completion

  issuance by the architect of a certificate of substantial completion with attached list of incomplete or unacceptable work

  after acceptance of the certificate of substantial completion by the practice and architect-engineer, the project manager monitors the guarantee period, identified in the certificate of substantial completion, while coordinating the practice occupancy and assuming responsibility for zone coordination and start-up integration.

  confirmation that the work has been completed and processing, in concert with the architect-engineer firm, the final payment application

With the client's acceptance of the certificate of final payment, the project is completed.

When necessary, the project manager can arrange for additional work that is not within the trade contract but that is within the scope of work and within the budget of the project.

Pricing Design

The introduction of a project manager to the veterinary facility planning team has broken with tradition, as described earlier. With someone else to talk to subcontractors, review construction details in an office, and get the advice of the people who will actually work on the job, the architect can go back to his or her original profession as a designer who defines quality, quantity, and form. Architects should not dictate every final construction technique or they will become inhibited in their ability to create things "that "can't be built." With a project manager, the hospital ownership can go back to client education and patient treatment, instead of just being an expensive absentee doctor not producing income because he or she is at the job site worrying. In the case of design-build architects, some practices have found cost overruns to be caused by the "fox supervising the hen house" syndrome, where the design-build oversight procures construction elements from preferred vendors, thereby increasing the supplies and equipment costs to the practice. The difference between theory and actual cost of a design must be worked out between a creative design team and the expert craftsman who got the bid for construction. Trying to be both can eliminate creative, economical design.

Pricing design is that interchange between craftsman and design team that can produce the most creative economics for the practice. Rather than final details, outlines are prepared and discussed. Once this interchange has produced the desired approach, the details are sketched in and specified for quality and quantity only. The final shop drawing submitted by the contractor keeps this interchange alive, and a design can be reviewed up until the moment before it is manufactured. This approach is applied to every item and then details are sketched for each room in the hospital. For the first time, because the project manager is now doing the required integration tasks, the practice manager/hospital administrator/practice owner can review every item in a room at once. The benefits are immense: The practice ownership can make budget and design decisions by having one simple document. Other benefits of pricing design include

- guaranteed price can be reached sooner because drafted detailed drawings are not required
- sole source procurement can be verified as essential, or competitive bidding can be initiated by the contractor/subcontractor
- the design/equipment vendor can make all form, quality, and quantity recommendations for each room, thus benefiting client, patient, and staff and encouraging innovation

- the contractor can estimate the job more easily with the freedom of an open line to discuss each item
- construction details can be changed quickly
- municipality and local review time is shorter because of the nature of the smaller document

As stated before, the ideas of project management and pricing are not new, but they must be understood in order to work in veterinary medicine. The pressures for social and economic change that now bear on every veterinary practice can be offset by a creative approach to construction and design. The voluntary effort that now applies to veterinary practices to provide affordable pet care also applies to the architectural, engineering, and contractor professions.

Conclusion

We have talked a lot about team makeup and the importance of understanding and integrity among the design team members. The reason that it is so important may be clear, but we would like to stress it. The planning and design team represents the client, patient, staff, and practice ownership, which is accountable to the public. The decisions and recommendations of the design team are presented to and approved by the practice's planning committee and the ownership, but the ideas formulated by the design team will affect thousands of clients and patients in the future. This makes it absolutely necessary to choose a first-rate design team and project manager in order that a mediocre project not be the final result.

Insights and Perspectives

From Start to Finish—Who Can Assist You
Sam Salahi, AIA

My first veterinary project right after college was assisting my parents with planning and construction of their veterinary clinic. Spending time with my parents and their architect prior to construction showed me the importance of proper planning, paying attention to details, and being organized. This experience, along with having worked at the clinic, has been instrumental in how I have approached various veterinary projects throughout the last fifteen years.

Plan and Build with Your Team

Every project starts with a dream due to a need or want. I firmly believe that you should at least have a basic plan in mind. If you are not quite sure of your needs or the extent of the plans, retain the services of a veterinary consultant to assist you. An appropriate plan and strategy can expedite progress and expansion of your business, and years down the road when you are ready to make your exit, it can enhance the value of your business and building.

When you think it is time to expand, remodel, or build a new facility, start by writing down your thoughts and dreams. Surround yourself with a good experienced team. Your team members—realtor, attorney, architect, contractors, etc.—should be on the same page because you gave them clear directions. They should work with you, for you, not around you. Establish a level of comfort with them. Experienced team members such as architects and contractors reduce your involvement during the length of the project, which allows you to spend more time with your business and personal lives.

Ask your potential team members to furnish you with a résumé, which outlines their philosophy, experience, a reference list, and fee schedule. Unfortunately, extra fees and extra costs have always been synonymous with every project. Therefore, fourteen years ago, we decided that all of our fees should be discussed up front for the scope of work set forth by our clients. Rather than looking at percentage of construction cost, we look at the time it takes to complete each phase. Our architectural and engineering fees never exceed 6 percent of construction cost unless our client increased or drastically changed the scope of work. This is an example of how you may have options for reducing your soft costs. Once you have your ideas, professional goals, finances, a location and your design team in place, you are ready to begin.

I would like to share with you my basic planner (see tables 2.1a–2.1e). Some parts of this planner may not be appropriate for your project, but for the most part, it outlines who can assist you with various tasks during planning and construction of your facility.

Table 2.1a. Site Planning

Task	Who Can Assist
• Selection of a Lot or a location	Consultant, realtor, architect*
• Purchasing	Realtor, real estate attorney, financial institution
• Proper zoning	Real estate attorney, architect
• Verifying setbacks, utility easements	Civil engineer, architect*
• Lot coverage, floor area ratio	Civil engineer, architect
• Special use or variance	Real estate attorney, architect
• Drainage and water runoff	Civil engineer
• Geotechnical studies (soil borings, etc.)	Soil/geotechnical engineer
• Environmental studies (contamination, etc.)	Environmental consultant/inspector
• Location of existing utilities	Local/city engineer, civil engineer
• Demography studies	Consultant, architect*
• Traffic studies	Consultant, architect*
• Site plan and surveys	Site/civil engineer
• Landscape planning	Landscape architect or contractor
• Parking lot layout	Site/civil engineer, architect*
• Building location	Architect, civil/site engineer
• Well & septic plans (if required)	Well & septic engineer/architect

Note: * designates a team member or his consultants.

Table 2.1b. Building Planning

Task	Who Can Assist
• Ultimate wish list	Consultant, architect, project manager
• Absolute needs	Consultant, architect, project manager
• Construction financing	Consultant, financial institution
• Predesign planning	Consultant, architect, site/civil engineer, project manager
• Design planning	Consultant, architect, site/civil engineer, project manager
• Cost estimating at design level	Contractor, architect*, project manager
• Meetings with the city design review board	Architect, project manager
• Construction documents	Architect*, civil/site engineer
• Interior and exterior specifications	Consultant, architect*, interior designer, project manager
• Establishing a construction schedule	Architect, project manager

Note: * designates a team member or his consultants.

Table 2.1c. Actual Site Work

Task	Who Can Assist
• Tree preservation or removal	Contractor*
• Well and septic	Well and septic contractor
• Utility hookup and installation	Various utility company contractors
• Grading	Contractor*
• Landscaping	Landscape contractor
• Fences, gates, exterior runs	Contractor* (per city/local codes)
• Parking lot	Contractor (per city/local codes)
• Exterior lighting and sign	Contractor* (per city/local codes)

Note: * designates a team member or his consultants.

A Few Sam Salahi Suggestions

• If you are planning to operate your practice during construction, hire a dedicated project manager, who, if they work out, will eventually become the practice manager after the transition into the new facility.
• Verify that the property or the location of the building is not in a flood plain.
• Water runoff from surrounding properties should not drain on your property or through your property.
• Verify that the site is big enough for your building, parking area, landscaping, and retention area as required by the local building department. (Variances and permits for conditional use take time and are costly).
• Verify that the site is zoned for the use and meets all other regulations.
• Check the soil condition around the construction area.

Table 2.1d. Actual Construction—Building

Task	Who Can Assist
• Building construction	Contractor, project manager
• Change orders, questions	Contractor, architect, project manager
• Credits or extra cost related to changes and revisions	Contractor, architect, project manager
• Unforeseen conditions	Contractor, architect, project manager
• Comparing actual construction to the plans	Architect, project manager
• Regular construction meetings	Contractor, architect, project manager
• Reviewing payouts	Architect, financial institution, project manager
• City inspections	Contractor
• Hospital equipment	Architect, project manager
• Data telecommunications setup	Consultant, project manager
• Furnishing	Interior designer, architect, project manager
• Final occupancy permit	Contractor
• Final punch-list	Architect, project manager
• Final payout approval	Architect, financial institution, project manager

Table 2.1e. Bidding and Contractor Selection and Permit

Task	Who Can Assist
• Prequalifying and selecting contractors	Colleagues, architect, project manager
• Establishing bid documents, bid forms, and deadline	Architect, project manager
• Receiving and reviewing bids	Architect, project manager
• Interviewing and selecting the contractor	Architect, project manager
• Finalizing construction schedule	Architect, contractor, project manager
• Construction contract with contractor	Architect, attorney, project manager
• Establishing payout schedule	Architect, contractor, project manager
• Insurance issues during construction	Contractor
• A chain of command to deal with changes and issues	Architect, contractor, project manager
• Actual start date	Architect, contractor, project manager
• Retaining required permits	Contractor, architect

• Verify that the demography of nearby population can support your practice and specific healthcare delivery goals.
• Verify the requirement of your financial institution or the city on traffic and environmental studies. (D&B [Dun & Bradstreet] in lieu of Environmental Phase 1 is often possible with established land that has had minimal use.)
• Establish a budget with an absolute cap for your project, and stay with it; ensure you overbuild to the future instead of underbuild to the past.

- Surround yourself with an experienced and competent team to assist you with the project. Negotiate all fees up front prior to retaining their services.
- Verify that your architect and contractor are familiar with local codes and ordinances, as they vary.
- Establish responsibilities and policies for your project manager and team members before an issue arises during the construction.
- If you think it is appropriate, involve your project manager and staff in planning and design reviews.
- Design and plan for your current and future needs.
- Make sure everybody understands and agrees with your schedules and deadlines.
- If time or your financing does not allow you to build your master plan, place the building on the property to allow for future expansion.
- If construction documents are somewhat overwhelming, ask your design team to walk you and your project manager through all layouts, finishes, etc., to verify that the plans meet all your needs and requirements.
- Ask your attorney to review or recommend all contracts.
- You don't have to hire the construction company with the lowest bid. Look at their promptness, experience, reference list, and demeanor.
- If you wish to implement penalties for missing deadlines, be prepared to offer bonuses if the construction is completed sooner than the established schedule.
- If you don't have the time or know how to perform a task, don't hesitate to ask the project manager or a team member to assist you.
- Meet on a regular basis with your project manager and team members. Take notes and ask questions if issues are not clear.
- Last, but not least, stay with your plan, stay organized, and ensure your project manager communicates with you and your team members.

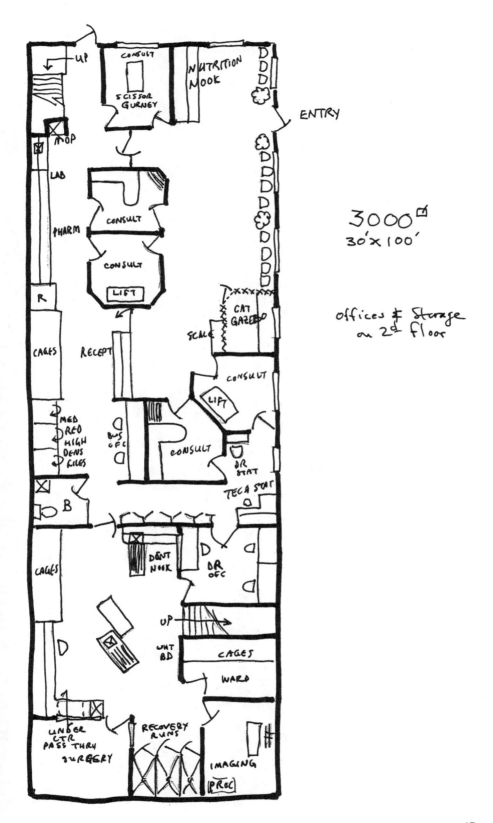

ENTRY

3000 ☐
30'x100'

Offices & Storage
on 2nd floor

UP

CONSULT

NUTRITION NOOK

SCISSOR GURNEY

MOP

LAB

PHARM

CONSULT

CONSULT

LIFT

R

CAGES

RECEPT

CAT GAZEBO

SCALE

CONSULT

LIFT

MED
RED
HIGH
DENS
FILES

BUS OFC

CONSULT

DR STAT

B

TECA STAT

CAGES

DENT NOOK

DR OFC

UP

WHT BD

CAGES

UNDER CTR
PASS THRU
SURGERY

RECOVERY RUNS

WARD

IMAGING

[PROC]

47

3

Design Scope and Fees

O NCE THE NEED for a construction project is determined, a game plan must be established—that is, an understanding by the entire design team of the scope of ideas contemplated for the project. At this point the veterinary-specific practice consultant, project manager, practice manager/hospital administrator, and ownership have been working on the projected and current needs of the community and catchment area. A facility master plan has been approved, in principle, by the ownership; a financial study of the practice liquidity has been completed; and an architect and engineers have now been added to fill out the team. The practice is now paying for a full team of design professionals.

It is at this time that understandings must be shared through brainstorming sessions or planning seminars. The architect and engineers should be on board within the scope of the budget and functional planning guidelines. A major part of the changes that will be produced in physical form will now be made. Irreversible cost determinations that develop now must be escalated to a schedule for the future. Each member of the design team will have ideas to offer, as will the veterinary-specific practice consultant, staff members, and project manager; the veterinary-specific practice consultant and project manager should be holding group sessions at this time—practice team buy in will be a key to success. If no such meetings are held, major conflicts can develop among the team members.

Engineering Plan

When cost overruns occur in the transition from programming to building, it is usually because there has been no clear engineering plan. At all phases of design planning, the engineering system's needs or desires must be identified. To do otherwise would be like buying a car without buying the motor.

An engineering plan may be only an engineering study with system description and loads. Existing mechanical and electrical systems for every facility zone should be studied. Existing mechanical systems that should be studied include

- domestic water
- sanitary storm sewers

- natural gas piping
- central oxygen
- nitrous oxide as indicated
- active waste gas exhaust system
- surgical vacuum
- compressed air
- deionized water
- fire protection
- steam requirements, if any
- condensate return and boiler feed water as applicable
- fuel oil/diesel oil as applicable
- heating, ventilating, and air-conditioning
- chilled water
- biomedical waste disposal +/- on-site Type IV biological waste incinerator
- central monitoring of mechanical systems

The following electrical systems should be checked:

- power supply
- emergency power systems
- telephones
- fire alarm and detection
- time clock in-and-out register
- radio/intercom/pager paging systems
- television cable/antenna
- loudspeaker paging
- intercom
- electronic client-patient tracking systems
- clocks
- surveillance, entry, and security alarms
- Internet access
- computer and CRT/LCD panel wiring and linkages
- physiological monitoring for patients
- exterior security and lighting
- power distribution
- secondary distribution feeders
- motor control centers
- branch circuit wiring
- receptacles (grounded, explosion proof, etc.)
- lighting (regular and emergency)

Envelope and Systems Building

The envelope is the building structure, skin, and mechanical systems. The way in which treatment is carried out, how receiving and discharge flow is done, and when special procedures are done are dependent on systems and space. The envelope defines this space for twenty to fifty years.

Flexible space has often been referred to in the planning of later expansions into attic and basement space, but without being well defined. The practice's planning team must know what is being developed versus what is being deferred.

Systems review takes into account the special training needed prior to utilizing a design capability within a particular facility. The methods of monitoring, reducing maintenance, supplying gases, plumbing, and carrying materials must be worked out by the design team, but utilized by the practice staff, so integrated planning is needed. This applies to any size veterinary facility and should be considered in the planning process. A good program states the internal mission focus of services, programs, and support systems as well as the broader mission of cage and run units and veterinary services to the community.

Energy Plan

The energy plan affects the long-range and yearly operational cost of any practice. It documents energy efficiency against current and projected fuel costs. The initial decision on what equipment to buy is studied against the equipment's life-cycle costs (i.e., when it will pay for itself and how much it will save). Solar energy, total energy, recycled energy, energy efficiency, recoverable energy, and potential energy can become feasible in the future, and these should not be ignored in the programming phase.

Operational Program

The operational program is a document that outlines the critical staffing patterns, zone utilization and locations, and major functional elements that will affect practice operations in the future. A detailed program is developed with the veterinary-specific practice consultant, ownership, practice manager/hospital administrator, key staff, and project manager. Appropriate protocols are written after the modern delivery systems are developed in the existing facility and then applied to the building project; these applied protocols may become a part of the documentation required by the design team if initiated far enough in advance of the team's identification. There is no standard veterinary practice operational program, and each practice must develop its system in different ways; building on existing practice and staff strengths is a consistent desire, as is using the expertise of a veterinary-specific practice consultant to assist in the development of alternatives. The practice programs should be written by the staff in concert with the consultant(s) who worked on the project scope. Concurrently, the consulting architect who completed the facility master plan should have adapted designs to the new delivery modalities (rather than past experiences or personal design habits). The practice manager/hospital administrator has a tremendous influence on this document and could write it him- or herself with enough time and a compatible team already operating under the new programs and delivery systems.

Writing the operational program will spur the creative ideas of the practice planning team and it is absolutely necessary that their knowledge and experience be involved. Although the architect and engineers do not write the final document, their ability to visualize design proposed by the veterinary-specific practice consultant, practice manager/hospital administrator, and practice ownership is important. As many meetings as necessary should be held, for there is no benefit to reducing the time spent during this creative period.

The following are goals of an operational program:

- to study the zone operations in regard to existing and projected number of clients, patients, staff, surgeries, dentistries, treatment tables, cages, runs, laboratory tests, imaging demands, and special procedures
- to continue to update the facility master plan each year
- to interview staff in order to establish personal and zone needs based on the proposed delivery systems
- to revise needs and operations in light of new AAHA hospital standards and emerging veterinary healthcare delivery programs

Many times operational and functional programming (that is, a room-by-room list of needs) is combined in an effort to determine the facility's size for cost estimating. It is important that input to the architectural design is begun before a final room-by-room size is decided; otherwise, the talents of a team member to create new space in order to meet unanticipated needs could be lost. Only after the team talks, writes, and draws its ideas can a functional program defining the exact size of the project be presented.

Once the ownership has approved the operational program, and the interzone functional elements are being discussed by the practice's planning team, the entire facility must be brought together as a single design. The creation of the hospital design centers on the architect and engineers with input from the veterinary-specific consulting team and practice planning team. Although architectural designers can create exciting shapes and forms, the scope of a hospital concept has certain limitations. At the same time, no standard design can ever be used for all veterinary hospitals. Because a veterinary practice is as complex as a city, individualized design is necessary. The economics of hospital construction indicate that more modular approaches must be developed around building systems, but the practice operation itself eliminates a pat approach.

Space Program

The *total area* of a hospital is expressed in gross square feet within a hospital (square meters in many countries outside the United States). *Net area* is the usable floor area of a space. *Gross area* of the building is the total enclosure as measured by, and including, the outside walls; it is the sum of the net areas and the nonassignable areas. Nonassignable areas include wall and partition thicknesses, vertical and horizontal circulation, and mechanical shafts. To convert net square feet to gross square feet, a multiple of 1.2-1.4 is usually used unless excessive hallways have been inserted.

In programming and planning a hospital, most architects and consulting architects use gross square footage per department plus circulation in order to properly size the real volume and cost of a proposed design. (*Note:* In this text, all zone needs and planning ratios are given in gross square feet. These numbers most often represent the needs of primary care general practices, and in a few places address the specialty practice complex supporting a veterinary community of practices. A teaching or tertiary care veterinary facility will usually require 20-50 percent more space because of specialty research and teaching space required within each department as well as separate expanded programs and will not be addressed in this text.)

Phasing and Expansion

The conversion of planning to capital improvements is carried out through phasing. Very seldom can all the needs and goals of a existing facility be met in one expansion project or expenditure. In fact, expansion may be limited by the practice liquidity, staffing, or patients-per-day access rates.

Expansion is most often dictated by the amount and type of land available and the existing facility condition. The number of entrances to a building and its footprint (the area of land covered by it at ground level) must be able to cope with an increasing barrage of people, patients, and vehicles. Future additions must be able to meet interior and exterior needs. To accomplish footprint growth, a phasing plan must be developed in the conceptual stage that defines future potential additions or any movement of either zones or the ancillary services base. This plan would also outline future spending needs and a proposed budget. A long-range plan must include future expansion phasing or it will be obsolete. In addition, each phase must stand alone, as if no other were ever to be built, for hospital zones can seldom close to accommodate remodel construction. This is also important in the engineering plan as relocating an entire engineering system is very expensive.

In many veterinary practices looking to remodel, we have promoted and implemented an outpatient wing expansion while the existing facility continues to operate (e.g., North Shore Animal Hospital [MN], Cleveland Heights Veterinary Hospital [FL], Lake Street Veterinary Clinic [IL], etc.). When the new outpatient wing opens, with a few cross connections to the old facility, the portal holes in the wall are covered while renovation of the existing original facility becomes the core of the new inpatient wing and office systems of the total renovation.

Additional Services

As previously stated, there is an "expert consultant" to be found on any conceivable subject; this is doubly true in veterinary hospital programs. The practice ownership must, therefore, actively determine the extent of additional services that must be employed to complete the project and review the published works and credentials of any veterinary consultant considered in the planning process.

The basic contract for architectural services has been defined for only the basic services. In the following list, basic services are noted as B, and extensive additional services that may be necessary and cost extra are noted as A.

1. Practice consultant or consulting architect:
   develop long-range plan and recommendations   A
   study of practice needs role   A
   staff questionnaire and assessment   A
   facility master plan   A
   space utilization review   B
   financial feasibility of construction budget   B
   operational programs   B
   special analysis of practice's needs   B
   personnel utilization review   A
   mobile and fixed equipment consulting   A
   materials-handling needs study, as applicable   A
   client access/catchment area profile   B
   negotiations with fiscal institutions   A
2. Architect:
   schematic design phase   B
   unit construction estimating   B
   design development   B
   construction documents   B
   normal engineering services   B
   specifications   B
   representative of client during construction   A or B
   periodic inspection   B
   extensive inspection   A
   architectural rendering   A or B
   scale models   A or B
   special analysis of practice's needs   A
   site evaluations   A or B
   design services for future facility expansion   A or B
   measured drawings or investigation of existing facility   B
   preparing documents for alternate bids   A
   detailed estimates and pro formas   B
   inventories of existing material or equipment   A
   changes in drawings beyond architect's control   A
   change orders   B
   consultation on replacing work damaged by fire or other
       cause during construction   A

services necessary through default of contractor	A
reproducible records drawings	A
operating manuals for installed equipment	B
inspection past construction time	A
serving as or briefing an expert witness for public hearing or legal proceedings	A
extra engineering studies (energy or existing conditions)	A
certified land survey	A
test borings (Environmental Phase 1)	A
soils engineer	A
laboratory tests (mechanical, electrical, structural, chemical)	A
legal and accounting services	A
reproduction costs above specified amounts	A
systems management	A
value engineering	A or B

3. Interior consultants:

interior design (textures and colors)	B
design display board (fabrics, floors, and colors)	A
furniture procurement	A
lighting design (fixtures and ambiances)	A
existing inventory	A

4. Graphics:

practice directional programs	A
practice logo (including "graphic standard" colors)	A
wall graphics and pictures	A
signage design (road attraction and practice colors)	B

5. Equipment design:

list of movable equipment	A
list of fixed equipment	B
dietary/feeding areas	A or B
cleaning systems, facility and animal areas	B
laboratory design	B
materials handling (linen, trash, foot supplies, people)	A
information technology needs	B
Ancillary service special requirements	A

6. Civil engineering:

site utility study	A or B
parking study	A or B
community master traffic plan integration	A or B

7. Construction:

project manager coordination	B
construction management	B
detailed construction estimating	B
critical-path scheduling with contractor	B
clerk-of-the-works	A

permits and bonds	A or B
utility companies liaison	A or B
insurance	A
8. Public relations:	
building programs	A
groundbreaking ceremony	A
employee manual	A
photography	A

This list illustrates the numerous variations available, variations that can amount to an additional 20 percent of the construction cost. An example of a total project construction budget with fees is shown in the appendix C. This budget does not include the legal, accounting, and hospital administration time involved in putting a project together.

The practice manager/hospital administrator and project manager should inform themselves and the practice planning committee of the vast possibilities that exist when developing a budget and should use professional services to their advantage. One of the most important aspects in a construction program is the project manager's ability to find and use professional services. When used properly, these services will more than pay for themselves in time saved and decisions made.

Costs

The final aspect of the game plan developed by the planning team is cost. It has been shown how operational costs are affected by design. No matter how much space is added above the amount programmed, it will be occupied by people and equipment and "empty" space will be used.

It must be stressed that every square foot of a hospital can become costly to the client and practice and therefore must be controlled. At this time, the cost per square foot of veterinary facilities in the United States ranges from $125 to $200, or even higher in certain parts of the country. This range is greatly affected by the fixed equipment, physical finishes, and quality of installed systems. The 2001 average of approximately $120 to $150 per square foot for new construction will probably escalate 8–15 percent per year until building industry restraints can be formulated. This average cost is for veterinary facility construction only and does not include land, contingency monies, municipality fees, equipment costs, and financing costs.

Discussion of realistic costs sets the mood for all further progress. There are many ways to estimate cost, as will be shown later, but the key issue here is the cost that the practice planning teams can project to build their concept. This will control the direction of the consultant, architect, and especially the project manager.

The responsibility for establishing a construction budget and developing a project that fits within that budget is shared by the practice planning team, the design team, and the professional veterinary-specific consultants available to the practice ownership. The budget (money available) and the cost (money required) should be reviewed, compared and made to match at scheduled intervals during the project. These reviews should be an integral part of the approval mechanism established by the ownership and project manager at the beginning of the job.

The design teams may have experienced highly publicized difficulties in the management of construction costs, and the importance and difficulty of establishing and maintaining a construction budget has not been given sufficient attention. Before work begins, design teams should be given, or should help to develop, an approved construction cost ceiling, together with a clear statement of the project's functional, aesthetic, and quality requirements. Planning a project involves thousands of decisions or choices that affect cost: A design team that is not working within clearly specified limits must rely solely on it's own sense of value, which may not be appropriate for the practice, the project, or even the owner(s). Costs for veterinary hospital construction have been inflating at the rate of 8–15 percent. This inflation may soon reach well over 20 percent per year.

The construction budget is usually established by subtracting all other costs, such as consultants, from the total projected cost. The difficulties of budgeting for construction usually arise from uncertainties about the availability of or the cost of obtaining the required funds. While it is not uncommon for planning and design to begin before sources of funding are finalized, the quality veterinary-specific consulting team should be available to expedite the term sheet development from potential financial institutions.

Where uncertainties remain, it is in the best interests of all concerned for the practice ownership, with the help of financial and design consultants, to make the necessary assumptions and establish a specific upper limit on construction cost. As the project and uncertainties are reduced, the status of the construction budget should be monitored and adjusted.

Cost estimates must be made and revised regularly from the conception of the program until the bid documents are at least half complete. Each time the construction cost is estimated, the project budget and associated project cost should also be updated for comparison. Discrepancies between projected budgets and costs should be resolved through the joint efforts of the practice, design team, and the project manager before design work proceeds.

Cost-estimating techniques are determined by the type of information used to describe the project and by the estimator. The accuracy of the estimate (pro forma) improves as the project becomes more specifically defined. In the earliest stages, experienced professionals can employ rule-of-thumb guidelines, such as cost per provider or cost per square foot, but the use of such techniques is extremely hazardous. Construction cost projections are not useful until they are based on reliable projections of space requirements and design characteristics (e.g., curved walls are more expensive than a four-corner rectangular building). Construction cost pro forma (estimate) revisions for a typical veterinary project might occur as the last step of each of the following tasks:

- preliminary space program by zone
- final space program by room
- preliminary schematic design (definition of building mass and zones only)
- final schematic design
- final elevations of exterior and interior design features
- design development
- contract document 50 percent complete
- contract document 80 percent complete

Pro formas and estimates made after the contract documents are more than 80 percent finished serve little practical purpose, since decisions made then have little impact on projected cost. Furthermore, any major structural changes made beyond the midpoint that would significantly alter the construction cost would also disrupt the project delivery schedule.

Construction cost pro formas (estimates) for the early phases (through preliminary schematic design) are made by the architect by projecting the probable cost per square foot of either the entire project or the project components. Additions to and renovations of existing veterinary hospitals should be analyzed between the ownership and the veterinary-specific consultant to determine the amount of space to be provided for each function or zone. Design teams and consultants who specialize in this type of project have learned to estimate the relative construction costs of veterinary hospital functions and zones with considerable confidence.

At the end of the schematic design stage, the project will be sufficiently well defined to permit more detailed cost estimates based on the actual quantities of materials or systems shown by the plans and outline specifications. By the time the design development is completed, all of the building systems and components will be described in sufficient detail for a full quantity takeoff to be prepared in much the same way a contractor prepares his bid. Further pro formas during contract document production consist of simply adjusting individual elements of the design development estimate as minor changes occur and greater detail is provided.

Veterinary-specific consultants and architects have traditionally prepared pro formas (estimates) for their own plans and designs, but it is becoming increasingly common for estimating to be done by a cost consultant. This specialized consultant is usually either a professional construction estimator or the construction manager for another veterinary project. In either case, the expertise of the cost consultant should be called upon whenever the project must be tailored to fit the current budget.

Two of the most costly items in a construction cost pro forma (estimate) are time and uncertainty. Time is taken into account by escalation: An inflation factor is incorporated into the estimate to adjust prices of labor and materials to the levels expected at the time bids will be received. At a 9 percent construction escalation rate, a large veterinary project that might not be bid for a year after the first program-based pro forma is made would cost almost 12 percent more than the current dollar estimate (escalation in construction, equipment, and contingency fees). Uncertainty is accounted for in the construction cost pro formas by including contingencies. The bid contingency is carried in the cost estimate to cover the unpredictability of responses when bids are invited. Ten percent is used as a bid contingency, but 5 percent is a more realistic expenditure when there is a project manager. In addition, a design contingency of 10 percent should be added to the early estimates to allow for unanticipated costs that might be necessary to satisfy all of the conditions and criteria of the building program. This design contingency can be progressively reduced to zero as the construction documents near completion since all significant costs will have been identified.

Another valuable means of managing the inevitable risk of the construction marketplace is to identify alternatives in the contract documents. Prices are quoted on the basic project (base bid), and the additional cost of the alternative is identified separately. The practice owner(s) can then choose to delete the alternative from the project if sufficient funds are not available. There can be several alternatives in a single bid package. The alternatives should not include any items that are critical to the success of the veterinary project, and they should add up to a least 5 percent of the estimated cost. Specifying alternatives will probably create more work for the design team members, who will expect to be paid for the additional services.

Cost of Money

The cost of money is a key factor for any building program. At this time, a program borrowing one million dollars for construction at an interest rate that may run as high as 12 percent will pay up to one million dollars in interest payments over the financing period. Construction costs will average 50-60 percent of the total project cost. The remainder goes for fees, contingencies, and financing costs.

Fees

The practice must anticipate the total fees and cost of a building program in order to prepare a realistic estimate for all time and costs. The traditional architect's pro forma process has suffered a black eye because of cost overruns so often applied for after the fact. With cost containment critical to program development, the total cost of construction, with all associated fees, must be most carefully considered by the ownership and project manager when assessing bids and pro formas.

Consulting Fees

There is no standard for consulting fees. Each study is costed out against a similar effort and is based upon work days times overhead plus profit. Travel costs and living expenses on the road are usually directly reimbursable and are in addition to the fee.

Studies for long-range plans in human healthcare vary from $40,000 to $300,000 in fees and expenses, depending on the scope of services to be performed. In veterinary medicine, this long-range planning has traditionally been ignored but should not be when building the larger multidisciplinary or multi-owner complexes. Facility master plans are also based upon the defined scope of services. For example, fees for a 400-bed facility in human healthcare could range from $40,000 to $250,000; fees for an 800-bed facility or medical center would cost $125,000 to $450,000. These fees include the cost of the supporting team of healthcare consultants, consulting architects, and consulting engineers.

Architect-Engineer Fees

Basic services for new construction are commonly split into two separate fees: schematics, design development, and contract documents; and design inspection of construction.

Total services range from 6–10 percent of the construction estimate plus contingency. If split, the fee packages for basic services can be estimated as follows: design accounts for 5.5–6 percent of construction; engineer costs account for another 1–2 percent of construction; inspection accounts for 1.2–2 percent of construction; and in some municipalities, grounds and outside image can be 30 percent over the construction cost. Because of the restraints placed on budgets, many practices now put professional design fees up for bid and negotiate a single price (lump-sum fee) that is not based on construction costs.

The architect-engineer firm that submits a single-price bid must base this on a well-defined scope of work that describes the veterinary project. Man-effort hours are calculated, and then overhead (direct and indirect) and profit are applied. A fixed effort is based upon an exact schedule. If the practice's scope (size or building program) changes, the architect must negotiate a change in fee based on a 2.6-3 multiplier of staff salary and range from $40 to $150 per hour.

Structural, mechanical, electrical, and civil engineering fees are included in the basic services or lump-sum fees and are paid by the architect. These fees are approximately as follows:

- Structural engineers receive 7-14 percent of total fee.
- Mechanical and electrical engineers get 5-6 percent of the estimated construction cost of the mechanical and engineering work.
- Civil engineers charge 1.5-2 percent of the total fee.
- The engineering systems within a veterinary facility construction pro forma can make up 5-25 percent of the total construction cost.
- Cost estimating is usually done for 2-3 percent of the total fee.

Because of the existing conditions and complex, detailed work to support phasing construction, renovation fees may be higher than those for new construction.

Additional Fees

Fees for interior design equal 10-15 percent of the interior furnishings cost. A fee of $1 to $2.50 per square foot of space is not unusual. The cost of interior furnishings can be estimated at 5–10 percent of the construction costs.

Fees for consulting on movable equipment can equal 6-7 percent of the cost of the equipment. The movable equipment constitutes 15-17 percent of estimated construction costs. For example:

- Graphic design will cost about twenty-five cents to seventy-five cents per square foot.
- Professional renderings will cost $1,500-$5,000 each.
  Scale models cost $500-$15,000 each.
- Topography and site surveys run $1,000–$15,000 depending on the size of the site.
- Fees for soils testing vary with the number of test holes and range from $6,000–$30,000.
- Value engineering will cost 0.1–0.3 percent of the total cost of construction.
- An equipment consultant may charge 5-6 percent of equipment costs.
- The clerk-of-the-works charges $25,000-$40,000 per year of construction.
- A materials-handling study runs $5,000-$30,000, based upon size and scope.
- As-built drawings cost $20-$30 per hour and require 30-50 hours per sheet.
- Trained project managers cost between $50,000 and $75,000 for a year.
- An engineering audit or study will cost $5,000-$30,000, depending on scope.
- Per-diem costs range from $50-$500 per day for specific consultants.

Schedule

The next step in formulating a project is a discussion of schedule. The only thing that can be predicted is the change in seasons, and even that has a large plus or minus factor. Defining a design and construction schedule is the first step the project manager takes on with the contractor; in turn, this step will involve the entire practice staff. It will be up to the project manager to set up and/or chair numerous meetings, reviews, committees, trips, ownership reviews, and operation phasing once construction starts. The schedule will depend on financing, zoning, municipality approval, environmental approval, practice approval, community public relations, and the tremendous amount of time spent with the design team and practice planning team. Construction becomes as time consuming for the project manager as does Saturday morning outpatient day for a doctor in a companion animal practice. The money the practice spends on construction will be the largest single contract that the project manager handles, and this can cause unanticipated pressure. An awareness of schedule for such an undertaking can only be gained through experience and knowledge of the construction field. A review by a veterinary-specific consultant would be helpful at this time since a construction project will probably occupy a over a full year of time and thought.

There are many services geared toward schedule estimating and time scheduling. Bar graphs and critical-path scheduling can be used to predict each step, but each step involves so many possibilities that it is very difficult to define a typical schedule.

Review of the proposed project with every possible authority and interest group at this stage cannot be overemphasized. Before the project goes into a design-development stage or is approved by the practice planning team, all operational and functional reviews should be completed. With the new veterinary extender delivery modalities, many projects cannot be effectively planned until the new delivery systems are experienced firsthand. This is often not possible on a full scale, but can be tested with the assistance of a veterinary practice consultant.

A listing of specific steps to take in the review process is impossible, but it is possible to tell you that missing a key review can be disastrous. The following list is only a beginning:

- review of other veterinary practice delivery systems
- review of previous architect and contractor performances
- city/county planning requirements
- municipality zoning requirements
- environmental or public health department requirements
- environmental impact reviews
- historic register or historic zoning review (D&B—Dun & Bradstreet)
- state or regulatory code or taxation issues
- *AAHA Standards for Veterinary Hospitals*
- any local animal codes
- any community review requirements
- public transportation considerations
- public utilities and access coordination requirements
- practice planning team review
- design team review
- financial institution reviews

The team of consultants, architects, and engineers will assist in, and in many cases handle, the total review. Each area, however, involves important people in the practice, and the greatest amount of project manager social, or diplomatic, time will be need to be spent here.

A final part of the project manager's work in setting up the project schedule is that of total payment and cash flow. All of the professionals involved in basic services, additional services, construction contracts, and projected operational budgets are interested in cash flow. From the schedules developed, each area of cost flow can be projected. It is important to all members of the design team that there be an even flow. It is the duty of the project manager to accomplish this in conjunction with the financial institution's guidelines. Payment schedules will be defined in the contracts of the consultants, architects, engineers, and contractors. A master plan should be drawn up to ensure a monthly cash flow.

Codes and Standards

Codes apply in two areas: public health and safety and minimum legal requirements. The design team architect and engineers must have a working knowledge and specific reference to various building codes and design standards requested by the practice. Various municipality and state building codes apply to each location and type of building. Municipal government agencies usually adopt a set of bureaucratic procedures to review proposals and plans and then form their own zoning and building construction codes. Zoning codes relate to the type and occupancy of the building and specify building setbacks; for example, parking requirement, lot coverage, height maximums, and use classification.

The national *Life Safety Code* outlines specific building type requirements: smoke control; fire rating separation for walls, doors, and exit stairs; smoke and fuel contribution standards for all interior materials; and all safety-related requirements.

The facility classification, fire and exit review, and safety standards must be reviewed and approved by the city and county before construction can proceed. A building construction permit and approved occupancy certificate must be obtained in the construction process. The property and improvements are then recorded into the city or county plats.

A review by various inspection agencies is also necessary in order to comply with health and safety standards. All health facilities must meet special fire and safety requirements for design and construction. Various national codes that apply to the handicapped and to staff operational safety must also be reviewed in order to conform. Barrier-free standards, Occupational Safety and Health Administration codes, and aids for the blind are a must in most healthcare facility designs.

Major codes for veterinary healthcare facility design are: (1) the *Life Safety Code* (National Fire Protection Association [NFPA], Code 101) and all other NFPA fire codes; (2) technical handbook for Facilities Engineering and Construction Manual, Part 4, Facilities Design and Construction (architectural section 412, Design of Barrier-Free Facilities); and (3) *Minimum Requirements of Construction and Equipment for Hospital and Medical Facilities.* If the hospital structure is deficient in any of these major areas of safety, fire, minimum function, barrier-free access, and public health standards, the facility may be determined not in conformance either in part or totally. Nonconformance implies that the deficiencies will be brought up to code before occupancy may occur. The ultimate threat is loss of access.

Insights and Perspectives

Project Economics

Lawrence A. Gates

How do you determine what you can spend on your facility and still make your business plan work? The answer to this question is found in the balance between your potential income and the cost of providing services.

On the income side, your income potential is based on your market, the services you offer, and the size and ability of your staff. One of the first steps to take in determining market potential is to establish for yourself the type of practice that would be ideal for you. This would include elements of practice personality and style, the types of services that you would like to offer, and target goals for overall size. Once you've defined your "dream practice," it's time to get realistic and see if you have the resources to make your dream happen.

Resources fall into a number of different categories: location, marketplace support, staff, and available equity.

Some locations are surefire winners. Some are losers. Most succeed based on the veterinarian having a feel for the temperament of the community, the relative value the community places on the veterinarian's services, and the competition.

The services you offer, to some extent, will be tailored to your market. Your practice may be high end, with a heavy emphasis on high-tech medical services and ancillary services, such as boarding, grooming, and training, or it might be a more traditional approach.

Market is generally defined by calculating the number of households, their demographic characteristics, income, and the competition within your market area. These are the numbers that you use to test your business plan and establish your income potential.

The success of your business strategy will depend on your costs. Even a business offering the best services will not survive if it can't make a profit. Your cost to provide services includes salaries, supplies, "rent," and other overhead costs.

Our focus here will be to demonstrate a method of determining the cost of rent.

Most real estate developers use a formula called a pro forma to evaluate the initial feasibility of an investment. Working with a pro forma is a balancing act with cost on one side and income potential on the other. It is used to help you optimize your yield on the resources you put into a project. Simply put, it is a standard way of tallying costs and calculating the facility cost, or rent. For our purposes, rent is defined as the amount you pay on a monthly or yearly basis for your facility. Whether the money goes to you, a holding company, or a third party, the formula will basically be the same.

A pro forma is divided into four parts:

1. Hard costs—tangible assets such as the land and the building
2. Soft costs—services such as architectural, engineering, legal, accounting, construction financing, and contingencies

3. Financing—principal and interest payments and return on equity
4. Operating expenses—taxes, insurance, utilities, maintenance, etc.

A quick explanation of the following pro forma example would be: Hard and soft costs are tallied to produce total project costs. Your equity requirements are subtracted from total project costs to establish the amount of money you need to borrow, which in turn tells you what your monthly payments will need to be. Loan payments added to operating expenses will give you the total amount you will have to pay for rent.

PRO FORMA

Hard Costs

Land costs		$150,000
Building costs		
Building sq. ft.		$4,000
Cost per sq. ft.		$150
Total building costs		$600,000
TOTAL HARD COSTS		$750,000

Soft Costs

Architectural		$42,000
Engineering		
Civil (survey, soils, drainage)		$7,500
Environmental (variable)		
Structural		$7,500
Mechanical		$9,000
Electrical		$4,500
Regulatory and utility		
Development fees (variable)		
Water/sewer tap fees		$3,000
Financing		
Appraisals		$4,000
Construction loan		
Points	1.00%	$6,000
Interest rate	8.25%	$12,375
Permanent loan commitment	1.5%	$9,000
Closing costs		$4,500
Contingency	3.00%	$21,280
TOTAL SOFT COSTS		$130,655
TOTAL PROJECT COSTS		$880,655

Financing

Equity	20.0%	$176,131

Permanent loan		
Loan amount		$704,525
Loan period in years	20	
Interest	8.25%	
Loan payment per month		$5,962
Loan payment per year		$71,544
Return on equity per month		$734

Operating Expenses (per year)	
Real estate taxes	$6,000
Building insurance	$3,000
Utilities	$4,000
Maintenance	$2,000
Total operating expenses per year	$15,000

REQUIRED CASH FLOW (RENT)	
Per Month	$7,212
Per Year	$86,544

Building Costs

Calculating a realistic budget for your facility is critical to developing a meaningful pro forma, simply because building costs are the single largest expenditure. The expenditure is large because veterinary hospitals have all the complexity of a human hospital, while adding the requirements of animal care and housing. They are custom, individualized endeavors designed to a specific set of requirements.

The national average construction cost for new, freestanding hospitals during the past year is reaching $150 per square foot. For leasehold/tenant finish facilities, the average cost is $90 per square foot.

The following should be taken into consideration when estimating cost:

1. Regional variations: Whereas the average construction cost is $150, the cost of construction varies across the country from a low of 74 percent (in rural Alabama) to a high of 136 percent (in New York City) based on data developed by the R. S. Means Company, a national clearinghouse for construction costs.
2. Inflation: Even if you assume that these costs are very current, there still could be as much as a six-month time lag between the date that you initiate the project and when bidding occurs and construction begins. According to R. S. Means, construction costs are increasing at a rate of 6–9 percent per year, once again depending on the region in which you are located.
3. Contingency: Rather than lock into a specific construction cost per square foot, it makes sense to determine a target range that would take into account factors as diverse as variations in project size, anticipated project complexity, contractor availability and pricing methods, code requirements, availability of utilities, site improvement, soil conditions, the price of labor, and a contin-

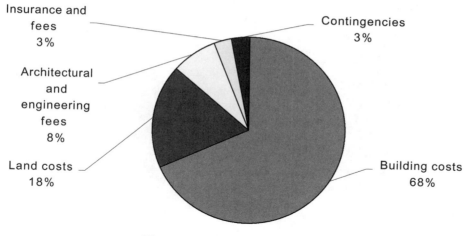

Total Project Costs

gency factor for the unforeseen costs. For these reasons, it is recommended that, at minimum, you set a range that would be plus or minus 5 percent.

Total Project Costs

While much discussion centers around the cost of the hospital structure, don't forget that you really need to keep focused on the *total project costs* as illustrated in figure 3.1. With a building cost of $150 per square foot, you might expect an *overall project cost* to run in the $220 range, based on average land costs and expenses.

Percentage of Total Project Cost

Building cost	68%
Land costs	18%
Architectural and engineering fees	8%
Interest, insurance, and fees	3%
Contingencies	3%

List of Possible Project Costs
I. Predesign services
    A. Site selection studies
    B Concept plan
    C. Legal fees
        1. Site acquisition negotiation
        2. Contract review
    D. Environmental studies
    E. Survey (meets and bounds, improvement, topo)
    F. Title commitment

    G. Planning and zoning review and application
       1. Filing fees
       2. Consultant coordination
       3. Legal fees
    H. Ground costs
  II. Financing/fund-raising
    A. Capital campaign
       1. Staff
       2. Advertising
       3. Consultants
    B. Government sponsored
       1. Legal
       2. Origination fees
 III. Site costs
    A. Soils report
    B. Additional hazardous waste studies
    C. Improvements to right of way
    D. Development fees
    E. Tap and utility fees
       1. Water
       2. Gas
       3. Electric
       4. Sewer
    F. Utility upgrade costs
 IV. Site and building costs
    A. Site development costs
       1. Landscape costs
       2. Fencing and screen walls
       3. Site demolition
    B. Building construction costs
    C. Building system equipment
       1. Emergency generator
       2. Cremation equipment
    D. Building department application
       1. Fees
       2. Consultant coordination
    E. Builder's risk insurance
    F. Owner-required testing and coordination
    G. Design fees
       1. Architectural
       2. Structural
       3. Mechanical
       4. Electrical
       5. Interiors
       6. Landscaping
       7. Civil engineering

V. Equipment
  A. Veterinary equipment built in
    1. Surgery/exam lights
    2. Tub/tables
    3. Cages and runs
    4. X-ray equipment
    5. Other
  B. Veterinary medical equipment
    1. Lab/processing
    2. Surgical
    3. Dental
    4. Prep
    5. Other
  C. Telephone and communication systems
  D. Computer systems
  E. Other
VI. Furnishings
  A. Furniture
  B. Signage
  C. Educational systems
  D. Retail display
VII. Relocation costs
  A. Moving
  B. Transition costs

Project Economics Review Issues

- Your income potential is based on your market, the services you offer, and the size and ability of your staff.
- Your resources will include location, marketplace support, staff, and available equity.
- You will probably adapt your services to fit the market your hospital serves.
- You can define your market by calculating the number of households in your area, their demographic characteristics and income, and the competition within your area.
- A formula called a pro forma can be used to determine the monthly payment you will need to pay for your hospital space.
- This pro forma is divided into four parts: hard costs, soft costs, financing, and operating expenses.
- Calculating a realistic budget for your hospital is critical to developing a meaningful pro forma because building costs are the single largest expenditure.
- The national average construction cost for new, freestanding hospitals during the past year is $150 per square foot. For leasehold/tenant finish facilities, the average cost is $90 per square foot.
- Average construction costs vary from region to region.

- It is important to figure the inflation that will happen during the lag time between bidding and the start of construction. Construction costs are increasing at a rate of 6–9 percent per year.
- A contingency of approximately 5 percent of the construction cost can help to pay for unforeseen costs.
- The total project cost includes building cost, land cost, architectural and engineering fees, interest, insurance, fees, and contingencies.

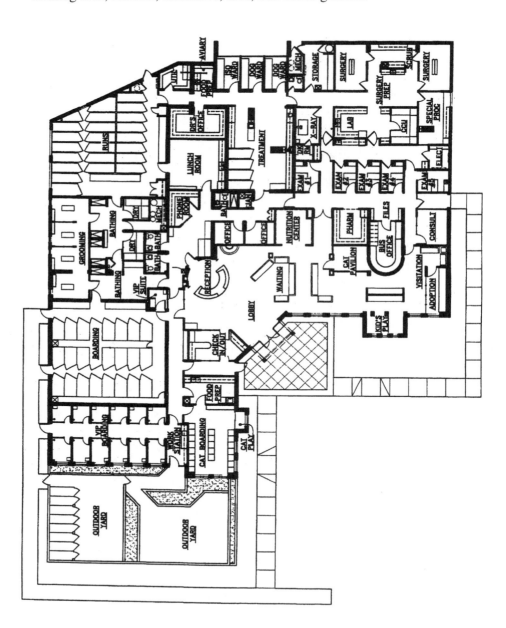

4

The Design Elements

THE DESIGN OF ANY given veterinary hospital must take into consideration a myriad of factors. In general, however, these factors fall into two categories: those features and problems that are common to all veterinary hospitals (though specific solutions vary), and those features and problems related to the specific vision, philosophies, and health-care delivery objectives of a given practice.

Common Factors

Factors common to all modern hospitals include

- veterinary design standards
- the elements in the architectural and engineering design process
- long-range facility plans
- structural systems
- functional adjacencies
- access, traffic, and transportation
- site and parking (including external traffic patterns and entrances)
- material-handling systems
- electronic, Internet, and security systems
- engineering systems (including plumbing and wastewater and lighting and electrical systems)
- heating, ventilation, air-conditioning

Design Standards

The design architect is bound by restrictions and codes that are absolutely necessary for public safety. Everyone agrees that the vast number of requirements must someday be coordinated and changed, but those who try to beat the intent of the codes are irresponsible.

The federal government's standards are listed in the Department of Health and Human Services Public Health Service document *General Standards of Construction and Equipment for Hospital and Medical Facilities,* which covers the steps involved in design and outlines minimum standards of size, program,

71

fire safety, and engineering systems as well as various trade and safety codes that control all areas of human hospital construction; these are seldom applicable to all aspects of a veterinary facility. The building design must meet all building codes, ordinances, and regulations enforced by the city, county, or state, and should meet the *AAHA Standards for Veterinary Hospitals*. Where specific codes do not exist, the national building codes will generally be in effect.

It is impossible to expect the practice manager/hospital administrator and/or practice owner to be familiar with all of the codes required in designing and building a structure. Meeting the national and local standards required of healthcare construction and operation is itself a full-time effort. However, the project manager should try to review the federal minimum standards, the AAHA standards, and local municipality codes and insist that his or her architect and engineer(s) observe them.

Another area of concern to the architect and to the project manager is that of human standards. The architect is responsible for size, space, and furniture— for every height, shape, weight, and mood of the human body (i.e., ergometrics). Ramsey and Sleeper's *Architectural Graphic Standards* and various publications on design for the handicapped are valuable for the project manager in understanding the design solutions of the architect. The project manager must ensure the hospital administrator/practice manager is involved in representing the staff when specific client, patient, and workflow decisions are being made in these ergometric areas.

Elements in the Design Process

The most important thing the architect brings to a project is design talent. Design affects the satisfaction of the client, the comfort of the patient, and the dignity and reputation of the practice as well as the efficiency and comfort of the staff. It applies to the function as well as the form of a building. Architectural and engineering design play an equal role in the success of a program. It is very difficult for the average practice staff member to judge design. Results can be measured in a market sense, but only once the veterinary facility is completed. Just the fact that a specific firm has designed many veterinary hospitals is not enough. Creative talent and broad public acceptance of their completed work are essential.

The ideal veterinary facility design starts with key functional planning, then adds a very clear, simple traffic configuration that includes the ability to expand the number of consultation rooms, treatment areas, patient holding areas, and diversity of the service zones in the future, as program growth and change within a practice structure are continuous. The need for cages or runs does not always grow at the same rate as the need for service programs, but both must have a master plan for direction. The long-range plan must also be flexible enough to allow for technological changes in all areas of veterinary healthcare delivery.

In the design process, the footprint (the land covered by the building) of the practice must be considered first, though it does not occupy the largest portion of the land. (Parking and multiple entries, discussed below, constitute a larger land use.) There are various approaches to designing the veterinary facility footprint and the patient holding units and service zones that make it up.

Base

Base services fall into two categories: ancillary services (oriented toward patient comfort care, often including retail areas, laundry, dietary, housekeeping, and so forth) and service zones (inpatient and outpatient, as well as pharmacy, laboratory, imaging, and related healthcare delivery areas). These elements can be combined into one base structure or they can be housed independently (as when an "animal mall" is developed by a practice). Different fire ratings for enclosures may determine the approach. The base can occupy 1,500 gross sq. ft. in shopping center practices to 30,000-plus sq. ft. in a multispecialty practice; the budget and community demographics help identify the potential size of the veterinary facility being considered.

Patient Units

Virtually every possible configuration for cage units has been designed: stainless steel, injected PVC, fiberboard, laminates, round, triangular, oval, square, horizontal, vertical, L-shaped, cross-shaped, Y-shaped, H-shaped, T-shaped, and hexagonal. The design chosen should meet the optimum patient nursing surveillance pattern for organization and staffing. Usually one cage bank is placed in each nursing ward to prevent gate fighting. The mix of private VIP suites and runs also determines floor and door design, as do minimum municipal standards, such as the distance from the property line to the door, or commonsense factors, such as the distance from the nurses' station to the ICU units. This is above and beyond the appropriate life safety codes. Specialty units and intensive care units vary in size based upon different species, programs, and levels of care. A pet resort unit may contain more than a hospital ward and an intensive care unit should contain only as many as visible and monitorable by the treatment room inpatient staff. Since the patient holding unit is basically a modular structure, its design may not be compatible with that of the generic base habits of the architect, so different structure and support concepts may be applied to the design of the wards, resort, and other patient holding areas. Interstitial space has recently been incorporated into some veterinary hospital designs, but the debate over whether the increased building flexibility justifies the higher cost must be settled on an individual basis.

The current ratio of inpatient to outpatient for a general companion animal practice is not stated in square feet but rather in a cost-income relationship; outpatient space costs 30 percent of the expenses for about 70 percent of the income, while inpatient space costs 70 percent of the expenses for only about 30 percent of the income. If the functional planning has addressed doctor "day admits" rates (~40 percent of all outpatients deserve the reduced stress of inpatient care), these ratios will begin to become more reasonable. These same ratios have caused consultants and design teams to discuss affiliation and networking within a community for sharing capital expense equipment between practices instead of every practice having their own ultrasound, computerized ECG, 500 mA X-ray, dry chemistry laboratory, and so on. A research or teaching facility may need double or triple the space, and some have even used Hermann-Miller walls to adjust space based on size of the grant/research dollars. University teaching hospitals require even more square feet due to the need for additional circulation space, since hordes of students must congregate and absorb knowledge at the feet of their clinical mentors.

The long-range cost implications of fuel also play a key role in design. Solar and reclaimed energy systems may be economically advantageous but they require more building and site space than do conventional systems. Future comfort and space depend upon a great deal of creative engineering now, and this part of the process is of the highest priority.

Long-Range Facility Planning

One of the major problems with many existing veterinary facilities is that they were built as end-stage facilities and therefore lack a long-range plan for expanding or adjusting to new programs. The concept of shared services and levels of care will someday be required, and a good long-range plan will enable the practice leadership to adjust. Adjustment can require remodeling, expansion, or both, and many older facilities have had to relocate when expansion became necessary due to their total physical obsolescence or the lack of available land. The veterinary-specific consultant's program and recommended long-range plan of animal healthcare needs and practice delivery systems are important factors in the building scope and future requirements. This is why the facility master plan should be developed before zone locations and facility flow are fixed. The future cost of phasing, relocation, and additions is a critical part of all design, and without a plan or map for the future, the practice facility may face delayed growth, cost overrun, and obsolescence.

Structural Elements

Potential vertical or horizontal expansion of the building is one of the most critical issues in the planning stage. Currently, the most popular term in the hospital structural systems market is "interstitial space." The idea is to construct mechanical spaces above occupied areas so that heating, plumbing, and electrical systems can be easily changed when the area below them is reprogrammed. Combined with this, a system of long-span structural elements will allow fewer fixed column locations and, therefore, easier modification of the occupied spaces in the future. Both elements, however, carry a high initial construction cost. Other systems designed to head off high remodeling and maintenance costs in the future have been developed on individual projects. The point is that future remodeling and expansion must be thought out for each new structure in its planning stage, and the long-term cost of the building's operational life must be given high priority. Not everyone will be able to afford the initial costs of advanced systems, even though the operations cost might someday be smaller; but unless these key factors of future change are considered, the neglected long-range plan will lead a short-range life.

Interstitial space is an excellent concept for the hospital inpatient and outpatient areas, and practice managers/hospital administrators and practice owners should review the idea before setting service zone locations, heights, and functions. Interstitial space use for nursing ward design and boarding facilities, however, is carrying the system too far and cannot be justified. Major changes in the patient holding units are not as likely as they are in the service zones, and a much more economical approach, such as flexible vertical mechanical shafts and individual air systems per zone, will allow for reasonable, predictable changes throughout the facility's life.

Comparisons should also be made in structural system difference, potential, and cost: concrete versus steel versus precast concrete and long-span systems and space frames versus the more conventional spans and erection (these analyses are a part of design and need to be reviewed closely by the practice's planning team). A full picture of the structural system(s) and the applicable cost(s) should be presented to the hospital ownership by the design team.

Functional Adjacencies

A very important example of functional adjacency is that of the radiology and emergency zones. The radiology zone has traditionally been a room off the treatment area, but when it is realized that "imaging" is responsible for the total X-ray and ultrasound (and maybe endoscopy) needs of an entire veterinary facility, and there are multispecialties within the facility, mediation and flow control must be addressed, often at the board level, to establish policy and operational precedence. Though the entire radiology staff is not on duty twenty-four hours a day, the emergency services often are. It is important, therefore, that the functional area of imaging/radiology can be available at night for emergency use. By designing these two areas adjacent to one another, both the operational cost and the critical time of travel can be reduced.

Other factors that affect the location include

- outpatient "day care" X-ray procedures
- admission procedures
- intensive and cardiac care procedures
- therapy procedures for extended-care patients
- surgery procedures
- special procedures
- inpatient movement and monitoring
- outpatient "day admit," holding, and RTG procedures
- operational relationship to nuclear medicine and isotopes
- in specialty hospitals, physical confinement of mass therapy wall design (X-ray shielding, floor loading, and electrical sources)

The final decision on the location of the imaging zone will require compromise in some areas, but the major factor must be the cost of operations for staff, patient movement, and equipment use throughout the life of the structure. Secondary factors in deciding zone adjacencies are building design, structural economics, future expansion, and site plan. Coming in last in this design planning sequence is the "turf protection" often exhibited by specific specialists within a multidisciplinary group; this is where the core values of the governance board stops the griping and gossip immediately.

Traffic, Transportation, and Adjacencies

Subsequent chapters and illustrations will address the multiple entrances, exits, and windows requested within facility design projects, but the arrangement of zones within the structure and their access/egress requirements must be considered together before ultimate zone adjacencies can be designed. Zone adjacencies are extremely important because they determine the operational costs of staff time and travel throughout the life of the building. One key to a successful functional plan and cost-efficient operation is a simple traffic flow. Maximum separation between public access zones and the staff/patient zones reduces confusion as well as staff and patient transit time. Material supply and trash removal should also have defined routes that do not interfere with the movement of people or patients. It is likewise very important that a veterinary hospital be designed so that clients can easily orient themselves within the building. If it is difficult to find consultation rooms and often will not be clear where to go, when the hallways were designed by mixed animal practitioners to be cattle chutes for people, it follows that staff and supply movement may also be confused and inefficient when there are too many hallways and "cubbyhole" rooms. The visual impact of travel distance and environment must be pleasant for the clients, staff, and patients. Zones and individual room adjacencies vary because of the variations in individual practice programs and providers. General outlines are given in the *AAHA Standards for Veterinary Hospitals*, but most doctors have personal preferences that seem to be inviolate; the veterinary-specific consultant must change these paradigms in the minds of the user *before* the design is locked into the 50-percent completion phase.

Site and Parking

The site plan involves all traffic and transportation access, parking, entry, exit, material, cost, topography, utilities, future expansion, form, shape, and size. City planning has been a profession since the first caveman occupied a cave, and a veterinary hospital contains every possible kind of cave and sensory excitement you can name. Every facet of government, industry, and social life is simulated in a veterinary hospital. Consequently, site consultants can be hired for landscaping, parking, directional signing, snow melting, truck docking, trash handling, air exhausting, air intaking, fencing, busing, and paving. The master site study by the consulting architect and/or design team should always be reviewed for any specialty areas that are practice or community specific (e.g., stock trailers are getting longer, so turnarounds and parking areas now have larger radiuses for mixed animal haul-in practices). Remember that the physical site size and topography place certain limitations upon potential growth and future expansion. The selection of a site and land acquisition must, therefore, involve long-range planning for fifty to a hundred years . . . one acre for a companion animal practice is therefore falling into disfavor when long-range panning is addressed early.

Three or four major entrances are required for a veterinary hospital facility; these entrances are determined by adjacencies and traffic flow inside the facility, and in turn will determine traffic flow outside and location of parking lots. The main hospital entrance is for clients entering with patients; it requires a lot for client parking. The ambulatory care entrance is for outpatient, emergency, and ambulance traffic; for a twenty-four-hour facility, it may be different than the main entrance. The service door(s) is for supply deliveries, rendering, crematorium pickup, and trash pickup; it may even have a dock that should be out of the client access traffic flow. The employee entrance is for current personnel to access the facility anytime; personal safety and security is a definite concern for this entrance. All of these entrances usually require some form of parking lot access. The type of parking required and an exact parking count for each entrance are extremely difficult to produce as both are related to the entrances' function, zoning expectations of the municipality, and colocation opportunities. Also, each veterinary facility has a different mix of transportation access and parking; the traffic patterns will vary accordingly. A downtown urban veterinary hospital that serves a walking population may require only one parking space for emergencies, whereas a suburban veterinary hospital may need two parking spaces per consultation room, plus one for each staff member. In general, the municipality will define the parking space requirements during the approval process. The following figures are a guide to initial design planning *before* the local zoning committee defines your new world:

- clients: one space for every three to five patient appointment slots
- ambulatory large animal: five spaces per doctor in outpatient receiving
- emergency and handicap parking
- practice staff: one space for every two employees during peak daytime shift
- doctor staff: one space for each doctor

The cost of parking lots varies greatly depending on whether the lot is on ground level, underground, or reinforced for production animal transport trailers. The overall amount of space allowed per car is usually 300 sq. ft., excluding access drives/ramps. The cost of a ground-level stall is approximately $750 per car, whereas underground lots must be mechanically ventilated and will cost between $8,000 and $12,000 per space. The cost of land plus excavation must also be considered in the parking costs.

Valet parking versus free parking must be worked out by each veterinary hospital facility based on the facility's own community location. The initial cost of construction for parking is a major element in the construction budget, and as much review time as required for each zone must be given to it.

Material Handling

Material management, storage, and handling affect every aspect of veterinary practice organization, operation, and facility design. Materials-handling systems and movable cabinet aids are fast becoming major cost considerations in the planning budget. The present state of the art relates very unevenly to veterinary practice needs and to the planning process; furthermore, there does not exist a universally accepted database or methodology for resolving the issues of whether to have manual or automated transport. Experience has revealed that there is little difference among the functional requirements of hospital material-handling systems, provided the materials are delivered to the user in the desired quantity and quality at the right place and at the right time.

To properly evaluate material-handling systems and other storage support devices, one must first develop the concept of materials management in the veterinary practice. While there are many definitions of materials management, it is more than the pack-prep area outside surgery; an organizational and functional concept should provide for efficient planning, coordination, and control of all materials before they are used and for the subsequent disposition of reusables, wastes, and soiled items. From the business management perspective, expense to income ratios are needed to determine shrinkage (theft) and loss; the days of "cigar box accounting" for expendables are over! To determine the most appropriate system(s) for a particular veterinary facility, the materials distribution program should first be planned with respect to specific schedules and user requirements. The job of implementing the handling system is then accomplished through further organization and space planning, equipment selection, engineering design, and training.

Materials management includes planning and anticipating commodity requirements, acquiring needed supplies and materials, storing them in a sanitary manner, introducing and moving them horizontally and sometimes vertically, monitoring their status as current assets, accounting for them as charges, and providing them at the right place and at the right time. Materials that fall within the system are medical treatment supplies; nonmedical, general use supplies; pharmaceuticals, biologicals, and drugs; linen (clean and soiled); food; mail; trash; body disposition; medical waste; gases; and reprocessibles (trays, litter pans, bowls, etc.). These commodities usually move within the veterinary practice as a bulk system (i.e., a quantity of supplies loaded aboard a single device going from point A to point B on a programmed basis) or as a small item. Items in the latter category are either nonprogrammable or very small, and they are needed immediately by the user. To meet the transport requirements of both systems, there is a wide choice of modes, from manual to highly sophisticated automation. Essential to the bulk system in multidiscipline specialty hospitals are carts or modular containers moved by an employee (or in some locations, by some type of automation). Moving small items falls within a much narrower range, such as pneumatic tubes and box conveyors.

Popular variations of materials-handling hardware and subsystems include

- bar code tracking systems
- selective vertical conveyor
- hand trucks and carts
- box conveyor systems
- dumbwaiter (cart size)
- elevator (primary patient/staff vertical transport)
- elevator (standard for freight)
- overhead rail (L.A. power and free)
- warehouse high-density storage shelf systems
- combinations of the above
- pneumatic tube (reception to accounting or pharmacy)
- slide chutes (subterranean laundry)

To determine the most efficient system for a facility, management options must first be considered and evaluated, then all expected movements (on a twenty-four-hour, weekly basis) must be simulated on paper. One accurate means of quantifying movement is to base the simulation on a cart-exchange system, even though this method primarily speaks to the bulk delivery requirements. Once this is clear, actual constraints on the most desirable pathways, either horizontal or vertical, become clear. However, engineering or building configurations should not be the deciding factors in achieving the most efficient patterns of movement; building system innovations such as prefabricated shaftways and interstitial spaces add great flexibility for the use of automated systems in larger facilities.

Paramount in the selection of any materials-handling system is a life-cycle cost analysis. While life-cycle cost analysis and value engineering have become very popular, there are certain pitfalls to be aware of when making comparisons. Each management method and individual item of equipment should be subjected to thorough cost analysis. To do so, each management principle and piece of equipment should represent solutions to a single problem. It is very easy to slip into comparisons of apples and oranges; be sure that each system is performing the same function under the same conditions.

Each life-cycle evaluation should include initial purchase price of the equipment, periodic overhaul costs, preventive maintenance costs, energy consumption costs, and labor costs. The costs of each of the systems to be evaluated should be derived by using the most appropriate and most recent market data for projections. Numerous methods are used in constructing a life-cycle analysis. The life-cycle analysis allows a manager to evaluate the method of delivery (for example, manual versus automation) as well as predict initial cost and operational cost to be consumed by the system over a predetermined period of time. Concurrent with this assessment are the alternatives to mass unit practice storage:

- vendor stocking
- outsource pharmacy

– warehouse/supply staff supporting multiple community facilities
– just-in-time deliveries

It is important, nonetheless, to develop a broader basis for selecting handling systems before preparing the life-cycle cost analysis. While the cost may be acceptable, other factors such as engineering impracticalities or environmental hazards may render the system unacceptable. Therefore, the basis of selection must be the benefit to patient care, as well as the cost of the system, compatibility with the building, healthcare delivery needs, and product reliability.

The field of veterinary practice materials handling is in the neophyte stages as this text is being written, so for the design team tasking this involves industrial engineering, mechanical engineering, production engineering, and architectural and equipment consulting. While it is virtually impossible for practice managers/hospital administrators to become experts in these fields, their contribution is most important to the project manager. Operational methods, staffing patterns, and management style must be translated by the materials-handling expert into sensible simulation models reflecting the most efficient system for each practice's facility. Only then can there be a comparison of equipment requirements for manual or automated handling systems, as opposed to outsourcing and vendor stocking options.

Electronic Systems

Electronic systems include intercommunications, paper and information flow, monitoring of patients, and, in the future, multiphasic screening. Although these systems do not usually affect the structural or functional layout of the veterinary hospital to the extent that the bulk materials system does, they must, nonetheless, be designed before individual service zones can be planned.

Modern Information Systems

Word processing and hard copy electronic record systems are under constant improvement and change. The future use of communications within the veterinary hospital and expansion into the home for veterinary medical use will dictate the staffing and utilization of hospital design. Even staff communications outside the hospital as well as home care or ambulance services are a major design field. Communications for a hospital project include

• intercom (intra- and interzone)
• telephone (incoming, modem, fax, credit card, courtesy, etc.)
• paging (intrastaff, client, and outside)
• staff zone call
• computerized visual display terminals
• closed-circuit and cable television
• pneumatic (monitoring systems)
• mechanical life system

- telephonic remote dictation systems for specialty hospitals
- Internet library and telemedicine consultations
- engineering controls and alarm systems
- physiological monitoring (contact, probes, as well as remote telemetry)
- space satellite hookups

Intercom and staff call systems have been greatly improved; many practices have gone to vibrating pagers. The cost of advanced manufactured systems, however, is a roadblock for the design team. Evaluations based on manufacturers' literature are dangerous because the life-cycle costs are very difficult to determine. Qualified engineers can do studies and equipment can be tested, but very few veterinary hospitals can afford to reevaluate these systems for each project. The task of comparing American Telephone and Telegraph's intercom against a privately owned one would be a tremendous effort, and the initial cost of such a study would make it out of the question. It would take a serious effort by a design team to compare the costs of systems. Also, space technology has affected electronic sensing and communications systems, and innovations hit the market each week; remote (Internet-based) patient telemetry will be seen in our lifetime. As a consequence, information systems and technology within the hospital will be dramatically improved in the future, and facilities design today should include features such as coaxial cable to every room in order to take advantage of two-way visual systems and multiple display and storage of computerized information.

Communications requirements and systems are extremely complex and come as close as any area of veterinary practice design to defying solution through the hiring of a technical designer. In this area, experience rather than analytical studies must take precedence. The following list sets out the choices of systems in major categories:

I. Intercommunication systems
  A. Hospital zones
  B. Telephone
  C. Private communications system
  D. Privately leased systems
  E. Computer links
  F. Nursing zones
  G. Audio intercom (to nurse station)
  H. Visual communication (patient to nurse station)
  I. Telephone (referral to nurse station)
II. Predesign services
  A. Site selection studies
  B Concept plan
  C. Legal fees
    1. Site acquisition negotiation
    2. Contract review
  D. Environmental studies

III. Medical and administrative departments
  A. Doctors' page
    1. Central audio
    2. Pocket frequency
  B. Doctors' register
    1. Visual
    2. Audio with message storage
  C. Central dictating
    1. Telephone
    2. Private
  D. Computer systems
    1. Billing
    2. Charting and addressing
    3. Visual display
    4. Medical records
  E. Emergency radio bands
  F. In-hospital paging
  G. Out-of-hospital paging
  H. Music systems
  I. Closed-circuit television
  J. Central clock system
  K. Television security system
IV. Physical monitoring
  A. EKG, pulse, respiration, etc. (including remote systems)
  B. Multiphasic screening tests
  C. Visual monitoring
  D. Biofeedback systems
V. Paper handling
  A. Pneumatic tube system
  B. Conveyor track
  C. Lifts
  D. Electronic sending
  E. Video
VI. Engineering systems
  A. Remote equipment monitoring (central control)
  B. Remote heat and lighting control
  C. Zone system sensing (heat, cool, light, sound)
  D. Timed switching
  E. Automatic snow melting
  F. Alarm wiring (smoke, emergency power, fire, and so on)
  G. Isolation grounding

Design of electronic systems will greatly affect the total design of the facility. Because life-cycle operational costs can save or cost millions of dollars over the life of a building, the importance of carrying out life-cycle analyses on every possible element of these systems in the initial design phase must be emphasized.

Engineering Systems

Materials handling and electronic systems are dealt with by the engineers on the design team who will detail the final systems that are approved by the practice's planning team. The engineer also takes the lead in the areas of heating, cooling, ventilating, plumbing, and electrical design. These mechanical and electrical systems and their construction may often account for almost half the cost of constructing a veterinary hospital. The practice manager/hospital administrator, therefore, must be well advised by the project manager in this highly technical but patient-oriented and staff-supported part of the total design.

The engineering profession has the responsibility for costing out the recommended system. Cost studies thus become a daily part of the engineer's life. Because it is possible to work with known fuel costs and detailed manufactured items, the engineer can justify each system recommended. Still, fuel studies, mechanical system studies, and use of computer analysis are an advanced art in the mechanical and electrical engineering fields and therefore the engineering team members' creative thoughts should be a major effort in the program conception.

Although static-quantity engineering has been described as a straightforward solution, let me warn you that a good engineer is as important to the final success of the building as any other member of the design team. Comfort control for every individual's thermostat is almost impossible, but it will be that one point that is criticized (never applauded) the most when the building is complete. The wrong decision can make the building shake, sweat, freeze, fry, smoke, leak, dark, dry, loud, smell, and even stop.

Heating, Ventilation, Air-Conditioning, and Electrical Systems

The design of the heating, ventilation, and air-conditioning (HVAC) system for a veterinary hospital is regulated by smell and sound, and while there will be municipality minimum standards, these two aesthetic requirements rule in a veterinary hospital design. The cost of the better systems can range from 15-30 percent of the total building cost. Any facility has two main areas of design for HVAC: the exterior walls (typically climate control concerns) and the interior areas (zones and sight/sound/smell concerns). A veterinary facility has three additional areas of design consideration for HVAC: client areas (reception and consultation areas, controlled within the sixty-eight- to seventy-two-degree range), treatment zone (inpatient, with separate thermostat and positive pressure for surgery, supplemental exhaust for film processor and dental area, lab hood, etc.), and animal holding areas (ten air exchanges per hour minimum for wards, boarding, boutique, and negative pressure isolation area).

Selecting the appropriate HVAC system for a veterinary hospital is a critical decision facing the architect and engineer, as is the number of "holes" they put in sound-retarding walls. On this decision rests the satisfaction of the entire hospital staff and the clients. Many factors must be analyzed, judged, screened, and coordinated. The desires of the practice staff, the practice manager/hospital administrator, and professional staff, as well as the economic aspects, are all considerations. The practice owner wants an HVAC installation that will provide maximum comfort and sound/odor prevention at a reasonable initial cost, with minimum operating costs. The engineer must be able to anticipate the behavior of the contemplated HVAC system. Complete air-conditioning HVAC provides an environment of correct temperature, humidity, air movement, air cleanliness, ventilation, and acoustical level. Anything less is a compromise and is not termed air-conditioning.

The patient holding units of a veterinary hospital should be considered like the treatment area, with the load requirements based on 100-percent occupancy with twenty-four-hour, year-round operation. Boarding facilities have a much wider ambient temperature tolerance (fifty-five degrees to eighty-five degrees, IAW Title 9, Chapter 1, Code of Federal Regulations). An important factor to remember is that air circulation must be contained within each room, but that does not mean each room needs an exhaust as well as a conditioned air intake source. Corridors, nurses' stations, and service zone areas must have a separate supply and exhaust system. Each patient ward must have an exhaust-creating negative pressure, and there should be no cross-contamination between various areas; specific temperature control must be maintained in client zones; and individual temperature, humidity, and ventilation control must be available in special treatment, therapeutic, exotic, surgical, and other service areas. Absolute cleanliness from duct-based odors and bacteria is essential; thus, rigid housekeeping procedures are required to ensure that the air-conditioning can be achieved if standard systems and equipment are utilized. They must be simple to operate and maintain, for equipment with extremely complicated control systems in confined spaces soon lacks proper care and attention.

Possibly the best low-maintenance control at the client zone is an all-air system. This is also the most expensive system for total design and cannot always be justified. Two common exterior systems are the fan-coil and the induction unit. With a fan-coil system, outside air and room air are circulated over a heating or cooling coil that is supplied with hot or cold water from a central source. This system can be modified in price and individual room control by having a two-or four-pipe supply. The main objection to the fan coil is the enclosed fan in the unit and the filter, which must be maintained and cleaned. The amount of air that can be recirculated in the room is spelled out in the construction specifications. Induction units are based on air that is warmed or cooled at a central source and that is sent to a room fast enough to cause the air to circulate within the room. This unit does not contain a fan, but it does cause a hissing noise that can be objectionable. Also, the cost is higher than that of a fan-coil unit. Other variations that have been used for veterinary facilities are radiant heat in the floor/ceiling (hot or cold water run through a grid in the floor/ceiling), electric radiant heat, and package electric units (at each window).

Because humidity control is needed in many of the interior zones, single or dual-duct air systems are often used. The dual-duct system supplies warm and cool air to a mixing box at the room, and thus individual room temperature control is gained along with humidity control. A single-duct system does not supply individual room control but rather a zoned area control.

HVAC equipment must be centrally located. Preferably, a utility room or central plant above the ceiling, separate from the main operating areas, should be constructed to house the HVAC system(s), chillers (cold water generation), and all auxiliary equipment needed for their operation. This steam, gas, or hot water and cold water should be piped through a service duct system to the main facility zones; balancing a system means that each zone is getting the volume it needs for temperature (and humidity) control. The central mechanical equipment room should be built to house the necessary air-handling units, secondary pumps, converters, and auxiliary equipment for distributing the air and heated and chilled water to meet the system requirements. In addition, a fan room could be located on the roof to house all the exhaust fans, instead of separate output points around the facility. The central plant concept includes the use of high-grade commercial equipment with longer life and more economical cost and maintenance.

An important concept in hospital design is that of "total energy." It involves an on-site plant where electric power is generated and the HVAC needs are supplied without using any outside fuel. Initial costs are very high, but if the rate structure for natural gas and oil in a given area is low, the life cycle of this system could possibly be justified. It cannot usually be justified for the normal-size general practice hospital.

The mechanical and electrical systems that must be designed in a veterinary hospital structure include

- energy source and solar energy considerations
- boiler-steam/heating system (with a standby fuel system)
- cooling tower/AC system
- gas (heating)
- water
- emergency power generators
- electrical
- electrical switchgear
- Internet and telemedicine circuitry and access
- special amp circuits for drying cages, radiology, washer/dryers, etc.
- lighting
- lightning protection
- X-ray power transformers
- electrical grounding
- plumbing
- domestic water
- hot and chilled water

- hypothermia system (piped heated or chilled water for a patient blanket system)
- compressed air (also oxygen generators as indicated)
- central vacuum
- central medical gases
- oxygen and nitrous oxide delivery and flow control systems
- mechanical
- elevator and lifts as indicated
- trash and biomedical waste disposal
- cadaver disposition
- central monitoring
- exhaust systems (air, boiler, emergency generator, vent)
- site drainage
- storm sewer
- sanitary sewer
- communication systems, internal and external
- telephone switchgear

Energy considerations for the life of the structure have an enormous effect on operating cost. All possible avenues for recovery of energy, new sources of energy, and energy efficiency should be considered in the design procedure. The design team's duty is to recommend the best possible concept, systems, and layouts to the hospital planning team and practice ownership. The engineering and the details for construction will be worked out by the engineer and coordinated by the architect. It is important that the project manager keep the hospital administrator/practice administrator well informed on the systems in order to answer questions by the staff.

Specific Factors

Factors that affect design but are specific to the philosophies and objectives of the individual project are found in the following facilities:

- freestanding ambulatory units (except for garage restocking points)
- university teaching hospitals
- industrial research clinics
- hospice services by veterinary hospitals
- international quarantine facilities
- pet resort facilities
- boutique (grooming and bathing) facilities
- some specialty facilities
- cancer treatment units

Ambulatory and Urgent Care

Ambulatory care includes multiple outpatient services in private residences for companion animals as well as mobile support of production, equine, and large exotic animals. In the search for better preventive care, the independent units, wellness programs, and alternative care therapies have been tested as to market and effect. Most comprehensive ambulatory care units are affiliated with a fixed veterinary facility in order to share advanced imaging, laboratory, advanced surgery, and other inpatient services.

The urgent care center may be aimed at a specific time period for a suburban population, or may serve as a feeder to a larger veterinary facility. Design of urgent care centers resembles that of an emergency or outpatient unit, depending on the philosophy, with holding cages and offices attached to consultation and treatment rooms. Emergency triage and treatment rooms serve for trauma and urgent care cases, while consultation rooms are used for outpatient visits. Support areas include records, administration office, sometimes an employee lounge and lockers, housekeeping area, storage, and entry waiting area. Full-time urgent care doctors and paraprofessional staff operate these facilities (not always the same as Veterinary Emergency and Critical Care Society (VECCS) board certified). The space allotment is based upon the characteristics of the service provided and predicted number of patient visits per year. No rule-of-thumb standards yet apply to these facilities.

Teaching Hospitals

The true university veterinary teaching hospital (VTH) offers a residency program that involves clinical staff and student medical education. The various technical teaching programs may even exist in multiple campus facilities. Some privately owned teaching hospitals are affiliated with universities so that interns and resident students in specialty programs may be sent to train with primary care access in the affiliated for-profit hospital. Another example would be the proliferation of multispecialty private practice facilities, where the residency or internship is involved in for-profit healthcare delivery while preparing for specialty boards. Even the private for-profit specialty practices may also have university affiliations so their boarded specialist(s) may carry the "real world" into academia. These alternative philosophies may alter the standard use of the multidisciplinary private practice, and the practice planning team and project manager must be sure that the design team understands the unique uses required with teaching and research in the private sector.

Veterinary teaching hospitals may require space to educate residents and interns in the clinical zones, in an academic department, in research and training laboratories, in specific referral clinics, and even near nurses' stations. Most VTH facilities need classrooms and some are adding living quarters. The size of the hospital depends on the number of residency programs or technical programs involved as well as the number and size of the specialties supported. Further, a technician training program, affiliated with an accredited schooling program, also affects the veterinary hospital's space needs. Although most technician programs provide most of the space needed within the school for didactic learning, affiliation with larger veterinary practices or specialty practices is used to accommodate the student's need for hands-on experience. The project manager must provide an exact calculation of space for program and functional areas to the design team, and future demands must be projected based upon individual training program support needs.

Hospices

The veterinary hospice is a new endeavor, most usually associated with a general veterinary practice. The inpatient section of a hospital has an area for the chronically ill animals, usually VIP-type suites, with a better staff-to-animal ratio than boarding and wards (one animal caretaker can handle thirty-three animals in a standard eight-hour day, yet hospice and ICU/CCU facilities are less than half this ratio). These chronic care patients have special needs in the areas of healthcare support, special staff training is needed, and specific programs of support are identified for establishing the cost of hospitalization. This type of facility use does not come under any approval at this time, AAHA has no standards established yet, and client fees vary greatly.

Very few hospice units have been in operation for a few years in the United States; we often recommend hospice programs when there is inadequate space for economy of scale boarding operations in an established companion animal practice. These programs, within companion animal facilities, have been successfully operated in some cases and not pursued in others. A hospice program is designed as an intense nursing support environment, with the staff surveillance highly increased. The "suites" are intended to be homelike, with beds, rugs, and televisions (just like the VIP suites in pet resorts), with each unit ensuring privacy and comfort (e.g., eight-foot-by-eight-foot room with window(s) and forty-eight-inch-high half door). The veterinary hospice programs usually emphasize frequent social interaction, psychological stimulation, and stress reduction management. The project manager for this type of high-touch/high-tech healthcare facility must "train" the engineers more than the architects.

International Quarantine Facilities

The disaster of 9-11-01 brought increased interest in quarantine facilities and bioterrorism. Occupational Safety and Health Administration (OSHA) consultants are being asked to assess the feedlots for bioterrorism threats and architectural and engineering consultants have been asked to look at the security access concurrent with their planning of international quarantine facilities. Many new firms are making a debut in veterinary and animal facility planning, flaunting expertise that does not exist. The project manager must ensure any such bioterrorism consultant employed by the design team has the credentials and expertise to warrant the additional expense.

In the field of veterinary healthcare delivery, planning has been underway at Plum Island for years, under security restrictions of the federal government. Fort Meade and Plum Island have some highly technical structures that have been operating for years; expertise is available, but in most general practices, and even specialty practices, this is not a requirement at this time. The quarantine system itself can be built as soon as the transportation system is ready to use it, and some veterinary hospitals have established lucrative support contracts with international airports just for this contingency.

The single most important feature of international quarantine planning is an understanding of the source country's culture and our country's restrictions (most of this information is readily available on the Internet). The emotions, social characteristics, environment, history, and desires of the animal owners must be addressed, and observation (and visiting privileges) should be incorporated into the facility design. Again, specialized education, training, technology, support service, and management must, however, precede international quarantine systems; the practice manager/hospital administrator must train the project manager in these areas so the project manager can represent the practice needs to the design team.

Production of Design Documents

Design taste is indefinable. A building that is functional and pleasing to those who use it follows no specific set of universal rules or standard veterinary procedures in its conception. The site, landscaping, building facade, and interior spaces are a variable mixture of materials designed to satisfy human emotions.

Concept

The concept of a building is the interpretation of the programs, education, operation, and unique identity it will embody as it evolves into its functional form. Block zone plans, traffic patterns, patient movement expectations, structural concepts, energy directions, material form, and client sitting concepts are developed to meet cost ideas as well as client and staff comfort desires.

The key to a successful project may be the ability of the planning team to read schematic drawings and project the volume represented in them. One of the best means of gaining an understanding of schematic drawings is to study drawings of a room the same size as an existing room. Another means is using full-size masking tape layouts of key zones and rooms on a large parking lot. The design architect has many ways of presenting the physical layouts and is extensively trained in such presentation; in most cases, the staff of the hospital has not attended these training sessions. The architect must rely on the practice manager/hospital administrator's assessment of staff learning, and the project manager must realign the architect's advice during this phase to give him or her the insight to reach the staff. This same architect needs the freedom to design space that will produce improved conditions for the patients, staff, and providers while minimizing the costs to the practice ownership.

Some explanation of terminology common to drawings developed during architectural design work may be helpful at this point.

- *Floor plan:* The plan is the top view of walls, doors, and windows.
- *Footprint:* The outline of the proposed facility is placed on the entire property, often showing drives, walks, and landscaping by the 80-percent design completion phase.

- *Elevation:* The elevation is the side view.
- *Section:* The section is similar to an elevation but shows what remains after an imaginary slice (section) has been cut through the facility.
- *Perspective:* Perspective is a three-dimensional drawing of an object.
- *Rendering:* A rendering is a finished architectural perspective drawing indicating materials and effects of light, shade, and shadow to help explain form or shape. Plans, elevations, and sections are also referred to as "rendered" when materials, light, shade, and shadow are shown.
- *Plan section:* The term "plan" is used interchangeably to refer to a top view and to what is actually a plan section. A plan section is a horizontal (rather than vertical) section of a building. It shows the top view of what remains after everything above the slice has been removed.

Plan, section, elevation, and perspective drawings are used to communicate architectural development in reviews with practice staff and municipality agents, as well as the contractor's craftsmen and subcontractors, throughout the course of the project. Once functional relationships among the zones, traffic patterns, material, site, and utilities have been established, schematic drawings of the design solution are presented for review and approval. Such drawings are the basis for fixing the scope of the project and for making the survey estimate of cost required to ensure that project scope and budget are compatible with the veterinary practice's healthcare delivery plans and vision.

Approved schematic drawings become the basis for further development of the project through a phase of the work referred to as preliminaries or design development. When schematic drawings have been approved, a rendered perspective drawing is usually made of the project. The rendering may be black and white, monochrome, or full color. It is usually delivered to and paid for by the practice owner and used with the practice's clients to start the word-of-mouth promotions. An architectural model of the project may also be commissioned; finished, detailed models are usually constructed by specialty stores and paid for by the practice owner. With many veterinary practices, an interior design texture and material board is more often displayed with the architect's rendering and placed in the client reception area of the existing practice.

Schematics

At this stage of planning, the overall concept and block drawings have produced general internal traffic and external access flow as well as addressed the adjacencies, expansion plan, and zone design criteria. It is now time to gather all the thoughts of the program and develop them into single-line schematic drawings. At this stage the project manager must rely heavily on the architect, who will draw up a single-line design showing the program scope and the budget in one concept.

The architect should take into account all of the elements that have stimulated the concept and produce the innovations and basic building that will meet the stated needs. The project manager should be totally involved in the results shown by the schematics, for he or she will be asked to approve, support, and present the final recommendations to the practice owner. The project manager must become familiar with the tools of the architect and with the drawings of what will someday be his or her physical plant.

At this stage of project development, detailed review and confirmation of the functional, operational, and architectural program is again required in order for physical plan development to represent consensus and current/projected practice needs. The practice staff and practice's planning team review the schematics together, providing any additional input in program review to the project manager. This is an important step because additional plan development and subsequent reviews will be based on approved schematics that support the healthcare delivery programs of the practice.

Careful attention must also be paid to the budget and how it is related to the scope of the practice programs. The budget can be checked by projecting the amount of space required to house a specific procedure or deliver a specific program (with appropriate allowances for equipment, site work, etc.) and applying a cost per square foot to the resulting area. In order to be realistic, these costs must be projected to the anticipated midpoint of construction. As a result of such a check, the direction to be taken in the development of schematic plans is established, and project scope, at the completion of schematics, should be on budget. In some situations, the practice may elect to design according to a program that is not adequately covered by the previous budget; this presents no problem as long as resources are available for increasing the budget.

Early schematic architectural development is normally diagrammatic in nature, with plan areas, or blocks, representing program elements being organized and reorganized in search of the best functional relationships, given necessary adjacencies. Drawings at this point are single line, often freehand or CAD developed, so that changes can be easily made with feedback from the practice planning team and from the existing practice staff.

Elevations

Exterior elevations, or drawings of how each face of the building will look, are the beginning of combining the function and the form. The building materials, windows, columns, roof lines, shadows, and color are all like notes in a beautiful symphony. Environmental factors of sun, shading, passive solar energy, insulation, cost, and beauty are elements of this creative effort.

There are several stages in the design of a building elevation. Elevations combine into three-dimensional form with the functions inside the structure, the topography of the land, and the land forms of trees, shrubs, flowers, parking lots, and human scale. Structural elements of the building are often exposed, converting function into form. The smallest details of shade and shadows, dark and light, and form and volume are studied and reflected in the design. Design carries through the entire building process, as each wall, ceiling, light, and floor is melded into the structure. The results are for everyone—

those who use it, those who spend their lives working in it, and the society it reflects.

The largest single problem with the elevations of a veterinary facility is the desire of zoning and architects to have a building that appears symmetrical on the outside while the inside is never symmetrical. If the practice can establish asymmetry as a standard facility appearance with the architect and municipality agencies, the elevations start to become more functional . . . form is supposed to follow function within any custom-designed facility, and it is especially important in a veterinary healthcare facility where natural light and structure security must coexist with client, patient, and staff acceptance.

Design Development

After schematics have been approved, architectural development becomes more technical and detailed. Virtually all work done during design development is an elaboration on concepts developed in the programming and schematics phases.

Site

If site survey, soils investigation, and utility information are still incomplete at this point, the project manager must ensure the necessary work is completed and information collected to support development of initial studies in foundation and structural framing, sanitary and storm sewer systems, site development and grading, and electrical power and energy services. Traffic access to the building entrances; separation of public, emergency, and service traffic elements; and parking provisions are further studied at this time. Site survey and soils investigation work are normally ordered and paid for by the practice, along with whatever legal services may be necessary in securing required easements, zoning waivers, and so on.

Building

Architectural development includes further study and decisions regarding materials, windows, exterior finishes, and architectural treatment and detail; refinement of space layout within the facility and selection of finishes and materials in keeping with maintenance and durability requirements; and comparative cost studies of methods and materials for partition systems and exterior walls, ceiling, and windows.

Engineering

Further development is also required on concepts of air handling, air-conditioning, electrical distribution-lighting-communications systems, and medical gas, plumbing, and piping systems. During design development these systems are worked out sufficiently to allow cost studies and basic interfacing decisions to be made. Drawings are normally single-line indications of piping or duct work. Total service requirements for electrical power, natural gas or fuel oil, sanitary and storm sewers, water, and solid waste disposal are now established.

Equipment

Transition planning requires careful attention to the fixed and movable equipment that will be needed to implement the operational program. Early in design development, equipment and room detail interviews are held with the veterinary professional and staff. In these sessions, equipment requirements (existing and proposed) are documented by the practice manager/hospital administrator. The information is used by the project manager and design team in coordinating room sizes, utility services, lighting, and work flow. Documentation usually takes the form of room-by-room equipment lists, or room data sheets, and is submitted for practice planning team review after compilation.

Systems

Complex systems of various types are often incorporated, in concept form, in the schematic design. Functionally, these include communications, information transmission, storage and retrieval, materials handling, security, food preparation, and others. Each system that is to be incorporated must be studied in detail and interfaced with equipment common to other building systems; space and structural requirements are often extensive. Justification of systems is critical because initial and maintenance costs are usually high.

Design development drawings normally show considerably greater detail than do schematic drawings. Major equipment and furniture are shown in the plans in order to facilitate engineering coordination of utilities and lighting. Plans show wall thickness, door and window function, and more detail regarding vertical circulation and materials. Sections and elevations at larger scale depict relationships between materials. Outline specifications to supplement the drawings are compiled for each material, system, and element of work. A room-by-room equipment list, or room data book, is included to record equipment requirements.

A design development is desirable to provide summary discussion of operational concepts, materials, special equipment, and environmental systems. When the design development documents are completed, a cost estimate is prepared and presented with the drawings, outline specifications, equipment information, and narrative for hospital review. The estimate provides a current check on project scope related to budget.

After approval, design development documents provide the basis for the working drawing or contract document phase of the project. The design development phase sets the detailed operation of each room and leads to approval of all systems, fixed equipment, material types, and building construction. This is the most important part of the project manager's role on the design team, as it sets all of the ideas, programs, needs, and designs into the final building plan. Anticipation of future needs is now fixed, as the following phases only detail and construct what is now the final design product.

Insights and Perspectives

Getting Started without Stumbling

Tony L. Cochrane, AIA

Veterinarians often ask why animal hospitals are so costly. The reality is that these buildings are unique and quite complicated.

For example, human medical clinics and dental offices are regularly used as comparable building types by banks, contractors, and others for determining the preliminary cost estimates for veterinary hospitals. However, veterinary facilities are more similar to human hospitals when you consider the complexity of the mechanical, plumbing, and electrical systems; the necessity of installing durable materials and finishes, and other similar features. Then when you add in radiology suites, surgery suites, and wards, veterinary facilities actually do become small-scale, self-contained hospitals.

So how do you get started?

The Predesign Phase

Whatever motivates the start of a project, there are common elements to establishing a workable "building program." In the simplest of terms, the building program is a written description of your wish list that has been condensed somewhat by the realities of budget, site limitations, and zoning restrictions. Often overlooked, the predesign phase is very important from the architect's perspective because everything is built on this foundation.

You will want to establish the project's scale, scope, quality, schedule, and budget. Time should be spent developing a program that answers the needs of your long-range plan as well as your immediate needs for the diverse functions required in your animal hospital. Once you have established a "vision" of what your hospital should be, the budget should be developed, financing options explored, and a schedule determined.

Demographic Studies

If you are new to a particular market, or if you are unsure if the local market can support the type of improvements you are planning, a demographic analysis may help. For example, the optimum location for an animal hospital can be determined by selecting a set of parameters, such as income level or the population most likely to own pets. Conversely, you can determine the demographics of the population around your existing facility, where there may be potential growth in the population and where your competition is located.

Site Studies

Once you have determined that your site has the capacity to meet your current and future needs—but prior to the initiation of the design process—site surveys, environmental impact, and soil reports should be ordered. They may reveal concerns that will affect the viability of the project, and they will certainly be necessary later in the construction documents phase.

Financing

With a building program established, the next step is to determine how you will capitalize your project. One of the more common ways veterinarians finance the construction of their hospitals is with a commercial loan through a bank where they have an established relationship. The bank can also help with securing a Small Business Administration (SBA) loan. There are also a number of banks and lending institutions that cater specifically to veterinarians. Many can be found in the back of veterinary trade magazines.

Your bank will assess the viability of your business and your proposed project. They will want to see a package that includes current financial statements and future projections, market data, and a detailed, well-thought-out business plan. When working with lenders, always check references and be cautious when deals seem too good to be true.

Planning Approvals

Most projects require regulatory approvals prior to construction.

In many locations there are a limited number of available building sites that are zoned for veterinary hospitals and/or boarding facilities. While some sites are zoned to include veterinary uses, they may be designated as a "conditional use" pending governmental approval. The approval process often takes a few weeks, but in some instances can take up to several months. Prior to starting the process, review with the appropriate agency the submittal schedule, the required paperwork, and the length of time required for approvals.

Delivery Process

This includes determining the design, consulting, and construction services you need. How you choose to work with a contractor and establish cost controls will have a significant impact on the success of your project.

The Team

Even the simplest building project requires the input of a great many people. As the owner, you have determined the need, or opportunity, for a new or renovated facility. You have selected a site, secured financing, and secured approvals to proceed. Architects and other design professionals have integrated your needs, resources, and ideas into appropriate solutions.

An army of contractors, fabricators, suppliers, manufacturers, and craftspeople will assemble the structure. The insurance, accounting, and legal professions are involved throughout, as are local, state, and federal regulatory agencies. Finally you, the public, and your staff will be involved with the building on a day-to-day basis. Teamwork, therefore, becomes critical.

Owner

The owner is ultimately in charge of establishing the project's priorities, building program, budget, and financing. In addition, surveys, soil reports, and other baseline information on the project must be provided. It is the responsibility of the owner to make the timely decisions that keep the design team progressing efficiently.

Architect

Your architect is the creator and coordinator of your facility's design. He or she has accomplished this by translating your requirements into drawings and specifications that will ultimately become bricks and mortar. The architect provides design services and project documentation, administers construction contracts, observes construction, and processes a variety of submissions for the project.

Engineers

Approximately half of the cost of a typical veterinary facility is in the structural, mechanical, plumbing, and electrical systems. Professional engineers have an in-depth knowledge and experience in these areas, and they understand the full range of design possibilities and details in their specific areas of expertise.

Contractors

The physical act of construction is accomplished by a virtual army of contractors, suppliers, and craftspeople. General contractors assemble the labor, materials, and management necessary to construct a project. They typically maintain small organizations, with the average firm having fewer than ten employees. Contractors are responsible for on-site equipment, such as tools, generators, temporary facilities, and other items that support the construction process but do not become part of the building. Most of the actual construction work is done by specialty contractors (subs) who are responsible for only a portion of the work, such as mechanical, plumbing, roofing, or drywall.

Suppliers

Building materials, components, and subsystems are manufactured, fabricated, and sometimes installed by suppliers.

Selecting Design Consultants

You and your staff bring a great deal to the design of your hospital: professional expertise, needs, desires, aspirations, and biases. In turn, your consultants should be more than just people who "draw up a building" for you. As the people who will help you turn your ideas into reality, they should challenge your preconceptions while not losing sight of the fact that they are designing for *you* and *your needs*. After the completion of the design stages, your consultants will also serve as your agents in dealing with the various government agencies and the contractor, ensuring that you are receiving the quality of workmanship and materials for which you have contracted.

Your architect will serve as your primary design consultant, and he or she will rely on the expertise of civil, structural, mechanical, and electrical engineers as well as acoustical consultants and landscape architects.

The American Institute of Architects has published a memo on selecting the architect. The following are some of the most important points:

- *Experience:* Look for a firm that will be able to show you projects of similar functional and design complexity. Each firm brings a different combination of skills, expertise, interest, and values to its projects. As important as experience is, you need to watch for "off-the-shelf" designs that may not fulfill your specific requirements. Select an architect who has the flexibility and imagination to provide you with the services that will best fulfill your needs.
- *References:* Find out how prospective architects do business, how responsible they are to their clients' needs, and how they stack up to their clients' expectations. The best way to do this is to talk with other veterinarians for whom the architect has provided services.
- *Fees:* Once you have selected the best firm for you, request a proposal for services and fees. If you cannot agree, begin negotiating with your second choice. Nationally known experts may charge more than inexperienced local architects. You will need to judge for yourself whether the experience and efficiency gained are worth the higher fee.
- *Rapport:* Having personal confidence in, and rapport with, your architect is critical. Find an architect who understands the importance of listening and who is also someone who you will enjoy working closely with throughout the life of your project.
- *Finally, be frank:* Tell your architect what you expect and what your capabilities are. Ask for an explanation of anything you don't understand. Discuss your needs and the architect's motivations. The result will be a better and more successful project for both of you.

The Design Phase

Architects will typically divide design into three phases: schematic (or preliminary) drawings, design development (detailed preliminary drawings), and construction documents (or working drawings). The schematic drawings are the initial drawings done by the architect based on the owner's vision of the project and the building program. They are then refined into the construction documents that are used by the contractor.

Schematic Drawings

These drawings represent the basic configuration and appearance of the building. They are often used by the owner to get preliminary pricing or to get governmental or financial approval. For the architect, they are the basic drawings that are, with refinement, later developed into the design development drawings. The actual time it takes for your architect to develop the schematic drawings is dependent on a realistic and well-considered program, your capacity to make timely and consistent decisions, your architect's ability to understand and translate your ideas onto paper, and the degree of familiarity your architect has with animal hospital design. This process will generally take four to six weeks.

Design Development

This phase refines the schematic drawings and in greater detail establishes the construction requirements for the building, including plans, elevations, sections, systems, materials, and equipment. This phase will take about six to eight weeks and will often be included in the construction documents phase on smaller projects.

Construction Documents

During the construction document phase, the architect creates the drawings necessary to cost and build your facility. These documents are also the legal basis for your contract with the contractor. Production and coordination of construction documents takes about eight to ten weeks.

The Construction Phase

Upon completion of the construction documents, a building permit is obtained and bids are obtained from contractors if the traditional owner/contractor relationship has been chosen. The time required to get a building permit varies greatly, from days to months, depending on where the project is located. With the design and permitting process complete, construction can finally begin! Construction time can change substantially based on the complexity of the job, whether or not the project has to be phased, the size and organizational skills of the contractor, and weather delays. As a general rule, a freestanding facility will take six to eight months.

Move In

With your building complete, it's time to move in. Care and attention to detail while preparing for the move will help to ease any moving challenges. While many of our clients are functioning within a couple of days, it is important to remember that it can take months to get well organized.

Go Out and Do It

Animal hospitals are unique and intricate facilities. When properly designed and executed, they can provide a friendly environment for animals and an inviting work place for you and your staff. So as you move through the building process, be prepared, be patient, and through all the ups and downs, try to keep your sense of humor.

Tony's Architectural Concerns for Site Selection

   I. Land costs
     A. Purchase price
     B. "Hidden development costs"
     C. Title search
  II. Site constraints
     A. Sufficient size to accommodate
       1. Building program
       2. Expansion requirements

      3. Parking requirements
      4. Landscaping requirements
      5. Setbacks
   B. Public rights-of-way
      1. Access
      2. Anticipated street improvements/restrictions
   C. Topographical constraints
   D. Soils
   E. Availability, capacity, and inverts for utilities
   F. Water
   G. Sewer
   H. Gas
   I. Electric
   J. Telephone
   K. Storm drainage
   L. Off-site requirements for street or utility work
III. Government regulations
   A. Zoning of property and adjacent properties
   B. Restrictions for shelters
   C. Anticipated changes in zoning or planning districts
   D. Development fees
IV. Special considerations
   A. Adjacent property owner or tenant opposition
   B. Neighborhood opposition

Getting Started Review Issues

- Veterinary hospitals are costly because they are similar to human hospitals when you consider the complexity of the mechanical, plumbing, and electrical systems; the necessity of installing durable materials and finishes; and the addition of radiology suites, surgery suites, and wards.
- Your building program is a written description of your practice healthcare delivery plan for the future, augmented by a wish list that has been condensed somewhat by the realities of budget, site limitations, and zoning restrictions.
- It is essential on anything more than a minor renovation that the practice ownership gets a dedicated project manager to represent them with the municipality, design team, contractor, and subcontractors. These people are school trained as healthcare administrators and are often referred to as facility planners in human healthcare. The VPC Brokerage, www.v-p-c.com, has been known to have some of these people available within their stable of professionals looking for a job in veterinary medicine.
- The predesign phase includes doing demographic studies, instigating site studies for surveys and soils reports, investigating how your project can be financed, finding out what your submittal schedule and time requirements for

approvals will be, and determining the design, consulting, and construction services you will need.

- An understanding of who comprises the design team (names of specific people who will be working together on your project) and the members' respective roles is essential. This design team will include your architect, engineers, contractors, suppliers, and craftspeople; insurance, accounting, and legal professionals; municipality agencies; your staff; a dedicated project manager; and you (practice ownership).

- In the operational and functional planning portions of veterinary hospital design, delivery modalities must be reassessed based on the emerging sciences of the profession. A veterinary practice consultant may be needed to facilitate the thought process and fine-tune the practice's delivery system as well as mentor the project manager and practice planning team and confront the design team when paradigms begin to outweigh practice desires. The AVPMCA web site (www.AVPMCA.org) has a consultant listing and an internal code of ethics that members must subscribe to when delivering support within this profession.

- When choosing an architect, some important points to consider are experience, including evidence of similar projects he or she has completed, and the flexibility to best fulfill your needs; references from other veterinarians; fees that can be slightly higher for nationally known experts than for inexperienced local architects; and a feeling of personal confidence and good rapport.

- The design phase of your project is divided into schematic drawings, which are the preliminary and basic appearance and configuration of the building; design development, which refines the schematics and establishes the construction requirements for the building; construction documents, which are the blueprints used to cost and build the facility; and the construction phase, which includes obtaining a building permit, bidding, and actually building the project.

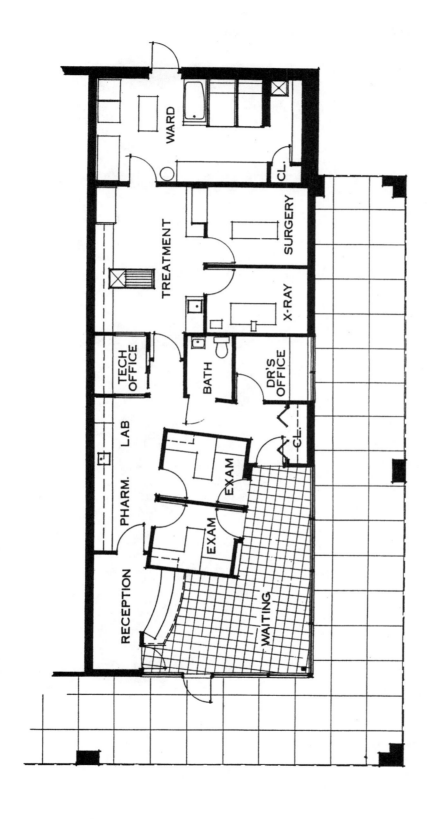

WARD

TREATMENT

SURGERY

CL.

X-RAY

TECH OFFICE

BATH

DR'S OFFICE

LAB

PHARM.

EXAM

EXAM

CL.

RECEPTION

WAITING

101

5

The Production Documents

THE PRODUCTION PHASE of a veterinary healthcare facility is much more than just the construction of the physical plant; in fact, it begins and ends with the execution of legal activities. From the production and execution of the owner-contractor agreement to the final inspections and acceptance of the completed structure, the project manager and practice ownership will find themselves involved with complex and critical legal documents and activities. In addition to these clearly legal activities, a new kind of architectural drawing must now be produced: the working drawings. The working drawings, along with written specifications, are in themselves a form of legal document as they describe in pictures and in words what the contractors have legally agreed to build and the purchaser has legally agreed to pay for.

Given these considerations, it is important that the project manager and practice ownership use the trusted practice attorney to develop and/or understand these documents and activities. What follows in this chapter is a brief discussion of what these documents are composed of, what they mean, and how to read them.

The contract documents consist of the practice owner-contractor agreement, general and supplementary conditions, drawings, specifications, and all addenda issued before the execution of the agreement. The practice owner-contractor agreement is considered the basic contract because it is the only one that requires the signature of both the practice owner and the contractor; it incorporates all other documents referred to in it. The agreement provides a statement of the contract sum, identifies the nature of the project, establishes the time of commencement and completion, and describes the manner wherein the contractor will be reimbursed for work performed.

The general conditions set forth the legal and regulatory requirements of the contract and are usually included as part of the contract through a standard form from the AIA—"General Conditions of the Contract for Construction," which is accepted by the construction industry as a standard. The supplementary conditions extend and modify the general conditions, defining the specific requirements of a particular veterinary facility project. The drawings are graphic representations of the work to be performed and contain information about design, location, and dimensions of the elements of the project. The specifications are a statement of particulars. Construction specifications are written instructions distinguishing or limiting and describing in detail the construction work to be undertaken; these specifications provide technical information about the materials indicated on the drawings.

The publication of a standard form that would reflect the studied approach of the architectural, construction, and legal professions was first undertaken by the AIA in 1888. Since then, the form has been revised at least twelve times. These modifications of format and content have resulted from thorough reviews of contract procedures and the desire for contract stipulations that are equally fair to, and protective of, the interests of the practice owner and the contractor. In order for the form to be used nationwide, some of its provisions had to be written in general, rather than specific, language. Provisions also allow for modifications to meet special circumstances. Although the standardized format has kept pace with the changes in construction practice, there developed the need for a supplement that would translate general provisions into specific project requirements. This led to two separate but related documents: the general and the supplementary conditions.

General Conditions

The "General Conditions of the Contract for Construction" is now the basis for a further review to determine whether supplementary conditions should be a part of the contract. Provisions are grouped into fourteen logically developed sequential articles.

- *Article 1: Contract Documents.* This article includes discussions of the following: contract documents, contract, work, execution, correlation, intent and interpretations, and copies furnished and their ownership. Also the components of the contract documents, the scope of the work to be included, and what constitutes the project are defined. The contractor is obligated by this article to familiarize himself with the site, local conditions affecting the work, and the requirements of the contract documents. The number of contract documents to be issued to the contractor is stated, together with the contingency that all such documents be returned to the architect.
- *Article 2: Architect.* This article has two sections: a definition and an explanation of the administration of the contract. The architect is defined as the person or firm licensed by the state to practice architecture and identified as such in the agreement. Notice is also provided that there exists no contractual obligation between the architect and the contractor for though the architect provides general administration of the construction contract he or she is not responsible for directing the work. The architect's authority to function as the owner's representative is outlined in the contract.
- *Article 3: Owner.* This article includes the following areas: definition, information, and services required by the practice owner; the owner's right to stop

the work; and the owner's right to carry out the work. The practice owner is defined as the person or firm executing the agreement with the contractor. The owner is obligated by this article to furnish all surveys, site investigation studies, easements, and legal access to the site. The right of the owner to stop the work or to have deficiencies resulting from the contractor's defaults or neglect corrected by others at the contractor's expense is spelled out. Ensure this section is amended to reflect that the project manager is the primary representative of the owner during construction and is the person who is responsible for reviewing daily progress of the work and the conduct of all those performing on the site.

- *Article 4: Contractor.* This article covers the following: definition, review of contract documents, supervision and construction procedures, labor and materials, warranty, taxes, permits, fees and notices, cash allowances, superintendent, responsibility for those performing the work, cleaning up, progress schedule, drawings and specifications at the site, shop drawings and samples, use of site, cutting and patching the work, communications, and indemnification. The contractor, defined as the person or firm executing the agreement with the owner, is obligated to review all contract documents carefully and report any deficiencies noted to the architect. He or she is to supervise the work and be responsible for construction methods, coordination, and procedures, using materials and workmanship that accord with contract requirements. By his or her execution of the contract, the contractor warrants that all work will be in conformance with the contract documents. The contractor is obliged to pay all taxes and to pay for all permits, fees, and licenses applicable at the time bids are received. The primary representative of the contractor during construction is the superintendent, who is responsible for daily progress of the work and the conduct of all those performing on the site. A schedule of anticipated progress leading to completion of the work is prepared by the contractor for distribution to everyone involved in the project. A set of drawings is provided to the contractor for recording all changes made during construction. These drawings will be surrendered to the owner to function as an "as-built" record. Shop drawings, which include drawings, diagrams, brochures, and other data sufficient to illustrate individual portions of the work, are prepared by the contractor and submitted to the architect for approval. Samples, where they serve the same purpose, are also submitted. All communications between practice owner and contractor should go through the architect. The indemnification provision requires that the contractor hold harmless the practice owner and architect in casualty situations where personal injury involves a contractor's employee or other member of the public, where property damage results from construction operations, and where either casualty is caused in whole or in part by negligent act or omission of the contractor or his/her forces.
- *Article 5: Subcontractors.* Subcontractors may be needed on the site to carry out work required by the contract. This article confirms that no contractual relationship exists between the practice owner and any subcontractor but that

the identity of all subcontractors is to be made known to the practice owner
so that he or she may express any reasonable cause for rejecting a subcontractor. While neither architect nor practice owner has any legal obligation
with respect to payments to subcontractors, the procedures relative to such
payments are spelled out in this article so that the contractor must assume
them as part of his or her contract obligation.

- *Article 6: Additional Contracts.* Article 6 reserves the right to award additional contracts to others who will pursue certain portions of the work simultaneously with the original contractor (e.g., cremation incinerators, capital
expense equipment technical installations, etc.). It then becomes necessary to
define mutual areas of responsibilities as they will apply to the separate contractors performing simultaneous work on the project.
- *Article 7: Miscellaneous Legal Provisions.* Included here are restrictions
against the assignment of the contract procedures related to processing claims
for damages, testing requirements to satisfy the orders of a public authority,
and the arbitration process that will be instituted in the event of an alleged
breach of contract.
- *Article 8: Time.* Article 8 is concerned with the definition of time as the term
will be employed in other contract provisions. The sections that apply to all
construction projects are those concerned with the commencement date and
the date of substantial completion. The latter is significant because it signals
the inauguration of the one-year guaranty period. The remaining sections,
which deal with delays and extensions of time, become particularly meaningful when the contract contains clauses entitling the owner to penalize the
contractor for delays in completing the project within an allocated period of
time.
- *Article 9: Periodic Payments Procedures.* This article elaborates the processes to be employed in confirming the basis on which payments are made to the
contractor as the work progresses. On projects in which large sums of money
and an extended period of construction are involved, progress payments are
normally made on a monthly basis to reflect work performed during the preceding month. The amount paid is usually 90 or 95 percent of the monies
earned with the remainder being retained by the practice owner to ensure
faithful completion of the project. Requests for payment are forwarded by the
contractor to the architect, who certifies their correctness and transmits them
to the practice owner with his or her endorsement that they be honored.
- *Article 10: Safety.* Article 10 delineates the responsibilities imposed on the
contractor to ensure protection of persons and property. Project safety is the
exclusive responsibility of the contractor, who must take all reasonable safety precautions necessary to protect the work, the people affected by the work,
the site, and the property adjacent to the site. Damage to the work or property resulting from inadequate protection is to be remedied by the contractor,
except where damage can be attributed to faulty drawings or specifications or
to the acts of the owner or architect not attributable to faults or negligence of
the contractor.

- *Article 11: Insurance.* This article identifies the type of insurance coverage to be provided by each of the parties to the contract. The contractor must secure worker's compensation coverage and bodily and property liability insurance. The practice owner must purchase and maintain property insurance that protects him or her and the contractor and his or her forces against fire, extended coverage, vandalism, and malicious mischief. The practice owner may also obtain liability insurance.
- *Article 12: Changes.* This article contains the details involved in formulating changes in the work defined in the original contract documents. Such changes, which normally will affect the contract sum, are formalized through a change order. Normally, the architect describes the intended change in writing or drawings and transmits the description to the contractor along with a request for the price of the work described. The contractor submits his or her proposal of the cost for such work to the architect, who recommends acceptance, rejection, or negotiation of the proposal to the owner. If the practice owner and contractor agree on the proposal, the architect prepares the change order for execution by all three parties.
- *Article 13: Uncovering and Correcting.* Article 13 is concerned with the uncovering and correcting of work performed by the contractor. If work is covered by the contract contrary to the request of the architect, the contractor must bear the expense of uncovering and recovering, even when the work is found to be in accordance with contract requirements. If the architect does not specifically request that the work be kept uncovered, then the contractor is liable only if the uncovered work is not in accordance with the contract documents. The cost of removing and correcting all work rejected by the architect as being defective is borne by the contractor, whether it occurs before substantial completion or within a year after substantial completion.
- *Article 14: Termination.* This article defines the circumstances under which the owner or contractor may legally terminate the contract before the project is completed.

Supplementary Conditions

The supplementary conditions contain amendments to the general conditions and are usually attached to them. Common modifications include the following:

- alteration of Article 1 by giving the number of sets of drawings and specifications the contractor will be furnished free of charge
- alteration of Article 7 to require that the contractor furnish performance and labor and material bonds in the amount of 100 percent of the contract sum
- alteration of Article 11 to establish the limit of liability in dollar amounts that must be covered in the insurance taken out by the contractor

Where guaranteed funds are involved in the project, the lending agency may require the inclusion of supplementary conditions concerning the right of access to and inspection of the work, compliance with equal opportunity requirements, adherence to a schedule of prevailing wages, extra compensation for overtime, and submission by the contractor of weekly affidavits certifying compliance with the fiscal institution's requirements.

Specifications

Specifications are written instructions describing in detail the construction work to be undertaken. Specifications and drawings serve complementary functions. The drawings represent, in graphic form, the size, shape, and location of the various building elements and the manner in which they relate to each other, thus defining the quantity and type of each building component. The specifications express the quality, performance standards, and end result expected from the assembly of the materials and equipment items identified on the drawings. Notes on the drawings are usually stated in general terms, with the more detailed information being incorporated in the specifications.

The preparation of specifications is an essential feature of the design process and proceeds most effectively when it is done concurrently with the drawings. During the evolution of the specifications, it is often necessary to confer with manufacturer's representatives and for contracting personnel to become fully conversant with materials and methods applicable to the project. The selection of materials and equipment is essentially the responsibility of the architect, and before being included in the specifications, products must be appraised by the architect as to their suitability for the use intended.

A working knowledge of the materials used in the building includes their basic composition, the manner of their fabrication and installation, and their suitability for the use intended. Such knowledge is vital to the development of the specifications. Because specifications are written, they are more readily comprehensible to persons not affiliated with the construction industry than are the drawings; thus, the practice owner, project manager, and their legal and financial counselors are better able to understand the nature of the building elements and their relative significance through reading the specifications.

Once the most suitable product is determined, the architect must specify it in such a manner as to allow competitive bidding. Four of the most common practices employed for this purpose can be briefly described as follows:

1. *Contractor's option:* This type of specification lists every acceptable trade name for each product. After execution of the contract, the contractor may use any product listed, but only products listed.
2. *Product approval:* This type of specification lists one or more trade names for each product; it includes a statement that any request for substitutions by a bidder must be made a given number of days before the opening of bids and that all approvals will be issued in the form of an addendum.
3. *Approved equal:* This type of specification lists one or more trade names for each product required and adds the phrase "or approved equal." After exe-

cution of the contract, the contractor may use any of the listed products or may request permission from the architect to substitute an unlisted one he considers equal. It is to be understood by the contractor that the phrase allowing substitution requires written approval of the architect and that no substitutions may be made without such written approval.

4. Product description: This type of specification describes completely all details, qualities, functions, and sizes of a product without mentioning a trade or a brand name. Any product that meets all of the detailed specifications will be approved.

It is sometimes advantageous to include within the specifications a request for alternative prices for a single element or for certain areas of the total project. There are two basic reasons why alternative prices are requested: (1) to reach a final decision between two different materials or methods on the basis of their comparative value; and (2) to adjust the bids received so that the contract sum can be made to fit within the budget established for the project. Alternatives should be held to a minimum, since an overabundance of them tends only to complicate the bidding process. Where alternative prices are requested, the form of proposal submitted by each bidder should identify alternative prices separately from the lump-sum proposal.

The specifications will be indexed and bound in book form by trade activities that have been accepted by the construction industry. In the final specifications, the technical sections will be preceded by documents that involve various aspects of project involvement but do not amplify or describe the work illustrated on the drawings. In addition to the title page and the table of contents, these sections will include bidding requirements, contract documents, and general requirements.

The bidding requirements section of the specifications is concerned with inviting firms to submit proposals and delineates a set of bidding requirements on the procedures for the preparation and submission of those proposals. The invitation identifies the project, owner, and architect; establishes the time and location for the receipt of bids; and tells where bidding documents may be obtained. The instructions define the format in which bids are to be tendered, for what period bids are to remain binding, how questions related to interpretation or bidding documents are to be formulated, what bonds are to be executed, and what actions are to be expected of the owner following his or her review of the bids.

The contract documents section of the specifications contains a sample form of the agreement to be executed by the owner and the winning contractor, general conditions of the contract, and supplementary conditions.

The general requirements section of the specifications includes general references to the contractor's work and resembles in content the supplementary conditions of the contract. However, since they are concerned with activities on the site once construction has begun, the requirements are traditionally isolated from the contract itself. A listing of typical general requirements would include

- temporary power
- temporary water
- temporary heat
- temporary ventilation
- temporary field offices
- temporary toilet facilities
- commencement and completion dates
- job meetings
- construction sign
- sequence of construction
- measurements where existing buildings are included
- access to existing buildings

It is customary to arrange the sections of the specifications in the order in which the respective trades normally begin their principal work at the site. In addition to the sequential evolution of the trade activity, current specification writing also dictates that no single section cover the work of more than one subcontractor or material supplier. Adherence to this principle will tend to minimize the chance of duplication, omission, or confusion. It is understood, however, that while the architect organizes the specification sections, he cannot assume responsibility for allotting portions of the work to specific subcontractors.

Specifications are currently subdivided by anticipated trade involvement on the site into sixteen headings:

- Division 1, general requirements
- Division 2, site work
- Division 3, concrete work
- Division 4, masonry work
- Division 5, metals
- Division 6, carpentry
- Division 7, moisture protection
- Division 8, doors, windows, and glass
- Division 9, finishes
- Division 10, specialties
- Division 11, equipment
- Division 12, furnishings
- Division 13, special construction
- Division 14, conveying equipment
- Division 15, mechanical
- Division 16, electrical

Each of these is further subdivided into a number of individual sections that progress from the general to the particular. For example, the heading for Division 9 is "finishes" and typical section headings would read "vinyl wall coverings," "resilient flooring," "acoustical ceilings," "painting," and so on.

In summary, a set of project specifications is the written material that accompanies the drawings for a construction project. This material has as its objectives the following:

- to describe what is shown on the drawings and to portray information and establish requirements that can be done best in writing rather than in graphic form
- to include all of the legal requirements that are to apply to the owner and contractor upon finalization of the contract
- to provide the necessary accompaniment to the drawings in establishing a firm base for the preparation of competitive bids and the execution of the work required by the contract
- to assist the contractor in organizing his or her bidding, purchasing, and construction procedures by classifying the various trade activities into the sixteen divisions identified previously
- to function as a guide for owner, contractor, and architect during construction and inspection of the work
- to regulate payments and to provide the basis for legal interpretations

Phasing and Remodeling

One of the key words in hospital construction is "phasing." When a project involves existing facilities or renovated facilities, a phasing plan for construction and operation must be worked out. The common notion that "we can just relocate our existing equipment in the new building to save cost" is one of the most difficult problems during construction. During hospital remodeling, the existing facility must usually be kept operational at all times. If an entire zone is to be replaced, the new zone must be ready before the existing one can move. This makes it almost impossible to relocate fixed equipment without shutting down the operation. Some fixed items, such as millwork, can only be reused in a zone that will be phased out later. By the time wood or metal cabinets are torn out, moved, refinished, and installed again, the cost of the old equipment will be very close to that of new items.

Phasing of operations and work flow involve the entire practice staff. Once a plan is coordinated with the contractor, the project manager must notify the practice manager/hospital administrator and assist in briefing the staff; equipment and utilities must be put in place; and traffic and time elements must be worked out. It may be necessary at many phases for the contractor to work at night or on weekends so that utilities can be disconnected and replaced. Time is critical on an hourly basis and takes a maximum effort by the project manager, architect, and contractor. The project manager must attempt to anticipate all of the problems that can occur. A phasing program connected with remodeling must be accomplished before the final plans are given to various contractors for bidding, and the time frames and temporary construction conditions must be clearly defined. Once a contractor is chosen, he or she should be made aware of the key areas of hospital operation concerned with the departments that will be remodeled.

Costs for major renovation can be as high as those for new construction, and hidden pipes and undocumented structures can cause disputes. The expertise of a remodeling contractor is as important, if not more so, as that of a new building contractor. Renovation design and operation is very difficult, and only experienced professionals should be employed to attempt it.

Alternatives and Costs

By this stage of the project development, the major decisions of the design team have been carried out and are very costly to change. The veterinary practice consultant completed his or her design assistance tasks before working drawings were started, and the architect is now 70 percent finished. The veterinary practice consultant still may be working with the practice team on learning new skills that will be essential in maximizing the use of the new facility. The zone coordinators have had their input on all fixed equipment and know the functional design has been set for months. The documents are by now supposed to contain every approval, thought, mood, change, and quality of all the various people involved over the design period. Construction prices, however, have been only estimates, and a final price can only be obtained with the complete scope of drawings, specifications, and conditions of the contract. It is at this point, before bidding, that *deductive* alternatives, *add-on* alternatives, or both should be included. Though most alternatives were conceived early in the design, because of budget, the formal proposal is only now drawn up.

What is an alternative and why is it necessary? An alternative is designed to meet the taste of the practice planning team or practice ownership on the day final prices are received. Anyone who has shopped for a major appliance for his or her home has faced the same situation: An estimated price is established on the basis of experience and advertisements, then the extras to be added on or features that may have to be taken care of are considered.

Typical deductive alternatives for a veterinary practice may be price for eliminating the proposed material-handling system, the dual laundry at pack prep and wards, or an above-the-ground kennel run system that makes individual run plumbing in the floor inappropriate. Add-on alternatives may include vinyl wall covering, wood paneling, parking structures, or extra landscaping. Furthermore, an anticipated labor problem, economy change, code enforcement, or even weather can vary the final price drastically. Therefore, the practice ownership should be prepared to face a situation in which its extra wants can be either deducted or added on. Deductible alternative estimates do not usually reflect a fair market price of the work items and construction; therefore, add-on alternatives must cover the real costs and are the preferred format.

In a system of scope set, pricing design, and guaranteed prices, alternatives are negotiated in or out of a project as the final prices are being put together. Quality control is absolutely necessary during the entire program and design stages, but a final decision on what items can be deducted or added must be made by the architect and project manager.

Working Drawings

Working drawings represent the culmination of the architect's efforts in interpreting the client's program requirements. They are intended to explain fully and in detail the volume of the building to be erected. This detail is necessary in bidding to determine total building cost; following receipt of bids and selection of the contractor, it is needed to erect the building.

Working drawings and specifications together are called the construction documents. The drawings graphically portray the design, while the specifications supply complementary verbal descriptions. As such, they are mutually extensive, and what is required by one is required by the other. In the event of conflict between the two documents, the architect is the interpreter. Another older definition states that the drawings tell the builders what to do, while the specifications tell him how to do it. Whereas this definition may once have been valid, it may be more accurate now to say, in layman's terms, that the drawings tell the builder where, what, and how to erect the building, and the specifications establish quality control.

The purpose of working drawings is to depict graphically the characteristics and extent of the project. Properly prepared drawings describe, locate, give dimensions, and give physical properties of, or specifically detail the assembly of, various materials. When issued, all working drawings, regardless of type, must represent a coordinated effort of the general construction trades and of structural, mechanical, and electrical designers and trades. Throughout the project's development, the architect has headed the efforts of all consulting engineers. Coordinating their design and project requirement implementation, as well as interpreting and complying with applicable codes, is the architect's responsibility. Specifications evolve concurrently with the development of working drawings. Ideally, the specifications define physical properties and performance criteria of each item to be incorporated into the structure. In addition, they identify acceptable materials, manufacturers, and materials and application standards. Regardless of the size of a project, the sequence of working drawings should be as follows.

1. The title sheet identifies the building or project. Supplemental sheets may enumerate the working drawings to follow, normally defined by trade and further trade-related by specific drawing enumeration such as A-1,2,3 for architectural (general construction) drawings; S-1,2,3 for structural drawings; P-1,2,3 for plumbing; M-1,2,3 for mechanical; and E-1,2,3 for electrical.
2. The site plan and detailed drawings illustrate how the building is situated on a real piece of ground; advise through an area location map as to community location and relationship; and delineate new and existing utilities, new

and existing grade, roads, improvements, retaining walls, outbuildings, and landscaping. In short, they delineate the scope of the project and the limits of the contract.

3. Architectural drawings typically include consecutive floor plans, the roof plan, elevations of the building, sections, details, and room finish and door schedule drawings.

4. Structural drawings generally consist of foundation plans, floor and roof forming plans, structural sections and details, column schedules, miscellaneous structural element schedules, and fireproofing requirements for the specific project.

5. Mechanical drawings usually begin with a site utilities drawing delineating incoming water supply service, a fire hydrant and underground fire protection water piping system, and storm water and sewer line networks. This drawing very closely follows the site plan. After this come the plumbing drawings, consisting of plans for normal plumbing fixtures, piping to and from them, medical gas systems, pneumatic tube systems, roof drainage systems, and sprinkler systems. Mechanical drawings also include plans illustrating heating, ventilating, and air-conditioning systems (especially equipment definitions, duct systems, and hot and cold water piping systems). Equipment schedules and details, along with system and fixture schedules and tack diagrams, complete this section.

6. Electrical drawings begin with a site plan that illustrates incoming power, its point of entry into the building, and site and exterior building lighting. Electrical plans are normally separate efforts designed to show interior lighting fixture arrangement; to define interior power (equipment and receptacle requirements); and to define other systems such as Internet access and intercommunications, telephones, electrostatic shielding, special grounding, and security and fire alarms. Plan drawings would be supplemented by fixture schedules, various system riser diagrams, and details.

In addition to these drawings the architect makes topographic survey drawings and test boring records available to the contractor. These are not usually included with the contract drawings, since they were not prepared by the architect or under his or her supervision or authority (they are provided directly to the practice owner by independent professionals).

Reading the Working Drawings

At first glance, working drawings are formidable, especially those of a typical veterinary facility project. Yet, if it is remembered that these documents tell the contractor exactly how the building is to be built, they become like a foreign language: The more one learns about them, the less mysterious they become. Taking part in the development of these drawings, from schematics to working drawings, for a single veterinary project would provide a complete education, but it would take from two to four years on the average.

Another approach is to analyze a small portion of the total drawing effort.

This limited approach can still be confusing because all the trades drawings rely heavily on standard material and equipment representations, on symbols, and on industry-accepted abbreviations.

Essentially, each trades drawing is meant to complement the others. The architect is responsible for coordinating the trades drawings, while the general contractor is charged with coordinating the work of subcontractors. In addition, the specifications require that all contractors study the work of other contractors as defined by the working drawings and specifications. Some architectural firms require composite drawings that lay out, on a large scale, the major elements of the plumbing, mechanical, and electrical systems. Such drawings not only force the engineers to coordinate their work in the field but also dictate the order in which system components are actually installed. Following completion of the work, the drawings are turned over to the client and become a valuable part of the as-built record of construction, enabling the in-house engineering personnel to more easily repair and control the systems. Should future alterations or additions be needed, these as-built records would be extremely useful.

Construction

Bidding Requirements and Procedures

As explained in the previous chapters, the system of construction management and guaranteed prices has become very popular in the hospital field and has been entering the veterinary market with some design-build firms. Traditionally, several building contractors submit sealed prices in competition for the total building project; competitive bidding will remain one of the most widely used methods of obtaining construction prices.

The discussion on general conditions outlined the responsibilities and conditions that a contractor must assume to complete a building project. The sections on specifications and working drawings define the materials produced by the architect. This phase of a building program now commits the hospital client to sign a separate contract with the construction contractor, with the architect acting as the client's representative. When using competitive bidding, it is wise to prequalify the contractors who will be involved. That is, the architect designs a form that asks each interested contractor to submit references and data on experience, financial condition, and the ability to be bonded.

An invitation to bid, or a request for bid, as described above, outlines the time, place, scope, and location of the final plans and actual bid. The sets of plans and specifications are usually very large rolls, and specification books must be distributed to the general contractors and kept at trade locations for the information of the subcontractors. The architect will supply a minimum number of bid sets, but it is the practice's responsibility to pay for additional sets (this responsibility should be verified by the project manager in the original architect-engineer contract, as the cost can annoy the practice ownership if they are not aware of it). Deposits can be collected to assure that the contractors who do not win the bid will return the sets.

The bidding contractors should be allowed approximately four weeks to come up with their final price. During this time, a conference may be held with the project manager and architect to make sure each bidder realizes the scope of the project; when so many people are looking at a set of plans and specifications there are bound to be questions. Clarifications and item changes should be worked up by the architect, and addendums issued showing each bidder the exact change. When bids are received, all addenda and alternatives are acknowledged. The final price submittals must be evaluated by the architect, who will advise the project manager and practice ownership as to technical accuracy. The contract can then be awarded. The lowest qualified bidder should not always receive the project if material substitutions or time-lines were bid as variances. At this time, the architect and the practice's legal counsel must draft a contract that is agreeable to the practice ownership and to the contractor.

In some mega-facility situations, as a financing mechanism, it is required that the general, mechanical, and electrical contracts be bid separately. The mechanical and electrical engineering contracts are then assigned to the successful general contractor so that one company is responsible for the project.

Once the bids are received and the contracts signed, the practice has very little control over the selection of subcontractors. The bid documents may require that a list of subcontractors be submitted, but this does not always come about. Whatever prices the general contractor used to formulate his or her total he or she can now negotiate; any savings that result will not be available to the practice. The contractor must, however, meet the quality and quantity as described in the drawings and specifications. Changes at this point will be very expensive.

Permits

The contractor must obtain the proper building permits from all local building and environmental authorities. Utility permits, site permits, and building permits have previously been approved according to the plan layouts, but they must be paid for before construction begins. These costs are usually in the contract, but the practice could have paid for them independently to avoid the contractor's markup.

General Contractor

The general conditions defined the liabilities and the role of all general contractors and subcontractors. The contractor must also understand the veterinary practice operations in order to disrupt routine as little as possible.

Construction touches special nerves of the doctors and hospital staff. The practice manager/hospital administrator will be blamed for the noise, site confusion, distractions, and labor strikes. These things are part of normal construction, but they place an unfamiliar burden on a practice's normal operation. The best advice that can be given to a practice manager/hospital administrator is to leave on vacation during construction, let the project manager handle it all, and come back when the project is finished! Of course, this is usually impossible, except when the project manager may become the new hospital administrator after the construction project is completed. The practice manager/hospital administrator should, however, leave construction problems up to the project manager and experienced professionals who have been hired to deal with them. Day-by-day construction seems like endless delay and problems to the average veterinary staff member; it is a way of life for the architect and the contractor.

The project manager must rely on the contractor and realize that the contractor's aim is to build an excellent facility that will carry his or her reputation in the community. The building contractor must be experienced in order to handle problem situations that occur every day. The contractor must, at one time, coordinate thirty to forty different trades (all with experience and advice), solve all labor problems, and build a complicated veterinary facility without creating noise, dust, delay, error, or sparks.

Inspection

One way to save the practice owner some of the headaches mentioned above is to employ a clerk-of-the-works or project manager. This dedicated person represents the practice; he or she is experienced in facility planning and is hired by the practice to check daily progress. Although the architect acts as the practice's representative during construction, he or she only performs inspection as it is required. The architect will not be on the site every day and, in fact, may negotiate extra fees for inspection services. The architect's duty here is to check shop drawings (detail of each item specified and submitted by the manufacturer for approval), verify the contractor's invoices to the owner, and see that quality and design are met. The architect does not tell the contractor how to build the building; he or she defines the size, shape, and quality of the building.

When the municipality does its inspection(s), the project manager accompanies the inspector, although the contractor is solely accountable for the safety, standards, and construction. If there is a variance between code and drawings, the contractor will forward the noncompliance to the architect, where the project manager's firsthand knowledge may prove very useful in mediating excess expenses and/or change orders.

Insights and Perspectives

Getting It Built—Construction Options
Paul Gladysz, AIA, CSI

So you've done your planning. You found an architect and you love their work. Now what? How do you take your paper dream and make it real?

Building your clinic will be one of the most memorable times of your life. At times exhilarating, at times draining. How much of each will depend in large part on how well you do your homework. The construction industry is changing. The recent boom years have been very good to contractors, subcontractors, and suppliers. With so much work to be had there is very little incentive to keep bids tight and costs down. Overhead and profit margins have been rising steadily. Increases in building materials and other costs have caused the construction cost index to rise more than 20 percent between 1995 and 2001, more than twice the inflation rate. Only those who understand their options will be able to take advantage of them. The business of design and construction is a mystery to most. Unless you've grown up in the business, it's hard to imagine how something so complex can be put together. So, how is it done?

In essence there are three methods the construction industry uses: design-bid-build, construction management, and design-build.

Design-Bid-Build

This is the traditional method most people associate with a new building. You hire an architect and together you design your building, and you solicit bids for the construction from local general contractors. With your architect's help you choose the best builder and sign a contract to do the work.

During construction your architect assists you in monitoring progress. Notice the number of times I said "you." The biggest misconception about the process of building or renovating your clinic is that the architect does everything and you mostly watch and sign checks. In reality you have a high level of involvement. Your first, and probably hardest, task is to establish a realistic budget and a building program, the document that defines your project: Will you build a new structure or renovate an existing one? How many exam rooms will it have? What equipment, exterior style, and so on? All the work to follow will be based on this building program, and reconciling the budget and the program is *the* essential first step. In 99.9 percent of the projects I've worked on the program has exceeded the budget. The hard part is finding out what your requirements will likely cost. It is, without doubt, the most difficult, and yet the most important part, of the process. This is where the experience of your designer is critical. You want one who has enough recent experience to compare similar completed projects to yours. If you don't get this part right, you are guaranteed to get bids all over budget. Make sure you discuss this before you hire your designer. The standard contract published by the AIA lists budgeting and programming as an owner's responsibility and an additional service (read: extra fee) if done by the architect.

Once the budget versus program issue is resolved your involvement is just beginning. Design is a collaborative process. It's also the fun part. Work with your architect; be creative. Design is usually an evolutionary process so there will be many versions and revisions. Just remember to stay within your program and budget limits. Above all beware of the evil "might as wells." Nothing will kill your budget faster than thinking, "As long as we are building we might as well put in a basement or an unfinished second floor or extra exams." If you need future expansion, program it into the budget. Adding things after will ruin all that hard work. In some instances, adding later might not be possible given the physical realities of what you have already designed and built.

Once the design is final, your architect, along with the appropriate engineers, will produce the construction plans, specifications, and bid documents. Other than periodic reviews your required involvement is minimal. Resist the impulse to make infinite minor improvements. With the possible exception of the Parthenon there has never been a perfect design. Everything can be improved, be tweaked, be made just a little better, but at some point you must stop designing and begin building.

When the construction documents are done the project goes out for bid, and in about four to five weeks you find out what it's really going to cost. Hopefully you did a careful job of programming and budgeting, your designer had accurate recent comparison projects, you stuck to the plan, and nothing major has changed the building climate in your area. No Florida hurricanes to drive up the cost of plywood, no trucker's strikes, OPEC production changes, or shortage of drywall. The reality is that there are so many unknowns that can affect the cost of construction that even the bid provided by the general contractors is their best guess. A well-educated guess, but a guess none the less. In fact, the biggest difference between your initial estimate and the bid you receive is that somebody is now willing to bet they can do the job for that price. They are taking a risk. A risk based on their experience, estimating abilities, and gut feel. Do they guess right? Not always. It's like a contractor friend once told me—sometimes you eat the bear, sometimes the bear eats you.

Construction Management

This method has been around for quite a while but has been used mostly for larger commercial projects. For the past ten years it has become more common for smaller (less than five-million-dollar) jobs. Construction management comes in several variations, but they all entail hiring a manager to be the go-between between you and the rest of the design and building groups. The idea is that you hire a professional, usually for a fee, who knows the process inside and out. The construction manager assists in programming, budgeting, design, bidding, and construction. He or she looks out for your best interests—keeping you from overprogramming, underestimating, overdesigning, and so on. This all sounds so good you wonder why all projects don't use one. The reason is that construction management represents an additional cost. Because it is so time consuming, it's not a small cost. Construction management fees range from 6 percent to as much as 15 percent of construction cost. That's on top of the designer's fee and the general contractor's overhead and profit. On a large enough project, a good construction manager may be able to save the amount of the fee in making sure you don't go over budget. However, sometimes it is difficult for a construction manager to find enough savings to pay the fee. The best reason to hire a construction manager is not to save money but to save time. You operate a thriving practice. You don't have the time to learn the construction process, do all the hundreds of things that it will demand of you, while you maintain your clinic and still have a family life. If that prospect has been keeping you from even starting, then a construction manager may be your answer. I said that construction managers *usually* work for a fee because there is one method that sometimes pays for the construction manager out of the construction cost. The construction manager can act as the constructor. In this scenario the construction manager does not bid to general contractors but directly to the subcontractors and suppliers. So instead of you signing a general contract you sign a series of subcontracts and purchase orders. The construction manager manages the construction site—scheduling, monitoring, and handling problems. In effect he or she acts in the same capacity as the general contractor except the construction manager's not taking the risk, you are. The cost of the fee is offset by the savings of eliminating the general contractor's overhead and profit. This way you get the best of both worlds—a construction manager's involvement and no additional fee. Remember, however, there is also no general contractor to take the financial risk of cost overruns. If the cost of drywall takes a big jump the extra cost comes out of your pocket. If you consider using this method make sure your budget has a healthy contingency fund—remember that bear!

Design-Build

Design-build is usually thought of as a new and innovative scheme: Having one group design a project and construct it. In fact it is the oldest method known. It's only in the past 150 years or so that the functions of design and construction diverged and moved away from the idea of the master builder. From the pyramids to the mechanical age the same person designed and directed construction, but with mechanization came specialization. As construction systems became more complex, even the work of design split between architecture and engineering.

What design-build does is recombine these back into a single entity, a sole source of responsibility. The usual situation is when a contractor and a designer form an alliance for a specific project. If the contractor specializes in design-build, he or she may even have designers on staff. More rare, but what I find personally more interesting, is when the designer takes on the task of construction. *That way the design controls the construction instead of the construction controlling the design.* Design becomes focused primarily on function rather than primarily on ease of construction.

Design-build usually involves a two-part contract. Part 1 includes predesign (your budget and programming), conceptual and schematic design, and the build proposal. The design-builder produces the design drawings in the same way as in the traditional design-bid-build method. Along with drawings are an outline; specifications, usually performance based; and a build proposal. The proposal gives a price to build the project along with what it includes. One of the big advantages of design-build is that you now have a fixed price to construct—before any engineering or architectural construction documents are started (which is Part 2). This usually occurs months sooner than in the other two methods. How can the price be fixed so early? Certainly the design-builder is taking a risk, but usually no greater than a general contractor would. Because the specifications are performance based, rather than product based, the design-builder has enough leeway to find materials that are in budget. For example, a product-based specification may say to use the following flooring in waiting:

> Crossville Ceramics 8″ × 8″ porcelain tile, color #502 with matching bullnose base cove: use Laticrete Sp-100 latipoxy grout, color #B7.

A performance-based specification would say:

> Reception flooring to be an "A" quality porcelain tile, 8″ × 8″ with matching bullnose base cove; grout to be 1st quality 2 part epoxy grout. Both to be in a color acceptable to the owner.

Both specifications accomplish the same result. The difference is that performance specifications give the design-builder leeway he or she needs to stay within budget. Performance specifications are a valuable tool and are slowly becoming more common on other types of projects, though they're still used on less than 10 percent of all jobs.

Another reason design-builders can quote a price so early is that the contractor is involved from the very beginning. Unlike the traditional design-bid-build method, here you have the experience of the builder to assist in budgeting. With more pricing experience to draw on, your initial budget should be more accurate. Design-build is a neat system, and the one that I feel provides the best value. However, this method is not for everyone. The structure of the project team is very different from the other two methods—design-build is collaborative, the others are competitive. With design-build you define your project and establish what you are willing to pay for it. Then you find the team that can do the best job. Dollars are not an unknown, price being established very early in the process. The other two methods are competitive—you define the project and make an educated guess at the cost. You count on a competitive bidding process to produce the best price. Unfortunately it's not until all design and engineering are done that you find out the real cost. Even so, some clients are reluctant to move away from competitive bidding. The perception, though not accurate, is that without it you don't know if you got the best price. Remember your goal is not the best price, it's the best value. Sometimes the most expensive building comes from the low bidder.

Making the Right Choice

It's always good to have options, but how can you decide which method is right for you? Start with a little soul-searching. Which one makes you feel the most comfortable? The last thing you need is to use a system that will keep you up at night, because this is a long process and a year is a long time to go without sleep.

Next look at the talent pool available to you. If there are no qualified or affordable construction managers in your area don't try to make do with a bad fit. There are firms that work nationally so don't forget to check them. Next look at experience. At a minimum you need a firm that is familiar with healthcare and is willing to learn the unique challenges of animal care. For example, most human clinics don't need soundproofing; veterinary facilities do. Make sure the firm you select understands that. Ideally you want a firm that has several successful veterinary projects under its belt. I don't mean to say that it's impossible to get a good project from a first timer. Many firms thrive on innovation and bring fresh ideas to the process. But after hundreds of projects, we still learn something on each new project. You might not want to be the first trial in somebody's trial-and-error education.

Next, check references. Besides the list of happy clients they will give you ask for the names of the last five completed clients, regardless of project size or type. These will provide a more accurate sampling of the firm's work. Key questions to ask the references: Was the schedule maintained? Did you move in within two weeks of the original estimated completion date? Did the firm stick to the price? All jobs will have a few change orders. If the cost grew by more than 2 percent of the original quote it could indicate a management problem. How were communications? Were you kept in the loop or did you have to chase them for answers? How did the project closeout go? Was the punch-list (the list of items remaining at occupancy) lengthy? How long did it take them to complete it? Have there been any warranty calls (things to be fixed under the standard general contractor's one-year warranty)? Were they responsive, were problems corrected quickly?

This research should result in a short list of candidates. The next step is to check the financial condition of each firm. Ask to see their balance sheet. Have your accountant review it and offer an opinion. Check with the local or state licensing agency for any claims that may have been filed. You are not necessarily looking for a spotless record as much as a history of problem resolution. All firms will, sooner or later, have a rough time on a job. The key is their ability to see it through.

Reviewing all of this should narrow your list to just a few. If you are going the traditional route and are looking for a general contractor, you now have prequalified your bidders list. If you are selecting a construction manager or design-builder, you have one more step to go. This one is subjective. Since all the firms left on your list are capable of doing a good job it comes down to instincts, your gut feel. Probably, as you were researching, there was one you just liked better, maybe for no reason you can quantify. It could be better chemistry with their people, a natural personal connection. You will be working closely with this group for more than a year and, all other things being equal, it helps if you like the people you work with.

Understanding Bids and Proposals

There is a truism lawyers like to use: If it's not in writing, it was never said. That is certainly true when it comes to construction bids and proposals. All the verbal promises and explanations don't mean anything if it's not put in writing. Learning to read and understand bids is a must if you are going to build. You can tell a lot about a company by reading their proposal. If you have done your prequalification properly, all your bids should be well thought out, concise, and thorough. They will describe the project in detail, identify what is included and, just as importantly, what's excluded.

The low bidder either missed something, has a lot of exclusions in his proposal, or is lowballing you. The bids in the middle represent the real cost of your building. You want to focus on those proposals. Take the time to read them. Your job now is to compare the price with what's in their scope. Compare their lists of exclusions. If everyone excludes the same things (such as permit fees, material testing services, or installing that koi pond you thought was such a cool idea) then you can compare the bid prices directly. If a bidder has an exclusion no one else has don't be shy about calling about it. Find out why, and get a value from them to put it back in.

Once you've compared the proposals you can now make your choice. You are safe picking the best price from this group. One last comment on exclusions: They come in two types, those things the contractor thinks are *probably* not required, and those that the contractor feels he or she can't do a good job on. If the contractor has never built a clinic before, he or she might be unsure about specialty items like O_2 systems, anesthesia and evacuation systems, and so on. Remember, the cost of this second group of exclusions will come out of your contingency fund, so make sure it's covered.

Summary

Reading all of this might give you an uneasy feeling in the pit of your stomach—there's so much to do, so much to know—and we've only scratched the surface. What your stomach is saying is you need a qualified team to make this project a reality. Unless you can dedicate twenty to thirty hours per week to this process, and you have a very high stress tolerance, you should not attempt to go solo. Know, going in, that you will have to be involved and, depending on which method you use, involved frequently. If you define your role early, and keep on top of the decisions you need to make, it is manageable. If there is one thing you take from this chapter, please remember this: You should pick the method and the team members you are comfortable with. Pick a level of involvement that allows the rest of your life to go on, pick professionals you have confidence in and trust, pick builders who know what they are doing. It might not be the cheapest way, but in the end you'll have a building and still have a practice, a marriage, and a life.

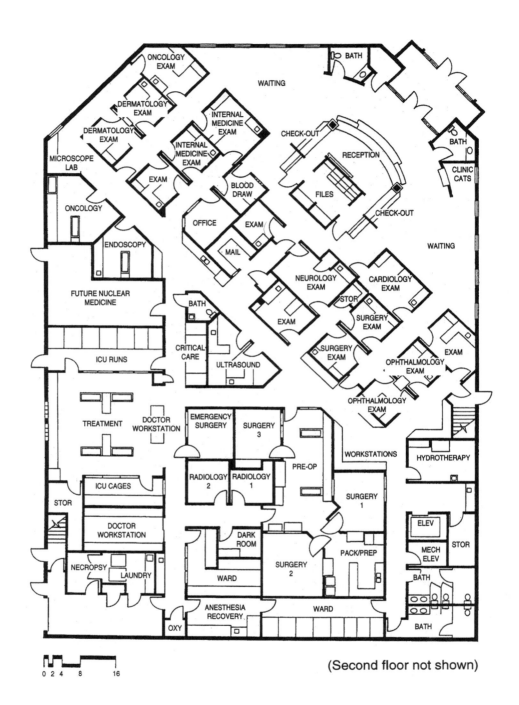

(Second floor not shown)

0 2 4 8 16

6

Public Affairs

PUBLIC AFFAIRS, OR veterinary practice design communications, is assuming important new roles in competitive veterinary healthcare delivery within a community. No longer the mere conveyor of publicity messages (e.g., public relations), the public relations mission is involved with the practice manager/hospital administrator developing a new community image during construction. By becoming the client's advocate and weighing the impact of new programs on the animals of the community, the public relations mission has become an important part of the veterinary healthcare delivery image, particularly in the vital areas of facility design and program delivery.

The new concept of veterinary facility design communications goes beyond communications with the conventional audiences within the practice—doctors, staff, administrative employees—and addresses the power structure in the area: It reaches out into the community and informs the potential clients as well as existing clients. The advantages and services of a new veterinary facility in the community should be presented to everyone who lives in the area. People should know how to get help before a condition becomes acute, how to get to the new facility, what services will be available, how to request urgent care assistance, and so on. A sound, concerned practice communications program will educate all the people in the community though various media, including newspaper, radio, television, and maybe even a practice-based speaker's bureau. New veterinary construction offers unique opportunities for the practice team involved to achieve excellent public and community relations. The practice manager/hospital administrator must be sensitive to, and knowledgeable about, the events that afford exceptional vehicles for communicating the philosophy, goals, and services of the center.

Communications: Internal

Internal communications have several audiences: the board in larger facilities, doctors and staff, paraprofessionals and animal caretakers, volunteers, contract employees, clients, and relief doctors (locums). Public information communicators should use all available practice healthcare literature as information media. News stories and features should be included in

- practice newsletters
- client health alerts
- information kits
- doctors' and staff bulletins
- special events brochures
- community meetings

Communications: External

External communications are aimed at the entire community and the wider public—legislators, government officials, opinion makers, social service and health organizations, and community groups. The media available for such communications include

- local newspapers
- wire services (Associated Press and United Press International)
- the local press
- local television stations
- local radio stations
- community magazines
- Chamber of Commerce and community bulletins
- health and social service organization newsletters
- pet stores and humane societies
- films, videotapes, closed-circuit television
- audiovisual slide presentations

A practice-specific speakers' bureau should be available for scheduled talks to luncheon and service clubs, the Chamber of Commerce, and community service, educational, and child care organizations. Other means of external communications include

- open-house tours
- press tours
- announcement of plans and programs
- booklets and newsletters
- anniversaries and birthdays
- volunteers
- school-to-work programs
- county and school publications

The following, in chronological order, are major building design events:

  - long-range plan and program development
  - zoning approval
  - announcement of architect's building plans
  - groundbreaking ceremonies
  - new staff personal profiles
  - openings and dedications

Additional opportunities present themselves at various stages of building and in expansion programs. It is at these important occasions in the life of a veterinary practice that the practice manager/hospital administrator should consult the design team and a local PR firm. In the public relations role, communications are considerably more complex than just planning a healthcare delivery program for animals in the community. To maximize the public relations potential of key events, there must be an integrated message being conveyed. The practice manager/hospital administrator must also be concerned about over-promising and underdelivering and become involved with many internal and external elements, including the staff and the community.

Red Hill Animal Medical Center

Demographically, the mountain valley could not support another veterinarian; the little one-doctor practices had proliferated in old houses and storefronts so there was far less than 4,000 population per FTE veterinarian in the valley.

Dr. Judi decided she wanted a practice in the valley, but had never practiced there. She looked around, and there were *no* substantial or quality-presenting facilities in the valley. She decided they needed an upscale 8,400-sq.-ft. hospital and boarding facility, so she committed to building one. Zoning was a nightmare, and even the other veterinary practices testified against her.

Once approved, she took her dogs to the center of the lot early on the ground-breaking morning and buried a couple of their favorite treats. Then at noon, when the press and community VIPs arrived for the groundbreaking, she came out with her dogs and told the audience as a progressive veterinary practice, she really wanted her patients to select where to break ground. As the dogs dug for their treats, the cameras snapped, and full-page pictures appeared in the community newspaper.

The boarding facility included a special area and access for the county impoundment needs, an inside exercise yard (snow gets deep in the mountains), and a two-story waterfall from stock tanks. She bought and publicized the first laser surgery in her half of the state, hired both an exotic doctor and an acupuncture doctor, and achieved triple certification by AAHA soon after opening. Without any previous valley practice time and an overpopulated veterinarian demographic, the gaining of 1,000 new clients in the first ninety days of operation was noteworthy. By her thirteenth month of operation, the new facility was doing $80,000 a month gross. Her practice was operating cleanly in the black by the twenty-third month of operation, and the money market account was growing.

She did it with public relations and self-belief, not demographic numbers!

Knowledgeable practice managers/hospital administrators and health design communicators should be familiar with the public relations program and goals of the American Veterinary Medical Association, American Animal Hospital Association, their state VMA, and even the county/regional VMA, all of which put the practice into the limelight as a key coordinator in providing veterinary healthcare delivery to the target animals of the practice. The educational roles of the practice team are further defined and encouraged; the public relations function is changed and becomes a planning and educational aid to the practice image in the community. In addition to defining the jobs of communicating to particular audiences and groups within and outside the practice's sphere of influence, public relations must ask such questions as, "How will we get cooperation and approval of the community, top opinion leaders, humane groups, and the Press?"

New Building Announcements

When announcing new construction or expansion plans, it is important to contact the architect. The architect is the person most able to articulate and interpret the structure. He should provide a reproducible photo of the rendering of the building. (When possible, a photo of a model of the structure can be very effective). A visit to the news editors and television and radio news directors can be most rewarding. The resulting scrapbook of press clippings can be valuable to the practice and staff memories. The veterinary practice manager/hospital administrator should delegate the outreach responsibility to an experienced public relations practitioner for best results.

Groundbreaking Ceremonies

Groundbreaking is almost a magic word—it means you have finally made it! It is the real beginning (see the Red Hill Animal Medical Center story in the preceding box). After the presentations, proposals, conferences, and approvals, groundbreaking calls for an appropriate community celebration. It is an ideal time to educate and communicate to the population about the practice's excitement. Everything should be geared to making the groundbreaking ceremony a successful event, one that has a positive impact on the community and its leaders as well as on the practice team and potential future staff residing in the community.

When planning groundbreaking ceremonies, one should

- *Create a theme:* Express the meaning of the new veterinary facility in terms of the animals of the community and elevate the awareness of the community about the veterinary services that can now be contributed to community resources.
- *Select the date:* Make it a convenient one for guests, the community, and the press.
- *Invite key speakers:* Choose community leaders who have something important to say and who can say it interestingly.

There are many details in setting up groundbreaking ceremonies, all of them important. One has to consider and evaluate the place, atmosphere, placement of speaker tables, audience, microphone, and podium. Arrangements have to be made for simple refreshments and for music, if desired. If the speeches are to be taped, preparations must be made in advance. If the weather is inclement, ceremonies will have to held indoors; guests can gather at the site afterward for digging and/or bulldozer (dog-dozer) ceremonies and photos. It is a good idea for the practice to have its own professional photographer, not only to document the event but to have immediate photos for press coverage.

Imagination is needed in invitation design and in the making up of the invitation list in order to reach the leaders in the community and the VIP guests. To accomplish this, the program brochure should be attractive. Also useful is an exhibit of plans, renderings, models, photographs, speakers, and unique and routine services of the new practice facility; all have to be planned well in advance. The guest list takes time to select, call, and refine. An established practice manager/hospital administrator should already have the community contacts to select key guests and speakers and to coordinate details. This person's follow-through work is vital in assuring that all the important people are invited and in making numerous day-before telephone calls reminding VIP guests, officials, and press to be present.

The Opening or Dedication

Openings and dedications of new veterinary facilities require the same intensive use of communications as do groundbreaking ceremonies, but they take place in the new building. New elements enter the picture and the logistics change. The following are important in creating a dedication program:

- a preview press tour (at which time a press kit should be distributed)
- a more elaborate program of ceremonies
- an open house for in-house staff first (doctors, nurses, paraprofessionals, animal caretakers, other employees, and their families) before the opening/dedication, followed by the community open house (opinion leaders, community officials, press, and a broad spectrum of community groups) after the opening/dedication
- television news coverage, if possible, and taping of the speeches for broadcast by a local radio station
- a more comprehensive speaker program, featuring leaders in the community or in the field of veterinary healthcare delivery, especially if the practice is offering a *new* service not previously offered in the community. The mayor, any senators or congressmen from the area, the county VMA president, the state VMA president, or even the practice owner is needed
- an attractively designed brochure (including the meaning of the new building or addition, its relation to existing programs, photographs, renderings, and the practice's community message; a page should be set aside for the architect's interpretation of the veterinary healthcare delivery design features)

The dedication program might proceed as follows:

– welcome
– invocation
– recognitions
– dedication remarks (maybe even a not-for-profit (e.g., IRS 501.c.3) fund for subsidized pet population control or emergency trauma cases)
– introduction of honored guests
– introduction of speakers
– principal speaker
– music
– tour of the facility (with large stuffed animals in surgery, X-ray, wards, etc.)
– refreshments at multiple locations throughout hospital

The techniques for making up a VIP guest list are similar to those used for the groundbreaking ceremonies. A public relations coordinator from the community can help make the event a greater success. Friendly telephone calls are needed to remind important guests and members of the press corps to attend.

Insights and Perspectives

Things to Consider After You Think You're Done— PR Issues Lurking in the Weeds to Bite You
Mark R. Hafen, AIA, NCARB

For all of us there has been a dramatic increase in governmental regulations and requirements that directly affect our professional lives. Conforming to these regulations and complying with the accompanying reviews has turned into a tremendous financial obligation for owners as they construct a building. The increase in the actual size and complexity of the building, along with the design fees incurred in designing and coordinating these regulations, all contribute to increased cost.

The best way to minimize the impact of these regulations on your project is to do your homework early and ask as many questions as possible before the start of the construction process. It is far less costly to anticipate and respond ahead of time than to scramble to fix problems after the fact.

Site Capacity

Your primary concern is whether or not your proposed building will fit on the site you have selected. To determine this, a simple site coverage formula can be used. Typically, a building will cover approximately 20–25 percent of your site. For example, if your building is 6,000 sq. ft., your site should be approximately 24,000–30,000 sq. ft.

If you consider that only 25 percent of your site is taken up by the actual structure, it is only natural to question what happens with the remainder of the space. Setbacks, landscaping, and parking account for this difference, with room for possible expansion.

Planning and Zoning

Virtually without exception, governing bodies in the country impose planning or zoning laws and ordinances that control

- how a site can be used
- the distance from the property line that a structure must sit
- the number of parking spaces required
- in some instances, what the structure must resemble
- the square footage maximum that can be on the site
- building height

Since planning and zoning ordinances can also specify how a site is titled and platted, it is critical to know prior to purchase what the planning or zoning requirements are. It is possible to apply for and receive a variance from specific zoning requirements. However, the primary goal is to buy a parcel where a veterinary hospital is a "use by right" and where the building you anticipate constructing will conform to the setback, parking, height, and area requirements. The application for a variance can be a time-consuming and costly process with no guarantee of success. In addition, there may be regulations that dictate landscaping, site access, availability of utilities, facility appearance, or funding of street or utility improvements.

The time involved in this application process has dramatically increased. Since time equals money, it is critical to research the regulations that may impact your site before you buy it.

Encumbrances and Easements and Zoning

Finding property that is not encumbered by easements, encroachments, deed restrictions, covenants, or "clouded" titles is becoming increasingly difficult due to the scarcity of land and increased governmental regulations. Always do your homework prior to purchasing any ground. Do not rely solely on the word of the existing owner or real estate agent. Check with the utility companies to determine if their services are available and if there are any easements against the property. Prior to the purchase of the ground, initiate a title search to determine if there are any other untold legal encumbrances on the property.

Topography and Soils

Often overlooked during the initial site selection process is the impact of topography and soils. A steep, sloping site can cause the driveways and sidewalks to be too vertical for handicap access, make it difficult to keep the site drainage away from the building, and increase the foundation costs.

Another dramatic impact on site development and building costs is soil geology. By commissioning a topographic survey and a soil report prior to the purchase of your site, you can avoid such concerns as needing to blast out bedrock or remove expansive clay, needing to remove and replace excessive fill dirt before you can build, or discovering high water tables or an excess of organic or peat material.

Environmental, Wetlands, and Storm Drainage Requirements

Environmental impact is without a doubt one of the fastest-growing areas of governmental regulations. It can include

- wetlands protection
- protection of watersheds, waterways, and aquifers, including storm drainage runoff
- protection of historic or natural vegetation, including heritage trees
- protection of wildlife
- mitigation of potential wildfire danger
- stabilization of slopes

There are stringent federal regulations regarding the protection of wetlands and wildlife. However, the majority of these regulations are local. Where there is a community commitment regarding the environment, the review and permitting process can be expensive and time consuming. Proving conformance can sometimes be difficult. Considering that environmental protection is a priority for today's society, it is imperative to have a basic assurance that the site you are considering does not have any hidden environmental concerns. This can be accomplished by commissioning an environmental assessment for the site. For the most part, a Level One Environmental Assessment can identify environmental conditions that may adversely impact the development of your site. There can be serious ramifications if you purchase a site that contains even a threshold level of environmental pollutants.

Other Constraints

In addition to the previously mentioned requirements, there can be other issues to take into consideration. Urban renewal, coastal commissions, and historic districts can also have an impact on your site location. Local and federal governmental agencies have earmarked certain areas for special consideration and additional regulation across the country. Thoroughly investigate any site you are considering to identify possible regulatory constraints.

Occupational Safety and Health Administration

In spite of the fact that OSHA inspectors have been known to drop in and close a facility, their regulations are not a significant part of the design, application, and permitting process. For the most part, OSHA deals with how a facility is used or how a facility is constructed, not how a facility is designed.

The design impact of OSHA requirements can be confined to

- eye wash stations
- proper shielding for X-ray and other imaging equipment
- ergonomically correct workstations, such as keyboards and computer monitors
- minimizing noise pollution
- controlling or eliminating hazardous air quality situations
- controlling access to hazardous materials

When a building is constructed, there is no formal OSHA review process.

Americans with Disabilities Act

The ADA, originally passed by Congress in 1992 as a civil law, has two purposes: to protect disabled employees from being discriminated against because a facility might not be accessible to them and to assure that the disabled public has reasonable and immediate access and use of public buildings. Most people are familiar with the "public" component of the act. However, the "employee" component often has the greater impact, because this means that an entire facility will most likely need to be accessible.

Virtually every municipality in the country has adopted and/or incorporated the essential requirements of this law as part of the building code review and application process. Unfortunately, different interpretations of what constitutes "accessible" and "reasonable" accommodations for the disabled can vary the requirements greatly from place to place. It is important to contact your local building department directly to learn what level of compliance will be required.

Life Safety and Building Codes

A building permit will be required for the construction of your facility in all but the most rural areas. The entity reviewing the drawings will, in most cases, be your local governmental agency. Design and construction requirements can vary from place to place. Keep in mind that most building codes look at life safety and health issues, including structural soundness, earthquake and hurricane resistance, exiting in case of emergency or fire, containment of fire, eliminating hazardous conditions, and providing necessary light, air supply, and exhaust.

Hazardous Wastes

Hazardous waste pollution and disposal that includes asbestos, hydrocarbon, heavy metal, and industrial wastes remains the area with the greatest potential for liability and cost. Dense urban development and heavy industry can often be indicators that a high number of sites are contaminated by hazardous wastes.

Many municipalities regulate the disposal of hazardous wastes from facilities such as veterinary hospitals. The disposal of silver (as a byproduct of X-ray film development) and radioactive isotopes (as a byproduct of radiation therapy) are just two examples. Some municipalities may want to know how much and what kind of biological waste your facility will be producing.

Health Department

Occasionally specific state health departments are required to review and approve facilities that are built to hold animals, whether it is for boarding or animal care. These inspections are rather cursory and usually occur after the facility is built.

State or local health departments also often require that the installation of X-ray equipment be inspected and that X-ray shielding be in place. These requirements have actually decreased in recent years due to the fact that more modern X-ray equipment has less "scatter" than the older equipment.

Conclusion

The regulations facing you as you begin to build or remodel a facility are many and varied. Some of them seem to be based on common sense, others don't. Regardless of how you view them, they all translate into increased time and cost as your hospital is being designed and built.

Things to Consider Review Issues

- The best way to minimize the impact of government regulations and requirements on your project is to do your homework early and ask as many questions as possible before the start of the construction process.
- When putting a building on your site, remember that a building will cover approximately 20 to 25 percent of the site, with the remainder being used for setbacks, landscaping, parking, and future expansion.
- Since planning and zoning ordinances can specify how a site is titled and platted, it is critical to know prior to purchase what the planning or zoning requirements are. It is also wise to comply with zoning, setback, parking, height, and area requirements from the outset rather than applying for a variance, which can be a time-consuming and costly process with no guarantee of success.
- When purchasing ground, do not rely solely on the word of the existing owner or real estate agent regarding such issues as easements, encroachments, deed restrictions, covenants, utility services, and legal encumbrances.
- During the initial site selection process, commission a topographic survey and a soil report to avoid any problems that could arise due to a steep or sloping site or problematic soil geology. It is also important to investigate protection issues of wetlands, watersheds and aquifers, historic or natural vegetation, and wildlife.
- A Level One Environmental Assessment can identify environmental conditions that may adversely impact the development of your site.
- Even though OSHA regulations are not a significant part of the design, application, and review process, their requirements make sense and should be incorporated into your design.
- The Americans with Disabilities Act has different interpretations from place to place of what constitutes "accessible" and "reasonable" accommodations for the disabled. It is important to contact your local building department directly to learn what level of compliance might be required in your building design.
- When applying for a building permit, keep in mind that building codes will look at life safety and health issues.
- Many municipalities regulate the disposal of such hazardous wastes as silver and radioactive isotopes from facilities such as veterinary hospitals.
- Occasionally specific state health departments review and approve facilities that are built to hold animals and inspect installation of X-ray equipment.

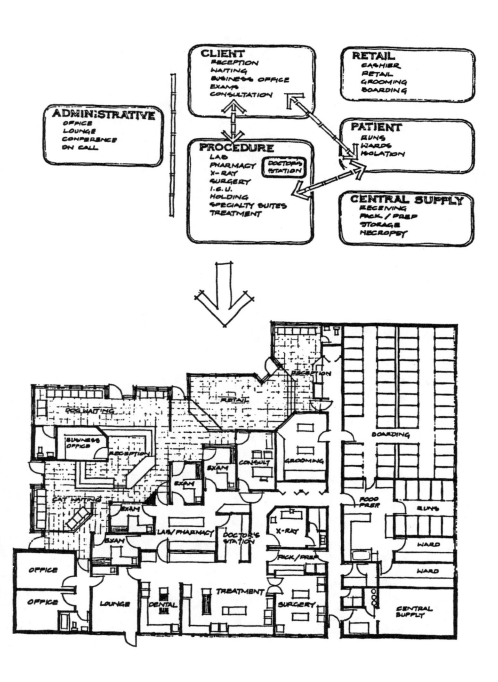

7

The Building of the Practice Team and Other Mega-Ideas

IN MOST EVERY SPECIALTY practice group or emergency practice, the traditional chain of command does not work. In chapter 1 of *Building the Successful Veterinary Practice: Volume 3: Innovation and Creativity,* we used a specialty practice scenario to illustrate the evolving perspectives of veterinary practice, including the new structures. In a specialty practice with many separate groups, or an emergency practice, usually with shareholders, the understanding of governance is essential (the entire chapter 2 of *Veterinary Management in Transition: Preparing for the Twenty-First Century*). In fact, *Building the Successful Veterinary Practice: Volume 3* shares the concept of hiring teams and finding the right people, while the text *Veterinary Management in Transition: Preparing for the Twenty-First Century* addresses the governance board, the administrator, and the methods used to ensure an effective fit and utilization of staff, so we will not repeat it here.

In this chapter, we want to look at the leadership structure. The legal options are discussed in *Beyond the Successful Veterinary Practice: Succession Planning and Other Legal Issues,* so the corporate structuring has already been covered. In short, a limited liability company (LLC) does not offer the tax advantages of a Sub-S, and a Sub-S does not afford the same investment potentials of a C-Corp. With the changing legal environment, a good corporate attorney who understands professional corporations is needed to guide the board through the choices based on economic plans of the shareholders and/or specialty practices. Ensure that everyone understands that while landlord shares are established by investment dollars, operational representation is based on participation within the board's core values and vision.

Regardless of the legal structure, and regardless of the organizational structure, the two critical elements must be *management* and *leadership*:

• Managers get work done through people and do things right.
• Leaders develop people through work and do the right things.

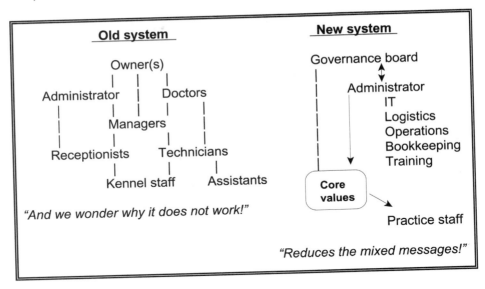

The text *Building the Successful Veterinary Practice: Volume 1: Leadership Tools* discusses the theory and structure of building a positive leadership environment and even shares fourteen basic leadership skills and meeting management concepts in the appendices. Let's apply those concepts to the practice team needed as the first-year income allows the hiring of staff.

Building the Practice Team

The vision and dream of a critical-care facility can only go so far; after that, the staff must believe in the core values of quality healthcare delivery, including

- no pain
- no puking
- help the clients feed their pets
- diagnostic medicine
- continual delivery and self-improvement

Think about a leader you respect, one who can get the job done and one everyone enjoys working with. What did the leader do that worked?

- Listened.
- Praised.
- Asked what others thought.
- Kept things moving.
- Made it fun.
- Facilitated discussion.
- Helped others draw conclusions.
- Provided clear direction.
- Worked in the background.

We like to say

- managers do things right, but leaders do the right things . . .
- managers get work done through people, while leaders develop people through work
- managers take credit and give blame, while leaders give credit and take blame
- moms are leaders and know that behavior rewarded is behavior repeated

Define an Effective Leader

With all this mind-set said, now please think about that leader you respect, the one who could get the job done and whom everyone enjoyed working with. What were the core leadership skills that were used, and what behaviors did you see?

Most are thinking of task behaviors. Task behaviors are what most veterinarians and many certified veterinary technicians have learned; they are the science of medicine and focus on getting the job done right, within the time and cost allocation and ensuring the expected outcome result. They include getting started, setting goals, and clearly defining expected task outcomes.

Here are some suggested procedures that initiate action:

- Seek the opinions of the group, but do not allow people to be made to feel "wrong" in their suggestions.
- Get the staff talking about what works.
- Leaders can give opinions as needed to help the group move forward but should not define the process.
- Clarify and elaborate the key issues and resources available.
- Clear up confusion by summarizing comments and validating the core values of the practice.
- Help others build on ideas to select potential alternatives.
- Allow discussion of issues affecting the various alternatives.
- Help the group envision how each alternative would work.
- Summarize frequently by putting various ideas together and then restating the multiple ideas in an outcome concept.
- Coordinate the flow of ideas or information to a Plan A and a Plan B, and maybe even a Plan C, D, or E.
- Help others set a clear course of action within each plan.
- Ensure the group develops the plans on how to measure success.
- Get the group's agreement on the time-line and outcome(s).
- Ensure the group makes specific accountability assignments.
- At implementation, ensure progress evaluations stay positive and outcome oriented.

Remember: Task behaviors, which provide direction, focus on what is needed to get the job done. An effective leader helps the group find solutions, make outcome-based decisions, and complete the work. Now that we have a plan and we are taking action, how do we keep it moving forward?

Maintenance Behaviors

What types of challenges could a practice encounter while developing and operating a new facility or a new healthcare delivery service? How do we get the whole team to deal with these problems, or better, what can we do to keep the challenges from becoming problems? We call these maintenance behaviors—those traits and actions that provide team support, help others focus on how well team members work together, and ensure the group stays together.

Here are some maintenance behaviors:

- Build accord while drawing out differing viewpoints.
- Work out disagreements by keeping the group harmony in focus.
- Admit errors and be willing to change bias, habits, and paradigms.
- Mediate conflicts and seek compromises and consensuses.
- Encourage participation by being responsive, friendly, and respectful.
- Acknowledge and praise.
- Be open to ideas of others and integrate at least 60 percent of the ideas received.
- Ease tensions and create an enjoyable atmosphere.
- Look for fun approaches to task that keep the group together.
- Take breaks when needed.
- Be an advocate; encourage the less talkative, control the more talkative.
- Look for ways to keep everyone involved.
- Look for the teachable moment of interest with each person.
- Diagnosing and facilitating:
  observe how the team is working together
  facilitate the group in examining its effectiveness
  actively listen; paraphrase and reflect feelings
  suspend judgment
  Respond nonverbally to what's said

Maintenance behaviors ensure good working relationships and maintain the vitality of the team; they keep the group together and wanting to continue. So now that you've got the skills, how do you make it click after hours or in your specialty practice?

Hint: Remember, in the group development cycle, with every new task, and with every new team member, the group cycle returns to "forming," and the leader who uses the early leadership skills (directive, persuasion, coaching) can accelerate the group through the "storming" phase, but it can *never* be totally avoided.

Hint: Once a function is delegated, a skilled leader will *never* take it back but instead will act as a mentor/consultant to bring more resources to bear on the needs of the group.

Hint: The high autonomy (low direction) that comes with performing is not without limits; a good leader establishes operation limitations/parameters for the group, concurrent with identifying clear outcome expectations, with measurements of success.

Situational Leadership

(Placed on group development flow.)

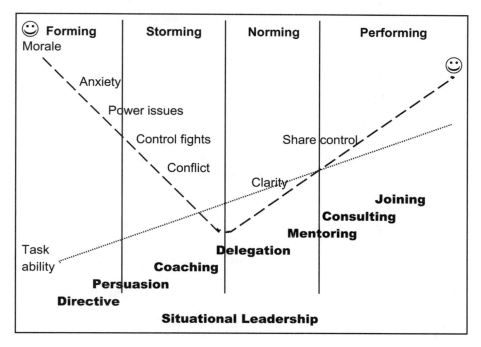

High direction . . . . Low direction
Low support . . . . High support . . . . High autonomy

The Leadership Style Sequence

Forming stages . . . . Performing stages
High direction . . . . Low direction
Low support . . . . High support . . . . High autonomy

        Directing ➡

           Persuading ➡

              Coaching ➡

                Delegating ➡

                      Mentoring ➡

                          Consulting ➡

                              Joining ➡ *

* Remember, when a new task or new person is added to the group, the group development cycle starts over. While the leadership and training plan can accelerate the process through "forming" and "storming," these phases cannot be skipped.

Observing and Timing

As you look at your team's stage of development and identify your team's needs for continued growth, you can use the team skills to provide the needed direction and support. The key is observation; observe the group and individuals.

- Keep in mind where the group is in the development stages.
  Orientation then forming.
  Dissatisfaction then storming.
  Resolution then norming.
  Production then performing.
- Look for the leadership skills that will facilitate each member through each phase and move him or her to the next phase (don't push it).
- Watch for individual needs and opportunities to meet those needs.
- Learn when to talk and when to let others talk.
  A poorly timed joke is not funny.
  Let the group and individuals experience the pain of learning without the suffering.
  Success is when they think they thought of it; leaders just need to plant the seeds.
- Be careful of things that gain you personal recognition and attention.

Pay attention to the task and maintenance behaviors that are occurring and to the absence of those behaviors. Use the leadership skills that the group needs at that point in time.

- Draw from what you have seen work, imitate those whom you respect as leaders.
- Focus on the task, set goals, get everyone involved, clarify points, get consensus, and assign tasks.
- Maintain the team and the individuals, build accord, encourage and praise individuals and the group, have fun, facilitate self-evaluation, and actively listen.
- Observe the group grow and think before you speak—timing is a key to success.
- Practice; you can't steer a parked car!
- Task behaviors:
  Initiating: Propose goals, tasks, and new definitions to problems. Suggest procedures for new ideas that initiate action within your team.
  Information/opinion seeking: Ask for relevant information, clarification, suggestions, or opinions from other team members to help the discussion.
  Information/opinion giving: Offer relevant facts, information, experiences, suggestions, or opinions to the team.
  Clarifying and elaborating: Clear up confusion. Interpret comments. Develop suggestions and build on ideas. Define terms. Envision how something might work.

Summarizing: Put various ideas and contributions together from relevant information. Restate content and ideas clearly and concisely.

Coordinating: Manage and sequence the flow of ideas or information. Pull together various ideas and activities toward a clear course of action. Develop plans on how to proceed, and keep team members focused on the task according to the team's agreements. Ensure that the team is satisfied with its procedure. Suggest new procedures when necessary.

- Maintenance behaviors:

Building accord: Elicit differing viewpoints. Explore and work out disagreements. Admit errors. Find common ground or communicate willingness to modify your own position. Work to resolve or mediate conflict among team members.

Encouraging: Acknowledge; praise others and their contributions. Encourage participation by being responsive, friendly, and respectful of others. Demonstrate acceptance and openness to others' ideas.

Reducing tension: Ease tension and help create an enjoyable atmosphere in which the team can stay focused on its tasks. Suggest fun approaches to tasks. Remind the team to take breaks when needed.

Gatekeeping: Increase participation and communication by encouraging less talkative members to contribute or by directly soliciting their opinions. Control airtime of more talkative members. Suggest procedures that encourage full participation and expression of ideas.

Diagnosing and facilitating: Observe the internal team processes (how team members are working together), and point out these processes to help the team examine its effectiveness. Express your own feelings, and ask others how they feel.

Active Listening: Suspend judgment to fully understand the ideas of others. Ensure understanding by paraphrasing and reflecting feelings. Respond nonverbally to what is being said.

When to Use Team Skills

All of the individual behaviors are constructive when used to help your team function more effectively. However, the same behaviors can hinder the team if used to gain personal recognition and attention. For example, telling a joke can be a maintenance behavior that breaks tension or helps team members enjoy their work. At another time, it could distract the team from its task.

Take a look at your team's stage of development and identify your team's needs for continued growth. Use the team skills to provide the needed direction and support. The key is observation. Pay attention to the task and maintenance behaviors that are occurring and to the absence of those behaviors that would help meet the team's needs at that point in time. The key is to be observant of the team's dynamics, to be aware of the team's needs and then be able to provide the leadership behavior needed for team functioning. Remember, in chapter 5 of *Building the Successful Veterinary Practice: Volume 3:*

Innovation and Creativity, we showed that task learning and change forces a group through four operational stages:

Clueless and comfortable
↘
    Clued in and uncomfortable
    ↘
        Awkward but trying
        ↘
            Proud and accomplished

So a leader needs to accelerate the group through the development and operational stages, but that is easier said than done. Let's look at a few common questions.

Q - *What is the basic style of leadership used when doing the initial training?*
A - Orientation/directive/instructive—set the performance standards and limits. Common understanding of purpose and ground rules of operation. We want an agreement, individually and by the group, on the roles, goals, standards, and behavior expectations . . . and an agreement on the decision-making authority and accountability.

Q - *What are the needs of the individuals in the group during this earliest stage?*
A - Agreement on boundaries—safe haven, what are the available resources, and who is accountable for what; knowledge/trust in each other to utilize the diverse talents and skills; and build personal connections

Q - *Think of the next stage, the clued-in and uncomfortable; think of T-ball— what is the principle?*
A - They are dissatisfied, they need to be persuaded, clarification of the big picture is needed; in T-ball, just getting them to swing at a ball without worrying about it flying at them is a significant step forward. Recommitment to values and norms, start to develop the team accountability for outcomes, improve the feedback communication process.

Q - *What are the needs of the individuals in the group during this storming stage?*
A - Value the differences in others; encouragement and reassurance; recognition of accomplishments; open and honest discussion of personality conflicts, coalitions, and other emotional blocks. Persuasion starts during this stage's onset, and it becomes coaching as we move them out of it . . . now we can tell them to swing flatter, or aim their hits, *after* they have tried to swing and succeeded.

Q - *As an individual and group leaves the dissatisfaction/storming phase, and enters the integration/norming stage, what is happening to the directive styles?*

A - The "directive styles" are reducing, the leader is becoming more support-ive; individuals are integrating into teams, skills are enhanced, problem solving becomes important . . . resolution is shifting to delegation of out-come accountabilities.

Q - *What are the group needs at this time?*
A - A focus on increased productivity (scoreboard), self-evaluation from each experience, shared responsibilities, mentoring, recognition, and celebration of successes.

Q - *When the group starts to exceed expectations, we call that producing; what are the group's needs now?*
A - The leader's validation is essential, as it reinforces the high standards and expectations; new challenges and learning must be forthcoming . . . to exceed expectations is to have *pride*—and others see pride as quality! Vali-dation includes decision-making autonomy within established boundaries, individual acknowledgment, recognition, and celebration of team accom-plishments.

Summary

Directing ➡ Persuading/coaching ➡ Supporting ➡ Delegating ➡ Mentoring/joining

Tom Cat's Tips

In the previous chapters, I discussed a practice planning team, the role of the project manager, and even how the practice manager/hospital administrator has a major role in new facility planning. This is the *new* American veterinary practice model, and it continues to build with zone accountability being held by working staff coordinators (accountability to ensure training to trust and competency are perceived within the practice leadership).

Some ask, Why a leadership chapter in a preconstruction design book? The answer is simple: I have seen too many veterinarians who believe they can be project managers as well as clinicians, and they watch their existing practice dry up and die because they were too cheap to hire a project manager. Then there is the other version, the veterinarian who expects his or her spouse to be an expert in everything about veterinary medicine just because he or she married a control freak veterinarian; the veterinarian gives all his or her personal "overflow" to the spouse, then blames him or her when things start to unravel.

We have about one in four veterinarians into some form of substance abuse, and about 50 percent of the marriages ending in divorce; the old curmudgeons in veterinary medicine usually took the practice on as a mistress and stole time from their families until the family ties were shattered beyond repair. We need to become leaders of team, not managers of people. A building project is the ulti-mate stress, and any veterinarian who has read the previous chapters and wants

(continued)

the construction stress, instead of hiring it done, should not only have his or her head examined, he or she should hire someone to show how many hours will be lost from clinical production during the project. At just $200 per hour outpatient and $300 per hour inpatient, two hours at the job site a day is a $500 loss of income, and over six months (~150 practice days), that is a $75,000 loss in income alone, not to mention the ulcer medicine, tranquilizers, and happy pills they will be taking to combat the effects of stress.

This important message is dedicated to Susie and other spouses who "tuck it up" and try to do it in spite of their personal needs"!

Insights and Perspectives
Business Planning Process for Veterinary Facility Development
Mark J. Schmidt, AIA

Introduction

Most of us agree that careful planning contributes to the success of any proposed project. Creating a standard process for business planning can help ensure that important factors are not forgotten along the way to creating successful building projects.

Animal medical services are generally offered in a business setting. Profitable financial transactions are essential for continuing to offer services. To have a successful veterinary practice, one must create profit by providing services at a cost that is less than the charges paid by the client. This is an obvious goal that all practices strive for and any that continue very long in business must achieve.

As architects, we create a process to analyze the development of changes within a practice and to identify and isolate the factors under our control that will have the most effect on the future success of the veterinary practice.

Architectural projects in the veterinary industry generally fall into two categories, each of which has particular needs. The first is expansion or change within a particular practice. This could involve reconstruction or addition to an existing veterinary facility or it could involve creation of an entirely new structure. The key point is that the client base remains constant. The second type of project is the creation of an entirely new practice. Although the veterinarian may bring some loyal clients from previous work, the majority of clients will have to be found within the local community. On occasion there may be some combination of the two project options, as in the case of an existing practice that creates a new satellite clinic with a proportion of clients from the original practice.

Architects have long provided feasibility analysis of projects. Most architects tend to specialize in particular project types. This is also true of the animal care industry in which there are numerous architectural firms specializing in veterinary, boarding, and shelter facilities. The advantage of such repeat business is that the firm can continue to expand its knowledge in the particulars of veterinary practice. Use of the specialists' skills and knowledge can prevent some typical problems and greatly increase the chances for success. The process that we have developed, and that is described in the following pages, helps our clients reach decisions that allow them to make the most of their assets in developing their hospital facilities. A team of expert consultants, such as architects, accountants, and management consultants, provides valuable counsel in achieving successful building projects.

The system Knapp Schmidt Architects (KSA) has assembled consists of three key components:

1. Demographic market analysis
2. Facility and site development cost analysis
3. Financial feasibility study

The following discussion details some of the goals we have in each of the three phases. If these issues are thoroughly analyzed, all team members can agree that the final business development plan presents the best solution for the client and business owner. Ideally, the team members who are involved in this business planning process are the owner(s) and his or her consultants, including accountant, architect, attorney, lender, sometimes the builder, and quite often family members. A consensus of all team members that the proposed development plan is the right one will get the project off to a confident start.

Step #1: Demographic Market Analysis

Demographic study is the analysis of the surrounding geographic area by studying the traits of the population within a given area. For our purposes we need to study the nearby population to quantify its likelihood to purchase animal care services. Although there are numerous sources of information, the simplest way to obtain data is to purchase it from national companies that collect data in many different areas.

The type of data that is pertinent for our purposes is the makeup of households in the market area of the animal care business under discussion. The obvious business is providing animal medical services, but other profit centers such as boarding, grooming, retail, and alternative therapies are an essential part of many practices. We want to know the local household composition. Is there an adequate number of households with children and likely to own pets? Are there households of older individuals who own fewer pets? We want to know the financial status of the community. Although families of modest means do spend significant portions of their income on veterinary services, there is no doubt that veterinary practices will experience different economic results in different communities. Other studies and analyses can be reviewed to obtain additional information on this subject.

The data companies will furnish data as you ask for it. We need to define the market that is being served. A judgment must be made about how far clients are likely to travel to use services from the subject business. There will be differences in market range among practices that are located in densely populated urban areas, small towns, and rural locations. Distance by miles has been used to define those areas. However, geographic formations like ocean bays, lakes, mesas, and mountains and man-made obstructions like shopping malls and highways, affect how easily clients can reach the practice. With the sophistication of computerized data, researchers can now use the drive time to reach a business as a basis for defining a market area. A six- to eight-minute drive time may be used in suburban areas. Drive time can be tested. Existing practices can analyze the zip codes of their existing client base to get a sense of the time spent reaching their facility.

Once the market area is defined, the data for that market is obtained. An analysis of household income and expenditures is done to determine the amount of spending that is expected for animal care, and particularly animal medical services.

The money spent to purchase veterinary care services will be shared among the veterinarians practicing in a particular market. Analysis and calculation must be performed to determine how much of the market is available on average for each veterinarian. Other practices near the proposed building site will offer stiffer competition than more distant ones. The calculation made by dividing the total veterinary spending in the defined market by the number of veterinarians working there can show what each practitioner can expect to earn. The results could predict that there is room for a number of additional veterinarians to work in the market before the earnings per doctor fall below acceptable standards. Areas with strong growth often show opportunities. The results could show that there are already so many practitioners that the current market is already saturated, with doctors only achieving average earnings. This occurs more often in stable or shrinking markets. Some practices move to the edge of a growth area, leaving other practices with a large market in stable older growth areas. Only a thorough analysis will allow the market to be quantified.

The knowledge about the percentage of a market available to a particular doctor should be used to make strategic business decisions. If there is a large market available, a decision could be made to seek veterinary partners or associates, to take advantage of market opportunity by creating a larger business. If the market is crowded, a business strategy might be to concentrate on particular services that are not offered by others or to seek acquisition of an existing practice rather than expanding or building a new practice.

Of course, two practices operating in the same market will not perform equally. Many factors such as staff competence, building location or image, and facility constraints affect the economic performance of the hospital.

Quantifying the market opportunity will not guarantee success, but it could provide the ability to avoid a critical mistake. By performing the same analysis on several potential locations, a judgment can be made as to which location might provide more opportunity.

The next section discusses the expenses that will be incurred in developing a new business. The largest factor is the construction of hospital space, and decisions made during building design will affect the facility function. Other facility issues, such as the business location, which will also have a great impact on the ability to capture the appropriate share of the market are discussed.

Some hospital owners will not be content to limit their earnings to the average share. Earnings goals may include attracting clients that otherwise go to other practices. The next step in the process is creating a specific business solution that will allow the business to succeed in the selected market.

Step #2: Facility and Site Development Cost Analysis

In the KSA office, the result of the facility and site development cost analysis is a written estimate of the costs involved in developing a particular project. The expense is divided into two categories, hard costs and soft costs. Hard costs are usually defined as the property purchase, the actual construction costs of both the building and the site development, and the furniture and medical equipment. This is the larger portion of development costs. Soft costs include financing costs; architectural, engineering, and legal fees; permit fees; and most other costs relating to the development of the project.

Many factors must be considered to arrive at a prediction of development costs. Following is a discussion of the major items related to building and site development.

Site Selection

Site selection is the first major decision. The two choices are selecting a new site or remaining on the site of an existing practice. The market analysis previously discussed is used to help make this decision. Existing practices can use the market information to judge whether the existing location is the best for the practice. New or relocated practices can use the market analysis to judge the value of various locations. However, even in the same market area will be building sites of differing quality. "Location, location, location" is true.

The market analysis views the veterinary practice as a retail service, so location on a major thoroughfare and visibility are important components in the success of the practice. Other factors, such as the cost of real estate and local zoning regulations, have a great impact on site selection. The goal is to choose the site that has the best public visibility that the owner can afford and that the local government will permit.

Typically the most visible site will cost more than a hidden site. However, the most visible site will usually provide the most business. Estimating the risk of spending a large sum on a high-quality site is part of the financial feasibility analysis. The risk in choosing a lower cost but less visible site should be part of the practice's marketing plan to address the problem of not having the building be seen by a large number of potential clients.

Zoning Ordinances

The legal ability to use a site for a particular use is paramount in determining the site's feasibility.

Zoning ordinances usually organize particular site uses in contiguous areas. Typical use categories or districts are residential, business or commercial, manufacturing or industrial, agricultural, and so on. These ordinances allow the community to have input into its overall development. Zoning ordinances are seen as beneficial because they can, for example, prevent noisy, smelly manufacturers from locating next to residential neighborhoods. Zoning can keep large volumes of traffic concentrated in commercial areas. As with most laws and regulations, people sometimes object to particular aspects of the rules. Unfortunately for animal care businesses, this use is often highly restricted in zoning ordinances, which are usually quite similar from one community to another. Historically, animal care businesses have had the reputation of being noisy and smelly. In recent years, the quality of these facilities has greatly improved, but it is likely to take years for zoning ordinances to respond to those changes. It is necessary to work within the current system.

As well as site use, zoning ordinances regulate aspects of site development such as the setback of buildings from property boundaries, the amount of parking required, the type and amount of landscaping, the height of buildings, and so forth. Planning departments usually conduct the process of development plan approvals. Zoning departments usually are part of the local building department. The building department enforces the zoning rules as well as any requirements placed by the planning department board.

Application to receive a building permit is normally a separate procedure from receiving planning department approval. However, before issuing a building permit, the building department will want plans that show compliance with zoning regulations and that are approved by the zoning and planning departments. The building inspector, who inspects buildings during construction, usually enforces zoning regulations. Zoning is part of the local legal system. In extreme cases enforcement involves the police and court system for resolution of noncompliance issues.

There are usually three categories of approval for use in a particular district:

1. *Permitted use:* The business is permitted within this district. With the appropriate construction plans, an owner can apply for and receive a building permit.
2. *Conditional use:* The business is permitted to operate in this district, but may have conditions placed upon its development or operation. These conditions are often based on the results of public hearings. A planning commission or board conducts these hearings. Each municipality has its own process of review, and there are various names for its committees or boards. Each municipality has its own standards of review that can include detailed information on site development or building design. In some jurisdictions or in certain districts, architectural review is part of the approval process. If a proposed project does not meet the zoning requirements, there is usually a process for appeal. The zoning board of appeals is likely to be part of a separate review process. If an owner can live with the conditions placed on the business, he or she can then apply for building permits.

3. *Not permitted:* The use is not allowed in the district. In most places this cannot be appealed. The usual remedy is to request to have the property rezoned. This would change the property district classification to one that would permit the proposed use. Often this is a difficult and lengthy process because planning boards make long-range plans for development and are reluctant to grant exceptions. Sometimes petitioning to change the zoning ordinance to allow a particular use is successful.

The plan approval process is political. In the United States we have local control of development, with some state and federal regulations of protected ecosystems. Not all units of local government have the same name, but most have similar structure. For the purpose of this chapter, we use the paradigm of village and city government. In some states, a "village" is called a "town." Regardless of the name, there are large municipalities, small municipalities, and rural areas. Often municipalities have extraterritorial zoning rights extending into neighboring rural areas.

Planning department staff members are hired to research and recommend approval or denial of projects that are submitted to the planning board or commission. The staff recommendation is based on the project's compliance with the zoning code. Final recommendations are made to the village board or city council by the planning board or commission. Typically the chairperson of the planning board is a member of the city council or village board, and members are political appointees. They try to carry out the wishes of the people.

If support is overwhelming for a particular project, it is likely to be approved, and solutions are found to create the legal means to carry it out. If there is overwhelming opposition, it is not likely that boards, commissions, or councils will go out of their way to approve a project. Any applicant who is serious about gaining approval will do his or her homework. The applicant should know ahead of time who is likely to show up at a public hearing and what their concerns are.

Planning a Building

Assuming that site use is approved, the physical conditions of a site must be evaluated to determine if the cost of site development is reasonable. If it is, planning the building can proceed.

Programming

The first work in the process of providing architectural services is called programming. First we tabulate the rooms needed and the area each would take. A total facility size is established. The size of the proposed building must be known in order to evaluate suitability of the chosen site.

Site Evaluation

Most owners will arrive at minimum area for the initial building project and may think that the business will grow and require future expansion. The market analysis should have helped bring those issues into focus. Some conceptual site planning may be necessary at this stage. Parking lots often occupy as much ground area as the building. Landscaping plus future expansion must be accounted for.

We recommend a site that is five to seven times the area of the first phase of the project, assuming the site is entirely usable. Many factors can limit the area of a site that is available for development. Underground utility lines and easements, flood plain areas, and unusual setback requirements can all affect a site's usability.

If the size of the site is adequate, the cost of development is the next issue to consider. Properties that have low purchase prices may have detrimental conditions that make development difficult. Some common problems are

- poor soil conditions that can't support a building foundation
- previous construction debris buried on site
- grade conditions that require fill to be brought in, or major excavation required to create a level building pad
- public utility services too far away to make connections at reasonable cost

The main goal at this phase of project planning is to determine the probable cost of proposed construction. Architects, construction managers, or contractors can prepare these costs. Not all projects are new construction. Evaluating existing structures is a regular architectural service. Architectural evaluation must be undertaken to make sure that reconstruction or renovation of an existing building is feasible. Considerations include structural conditions, mechanical systems conditions, physical dimensions, and site development issues.

In summary, *hard costs* include:

- property purchase cost
- site development construction costs
- building construction costs
- hospital medical equipment
- furniture and furnishings

Add to the estimated hard cost total the estimated *soft cost* items:

- professional fees for architectural, mechanical, and electrical engineering
- professional fees for survey, civil, and geotechnical engineering
- fees for attorneys and real estate purchase negotiations
- fees for practice management consultant
- fees for accounting and business planning services
- environmental studies, sometimes required for financing
- government permit fees for site use, building permits and inspections, and utility connections
- financing costs, including loan closing costs and construction loan interest

Step #3: Financial Feasibility

The third step in completing the business plan is to analyze the probable results of putting your plan into effect. This phase answers the question, "What will happen if we build this facility and provide these services in this market?"

The feasibility study, as any financial statement, has two components. First is income. If you did not anticipate income, you would not plan to incur expense. Income is expected as a return for providing services. At this stage, a veterinary practice manager can be a valuable consultant. Essentially, we want to estimate the services that will be provided and the volume of those services. These services usually are itemized as transactions, with a transaction rate established for each service type. The transaction rates are usually compared to existing practices in the same market area and perhaps based on an existing practice that will continue in the newly developed facility.

In most cases, the current plan assumes that additional services will be provided in the new facility, either with new services, such as adding boarding, grooming, and so on, or increased volume, such as the result of adding associates and exam rooms. You can see how interrelated the three portions of business planning are, because one can't expect to provide additional services if the market analysis shows that there is an insufficient number of households to purchase more services. Or, if a particular volume of services is anticipated, the size of the facility and staff must match appropriately. It is not unusual to modify the facility cost analysis to correspond to financial issues that are clarified in the financial feasibility study, or to modify the financial study to correspond to actual costs of development.

Once you have established the basic services and transaction rates and volumes, you need to think about how the services are affected by the market. Is growth anticipated in the market that will imply growth in the practice? The financial income projection should take these issues into account.

We like to project income for a ten-year period. The first five-year projections are probably most accurate, but strategic planning for the practice becomes a very important aspect of the financial feasibility. Think about the transition of ownership of the practice. Will new associates be brought into the practice? Will some associates retire or sell their interest? These issues are likely to have a great impact on financing commitments.

The expense side of the equation is equally important. Assuming anticipated income level, limiting of expenses determines profit. The cost analysis will determine the amount of money required for the proposed project. Assuming that the bulk of these expenses is borrowed from a lending institution, the mortgage payment is a significant issue. Practice management consultants and accounting consultants can determine safe proportions of mortgage cost to gross annual revenue. The mortgage cost is important, but far more significant is the operation of your new facility. In order to accurately predict expenses, one must plan how many employees will be hired, what their duties will be, and how much they will be paid. Note that if financial projections are made for a ten-year period, and growth of the practice is assumed based on market projections, there will be changes in staff during these ten years.

All of the normal costs of operation must be accounted for, such as building maintenance, utilities, purchase of hospital supplies, and so on. If the newly developed facility will house an existing practice, you probably already have an accountant as part of your development team. If this is a new practice, you may want to consult with an accountant who specializes in veterinary practice.

When the income projections are compared to the expense projections, it will become clear whether the proposed project can be profitable. If the project is a new practice, there is likely to be an initial time period of financial loss until the volume of business grows to a point of profitability. When the financial feasibility study is complete and acceptable, financing for the project can be pursued.

Note that the discussion of business planning is predicated on the concept that the proposed business activities and complementary income and expenses are the basis of analysis. Too many times practice development proceeds on another basis: figuring how much money can be borrowed at present financial conditions and deciding to proceed with a project with current borrowing capacity as a basis for development. Why would anyone spend a significant amount of money on a project unless there is a plan to earn enough money to pay for the cost of development and generate a profit besides? Basing a project on current borrowing capacity indicates shortsighted planning. There is no ability to respond to market conditions. Success is still possible, but it is uncertain and can't be quantified.

There is undoubtedly a limit to how much financial institutions will lend to an individual or a practice. However, in today's financial climate, there are lending institutions that will find a way to provide funds for a project that is shown to be successful. That is what a comprehensive business plan can accomplish.

We, as architects, are always ready to leap into a design project and let our creative instincts have full reign. However, our most successful projects are those in which the owner/client has a clear vision and places limits and constraints on the project. The clear vision provided by complete business planning will produce a design process that is efficient and clearly addresses the right challenges successfully.

Credits

Because of my position of ownership in Knapp Schmidt Architects, I have the privilege of being able to articulate the policies and theories we use to carry on our work. The previous discussion summarizes years of work by several individuals who have initiated many of the concepts described, and who have done the work to carry out these principles in our clients' interest. Architect and planner E. John Knapp, AIA, pioneered the use of demographic market analysis for the veterinary business. His speaking engagements and articles have kept location and financing options a priority in the industry.

Additionally and more recently, James Hornik has expanded the feasibility study by preparing financial models for clients. This work has helped to focus and standardize systems that can be repeated for many clients on a cost-efficient basis.

Business Planning Review Issues

- Advance business planning increases your chance of a successful building project.
- Demographic market analysis helps to evaluate current and prospective locations. Your clients' access to the site and its visibility make location important to profitability.
- Analyze present and future space needs to decide size of the building.
- Evaluate site itself for size, topography, and zoning.
- The local government planning board or commission recommends approval or denial of proposed building projects. Public opinion matters to them.
- The village board or city council makes the final decision. Public hearings are held on requests for zoning change or variance.
- The local building department enforces zoning rules and requirements placed by planning boards.
- Base your construction budget and borrowing on future income projections. Don't restrict yourself to borrowing based on current income.
- The most successful building projects result from plans made by owners who have a clear vision of their building program and are able to reconcile their wish list and their budget.
- The most efficient and cost-effective projects result when programming decisions are made early in the process and adhered to throughout. Major design changes made in midprocess will add to the cost.

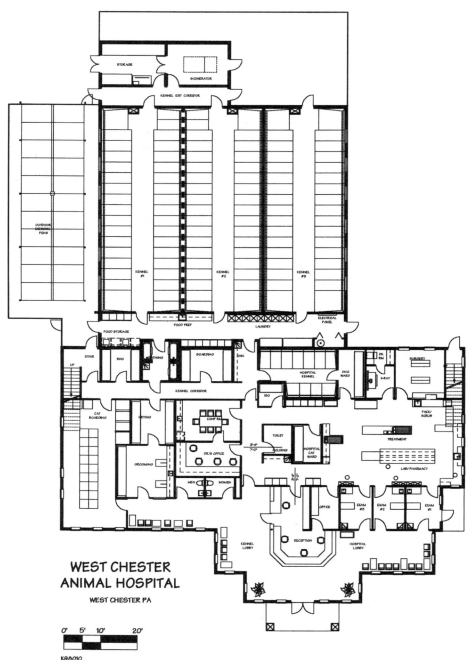

WEST CHESTER
ANIMAL HOSPITAL

WEST CHESTER PA

0' 5' 10'   20'

K98010
COPYRIGHT © 2000 KNAPP SCHMIDT ARCHITECTS, LLC

156

8

The Expanded Facility Planning Process

THE OPERATIONAL TRANSITION from old to new for staff will *always* be traumatic. I only put one page into the AAHA *Design Starter Kit* about this stress, but it has been the cause of many practice expansion derailments. As consultants, we often start a practice in the "new methods" six to twelve months *before* the move to ensure the new facility is not "blamed" for the changes. Now for the steps.

Step #1: Work Flow

The AAHA *Design Starter Kit* has scale drawings in the back, designed to be copied, cut out, and slid around the table until a flow becomes visible. Some other items to consider:

- waiting room cul-de-sacs with cat gazebo versus cat-dog areas, small seating areas to give visual privacy from others but not reception
- behavior center viewed from reception, high-density medical record cabinets down the hall, window to lab for high tech . . . image and image!
- paired exam rooms with doctor stations, since an outpatient doctor will *always* be working two out of sync with an outpatient nurse (OPN) in high-density scheduling, and the nursing staff can have the other ones for walk-ins and emergencies
- dental room (also a "stat" procedure room for outpatient) also acts as holding for morning admissions (reduces running), adds quiet, and allows negative pressure exhaust in small area to reduce aerosol contamination
- alternative medicine rooms near laboratory, so the laboratory technician can also be the alternative care nurse
- imaging area versus X-ray room (dark room allows multiple procedures to go concurrently) versus special procedures (ultrasound, endoscope, Vetronics, on rolling stock, under the film shelves)
- adequate staff lounge and storage downstairs, drop stairs to attic space, and effective use of cabinets and drawers

- respite care suites can lead into the geriatric care, oncology, arthritis, cardio-logical stress, diabetes patients, etc. (plan for inpatient capability, plus glass-surround recovery runs)
- lots of glass (double pane, unequal diameters, reduce sound) can add depth while adding light; lighting could also be augmented with skylights
- placement and flow considerations: telephone receptionist in business office (with headset), potential consult room checkout, consultation/grieving room, alternative care rooms, walk-in flow, emergency flow, etc.
- nursing station central to hospital (and doctor's station) with open hearing to reception
- family feeling of reception—woodlike floor covering coupled with molding, ceiling fans, art and decor, murals, warmth of layout and people
- knowledge center for wellness instead of curative medicine facility, selling peace of mind rather than products, offering initial courtesy nursing consults instead of doctor consults for high fees

Step #2: Operational Review

Form follows function—*always*—so use sample floor plans to walk through the common procedures with staff members. Staff members see themselves as equal to or above the team in most all "soft skills," which means they offer per-ceived strengths that can be called upon later. The following concepts, if they are appropriate to your design, need to be considered:

- Full-spectrum lighting is needed at most interior locations of the practice and resort—look at life against cost before deciding the cost.
- Pharmacy needs to be common to all consultation rooms and the terminal can have dual use for invoicing (a holistic pharmacy at alternative-care side?). Twelve-inch shelves between closets allow all reference files to be consoli-dated in outpatient (or other singular) area.
- Business office may have half glass walls for many reasons: team visibility and communication, checkout observation as a security system, provide for bookkeeper space or telephone receptionist space.
- Numerous workstations in treatment area allow one inpatient nurse (IPN) to orchestrate many areas as well as one doctor to float and mentor the staff.
- A cat gazebo is another draw for clients and very feline friendly. It could also allow retail space to be developed on an opposing wall, as long as the front shelf unit is only five feet high so the openness is not blocked.
- The medical records could be high-density files (two-sided rotating) and gain double the linear feet of shelves without being seen by clients.
- Medical records pulled for the OPN or IPN are stored where? If the front counter is too small for all nursing staff pickups, there may be buckets on the wall and/or vertical stacks under the counter.
- Plan for productive flow and eliminate hallway traffic before it starts.

- The treatment room could have a scissor gurney, maybe with below-counter storage space. Also, due to ADA and OSHA, a lift table will most likely be needed in treatment as well as at least between each pair of consultation/exam rooms. The lift table in treatment can have a built-in scale, and the dental area can have its own holding cages. A scale site in the reception counter will catch most incoming, but any animal with a length of stay needs sequential weights while an inpatient. Recovery runs in treatment are a great idea. A nurse's station in treatment should hold the priority list and medical records for all inpatients (and drop-offs) and will be monitored by the inpatient nurse for changes and additions; the white board will show all animals and priorities for inpatient care (established at 8 A.M. and 1 P.M. by the inpatient doctor and shift IPN).
- A bathing tub needs to be addressed—all discharges need to smell good. New fiberboard-laminated Clark-Cote or Snyder cages installed for cats and ICU will reduce noise and add "softness."
- HVAC and plumbing challenges need to be planned for: special exhaust required in dentistry; pharmacy and laboratory for oncology drugs; ICU circulation; positive pressure in surgery and negative pressure in the isolation area; plus the conditioned air ducts should be designed not to break the sound barriers. Bathing and recovery runs, as well as K-9 and isolation wards, need a high air exchange (greater than ten times per hour).
- The 3Rs need to be revisited: *recall, recheck,* and *remind.* Recall and recheck should be coded to nurses in more than 70 percent of the cases and tracked by computer, so a printout each morning can be nurse specific for handouts and callback activities.
- Schedule zones, plan triad teams, stick to the schedule (no getting distracted by outside calls, excessive client schmoozing, etc.), and avoid a staff feeding frenzy trying to catch up.
- Form follows function—"one picture is worth a thousand words"—review of floor plans by the staff. Each set of key team members must walk their day through the process of client and patient access scenarios with specific interest in storage sites, reporting methods, tracking methods, critter flow, and day-to-day operational needs for resources. Form must follow function, so define and test the functions based on the *new* operational areas: outpatient triad, inpatient triad, surgery triad, day patient check-in, drop-off patient admission, play and people time, etc.

Step #3: Contractor Construction Estimates

Estimates are "bang for buck" investment concerns and expand the historical-based budget projections; these need to be discussed with your accountant *before* going to bankers and other lenders.

- May need a contractor search and pro forma with time-line at this point.
- Should have multiple sources for runs, cages, lights, and fixtures.

- Computer upgrades need to be considered in budget.
- Self-search for scope of services to be offered at new facility.
- Is a "new face" for reception/waiting areas essential? If so, don't plan to salvage anything from the existing facility for client areas.

Step #4: Financing Sources

Bankers, lending group, SBA . . . and yes, this is slow up to this point . . . and you will need a contractor's pro forma with time-line before this phase is completed.

Step #5: Staff and Client Involvement

Staff involvement for needed services, colors, and textures is important. Utilize a council of clients for feedback of perceptions. There are also operational areas that need testing and evaluation before moving to the new facility (tested for four to eight hours and then evaluated by the players), then retest and evaluate with a new mix of players, then recycle until all the different groupings and permeations have been tested. This includes testing and discussing:

- Do you have a manager on staff? If not, you probably need one now! With expansion concerns, do they have personal "extenders" on board to mediate their duties and support IPN and OPN rotations?
- High-density scheduling (see *Zoned Systems & Schedules for Multi-Doctor Practices* Signature Series Monograph from VPC).
- Schedule rooms, not doctors, and get clients in and out in 30 minutes or less since 87 percent want twenty minutes or less (Pfizer study of 37,000 clients; see *Zoned Systems & Schedules for Multi-Doctor Practices Signature Series* monograph from VPC).
- Utilize outpatient nursing (see chapter 3 of *Building the Successful Veterinary Practice: Volume 2: Programs and Procedures*).
- Internal referral systems to other provider triads.
- Inpatient triad for drop-offs, walk-ins, and emergencies.
- Surgery triad times.
- What cases deserve admission rather than extended outpatient time?
- Thirty-minute appointments maximum (new client, exotics, or two pets), except three or four dogs, who can get forty minutes . . . use the ten-minute unit plan to allow for suture removal and other fast procedures to be scheduled.
- Receptionists *never* run laps; use an intercom or other means to get prescriptions and assistance from nursing staff.
- Address client concerns *before* doing anything else—wellness screen for asymmetry in three to five minutes, doctor prioritizes care, then returns the client to OPN for client education, pharmacy, and other services.

- Use color codes on some computerized appointment log systems and appointment formatting to schedule pairs of rooms, rather than just doctors, in horizontal format for high-density schedule.
- Totally computerize tracking operations, including the cage card by computer entry.
- Separate companies for building/property versus general practice, separate profit and loss (P&L) (see *Building the Successful Veterinary Practice: Volume 2: Programs and Procedures*, appendixes E and F and chapter 4, "Program-Based Budgeting").
- Research Sunday hours and ensure evening and extended Saturday hours.
- Research transfer between activities (TBA) effort (see *Building the Successful Veterinary Practice: Volume 2: Programs and Procedures*) to ensure proper resale-to-wholesale transfer of property and products.
- Informed consent for procedures includes the statement of needed care that is being authorized and the fair fee assessed; the agent authorized to decide the animal's rights signs the rights waiver. Clients don't waive care, they don't have the knowledge; just the animal's right to care can be waived. Change your forms and approach to *needed* care now!
- Medical records should be end-tabbed manila; use dividers and one prong per animal format (see appendix C of *Building the Successful Veterinary Practice: Volume 2: Programs and Procedures* for forms, chapter 3 for methods); if you have divergent clients, such as alternative medicine clients versus traditional clients, consider placing alternative care medical records in different color manila folders.
- Progress notes need to be simple, as does the new client welcome form. Removing redundancies adds clarity of purpose.
- Test healthcare bundles (see *Building the Successful Veterinary Practice: Volume 3: Innovation and Creativity* text) and preferred client programs as the community situation dictates, but talk the programs through in current facility and start testing them immediately so your leadership team can be aware of when they need to be initiated.
- Start testing and shifting the nomenclature and titles, including:
  Animal caretaker versus kennel kid
  Wellness care and asymmetry screens by OPN
  Admission versus check-in
  Prioritize/sequence inpatient care twice a day
  Behavior management programs
  Nutritional counselors
  Parasite prevention/control specialists
  Outpatient nurses
  Inpatient nurses
  Technical assistants
  Walk-ins welcomed versus squeezed in
  Dental hygiene nurses versus technicians
  Surgical nurse
  Other staff ideas

Step #6: The Contracting and Building Phase

This phase will have change orders and great stresses, and if you don't have someone you can trust (at practice and at construction site), look for the practice liquidity to take a hit due to your personal distractions.

- Strategic assessment of community, announcement door hangers for subdivisions that feed your demographic area.
- Target announcements and external image enhancements with surrounding Chamber of Commerce sources and local media (use elevations, not floor plans, for better female awareness).
- Make most of the operational changes in your current facility (new appointment logs, revised medical record formats, new informed consent systems, new healthcare standards, etc.).
- Alternative or additional services should open; possible delays in construction should not affect this word-of-mouth promotion.
- Buy-against contract and bonus for early completion are reciprocal requirements; ensure these and other construction parameters are included in any contract deal.
- A manager needs to have "extenders" on board by now to mediate their duties and allow them contractor review time

Step #7: The Move-In Phase

This is the pride-building phase, and that must start *today* by catching people doing things right on a daily basis and telling them *very specifically* exactly which behaviors you are impressed by (each doctor must start doing this now). Then move in with a smile.

- Leave bad habits at your old facility.
- Relook at the new flow—walk everyone through the physical facility and explain new zones. Big increases in floor space will prevent everyone from being everywhere all the time as in tight facilities (and doctors will have less control).
- Look at new areas of accountability and release the resource access so the appropriate staff member(s) can resolve emerging issues without doctor or manager permission.
- Open house *after* contractor leaves—hopefully in the first month

Note: If you have not yet figured it out, you are not expanding the old facility operations, you are creating a new culture and a revised team approach to veterinary healthcare delivery! The trauma and stress will be worth it, but probably will be felt for many months after the move *unless* you start the move in the current facility by addressing the new programs and procedures *now*! See the fun? Trust me, it will be worth it.

New Resort Options
Included at check-in for each guest:
• External parasite screen
• Wellness physical (nose to tail check for asymmetry)
• Twice a day outside walk (under cover if bad weather)
• Spacious guest unit (no cages are used for resort guests)

Options offered each guest:
• VIP suites with television and pet partner people (advanced registration only)
• Pet partner people time (exploration zone)
• Play time
• Afternoon chilled snack (animal-formulated yogurt)

Ancillary care offered to all guests:
• Dental hygiene screen
• Nutritional assessments
• Extended stay fat farm program, with refeeding program
• Behavior management evaluation
• Boutique grooming
• Bath
• Pedicure (nail trim)

Insights and Perspectives

Team Roles and Expectations
Daniel D. Chapel, AIA

Building your own animal care facility is a vast undertaking, but there is a range of professionals out there whose jobs are to help you create the custom facility you are dreaming about. Choosing which kind of and how many professionals you work with—architects, contractors, engineers, interior designers—depends on your budget and what you wish to accomplish. Architects and engineers are trained to deal with spatial and structural questions and may also help with the material and product specifications for your facility. Designers vary in expertise—some are best at decorating, others at space planning. A general contractor, in addition to dealing with construction issues, may recommend local subcontractors and specialists with whom they've worked.

Why Work with a Pro?

Why should you hire a professional building team at all? Design and building professionals have learned from their experiences what works and what does not work functionally, aesthetically, and financially. Their expertise can keep you from making costly mistakes. After all, they have probably been through the building process hundreds of times, whereas you may be going through it for only the first or second time.

A professional will also have more access to and knowledge of state-of-the-art products, services, and techniques than you would. Whether it's outfitting your closets with the storage systems that suit your practice best or investing in the best quality flooring for your money, a professional can help you make wise design choices that suit your special needs.

If you have only a vague idea of what you want your new facility to look like but aren't sure of all the details, a professional architect or designer can help you clarify the vision you want—and fit the budget you have available.

How Do I Find a Professional Building Team?

Every team has to have a leader, and the leader of a professional building team is the architect. The architect is your representative, your liaison to the contractors, subcontractors, interior designers, and engineers.

Ask fellow veterinarians, friends, coworkers, and area builders you trust whom they would recommend. Ask for and review the architect's entire portfolio—not just one project. Ask for and check out references and professional affiliations.

It's important that you choose someone you can talk to and not feel intimidated by and someone whose opinion you will respect. Architects are there to make your vision a reality, not to create a vision of their own.

The architect, in turn, can recommend contractors, engineers, and other building professionals based on past experience.

Clear communication between you and your architect is the key ingredient in smooth and successful facility construction. After you have selected an architect and the architect has accepted the project, he or she will expect you to give as much specific information as you can about the kind of facility you want, inside and out.

How Do I Prepare?

Planning your animal care facility should be the result of careful, thorough thought. Many details may require research on your part. Design and building professionals are not in business to build and design what they want, but are hired by you to realize your vision. To make the most of this opportunity, you need to prepare as best you can for your collaboration with them. Here is a sampling of some of the elements you need to decide upon and communicate to your architect early in the process:

1. *Budget:* One of the most important pieces of information you can give the architect is your budget. How much money can you afford to spend? Be honest and realistic about that figure. Most architects, through experience, can look at facility plans and estimate how much the facility will cost to build in a particular square footage. Be prepared to tell the architect up front how much you want to spend. If the plans you have go over your budget, a good architect will work with you to modify them to meet your needs or set you in the right direction as to what type of facility you should look for that you can really afford.

2. *The kind of facility you want:* Take six to nine months to decide what you want the facility to look like and include in the way of equipment, flooring, storage, fixtures, furnishings, and so forth. Tour other facilities for ideas, and collect examples of what you do and don't like from magazines and other photo sources. Think about how you currently use your rooms and write down what you would like to see changed. Note any problems you have in your existing facility. Is there too little storage? Not enough ventilation? Poor noise reduction? List what features you'd like most if it all isn't possible or affordable. Put function first. No matter how wonderful a fixture or feature looks, if it isn't useful, you'll eventually be unhappy with it. Think about traffic patterns, client considerations and ample lighting. Be flexible. Be open to substitutions and ideas offered by your professional building team that might achieve your goal in a better way than you had originally imagined.

3. *Special requirements:* What will your practice require several years from now? Will you need extra phone lines for a computer or fax machine? All too often owners of new facilities don't think far enough ahead. Try to identify any special requirements you have now and try to anticipate future needs for at least five years in advance.

4. *Selections you can stick to:* Changing material choices or other selections can incur additional expenses or create delays. For example, cabinets may be ordered in a specific configuration to surround the new business area you have selected. But if you change your mind and decide to bring a piece of furniture from your old facility instead of purchasing a new one, the old item may be the wrong size and not fit into the space between your new cabinets. Also keep in mind that just because items haven't arrived yet doesn't mean there is time to change your selection. In many cases, components are ordered several weeks in advance of when they will be installed. Changing one component to a different size or shape may have a domino effect and necessitate a string of other change orders—resulting in potentially disastrous expense and delay.

5. *Let the architect know who's in charge:* Who makes the decisions? If there is more than one veterinarian in your practice, it should be clear who has the final say. If a dual practice team makes decisions jointly, the architect must respect that arrangement. The goal is to work together to realize the dreams of the facility owner or owners.

6. *Trust and respect your architect:* Veterinarians new to the building process sometimes dislike talking to architects about money because they fear being taken advantage of. Without trust and respect, antagonism between you and your architect can grow to be an unpleasant subtext in the relationship. Honest communication is the best remedy against it.

Who Does What?

Understanding the roles that members of your building team play in the design and construction of your veterinary facility is essential. Let's take a closer look at the function of the various team members and how the chain of command works.

Your building team will likely consist of you, your architect, an interior designer, a general contractor, and various engineers, subcontractors and specialists.

Building a new facility is, of course, an expensive and exciting undertaking for the veterinary practice, and it's perfectly understandable that the owner may have a tendency to micromanage the process. The temptation to visit the site often and become personally involved in the day-to-day construction process is almost irresistible.

There's nothing wrong with visiting and overseeing the process, but there are some inherent dangers.

Too much or too active supervision can distract, annoy, or intimidate the professional builders. Who, after all, enjoys working with someone looking over his or her shoulder? Just as animal care specialists are plagued by amateur veterinarians who gleaned their "knowledge" from cable television, design and building professionals must put up with "sidewalk superintendents" and other amateur builders.

To resist the urge, work through your contractual representative—your architect. Let him or her be your voice. After all, the architect is a trained professional conversant with the jargon of the various building trades. Let the architect's experience work for you. The architect functions as your general, designing and planning the facility, supervising the overall process, translating your desires and dreams into practical and functional reality.

Another building professional who works closely with the owner is the interior design specialist. Again, the professional's job is to understand and actualize your vision of the facility. All too often, "champagne" facilities are ruined by "beer" interior design. Allow the professionals to advise you on color choices, lighting, furnishings, and so forth.

The various engineers are experts in specialized areas like electrical or mechanical engineering. Their knowledge in such matters as the kind and size of air-conditioning units, wiring, and the like should be respected.

The general contractor acts as the owner's hands, managing and supervising the actual construction. He or she will hire the various subcontractors based on experience and association.

Perhaps the most important member of the building team is the owner. The owner's role is vision creation. He or she must predict needs, think about the growth of the practice, and generally make the decisions about what type of facility is wanted and needed. Building a new animal care facility is an opportunity. The veterinarian can adapt the facility to the practice rather than adapting the practice to the existing facility.

How Do I Hire an Architect?

There are many qualities to look for in an architect. You will, of course, want someone who can successfully manage a building team skilled at constructing a quality animal care facility. Other characteristics are more difficult to evaluate. These include the ability to listen, to be a partner with you in solving problems as they arise, and to be honest and fair. Here are some paths to follow to help you select the architect who is right for you:

1. *Check references:* Thoroughly investigate three or four references for each architect you consider. The references should be people for whom the architect has completed construction of a facility. Spend time either in person or on the telephone with the references to discuss the architect's honesty, professionalism, patience, ability to listen, and problem-solving capability. Be sure to do this when the architect isn't there, as his or her presence might inhibit the facility owners from giving you the frank and candid answers you need. Just phoning and asking a few questions may not be enough. If possible, arrange to visit facilities designed and completed by the architect in question. Specific questions might include: Did the project run smoothly? If not, what went wrong? Did the job finish on schedule? If not, what held it up? Were the cost estimates accurate? If they went over budget, where and why? Was the architect helpful in solving budget and construction problems? Did the architect make helpful suggestions or bring up ideas the owner hadn't thought of? Were his or her explanations clear and logical? Was he or she available? Did he or she visit the site? Have there been any major problems with the facility since its construction? If there has been a problem, was the architect efficient in answering calls and following up?

2. *Check credentials:* Ask your prospective architects if they belong to the American Institute of Architects or any other national or local organization. Then you can check with that organization to see if the architect is a member in good standing. Keep in mind that there are some good architects who choose not to affiliate themselves with any professional organization. Your decision on which architect to select should not be based on this type of credential alone.

3. *Match the architect to your needs:* Look for an architect who is familiar with the type and size of facility you want built. Architects often have areas of expertise. If you want to build a no-frills, budget facility, don't hire an architect who designs high-end facilities. Experience counts. There's nothing wrong with new architects in the field, but let someone else hire them. This may be your once-in-a-lifetime chance to build your dream facility. Choose someone with proven experience.

4. *Ask the architect how available he or she will be:* As noted above, it's important to hire an architect who can devote the proper amount of time to your project. Check with the architect's references to verify that he or she will give you the time and attention you deserve and are paying for. If the architect's presence on-site is particularly important to you, you might consider selecting an architect with a small practice. Such architects often are able to devote more time, since your project will be a major one for him or her.

5. *Investigate fees:* Different architects have differing fee schedules. Of course, everyone would like to save as much money as possible, but beware of architecture firms whose fees are far below the norm. After all, you usually get what you pay for. Architects with bargain-basement fees may not be a bargain in the long run.

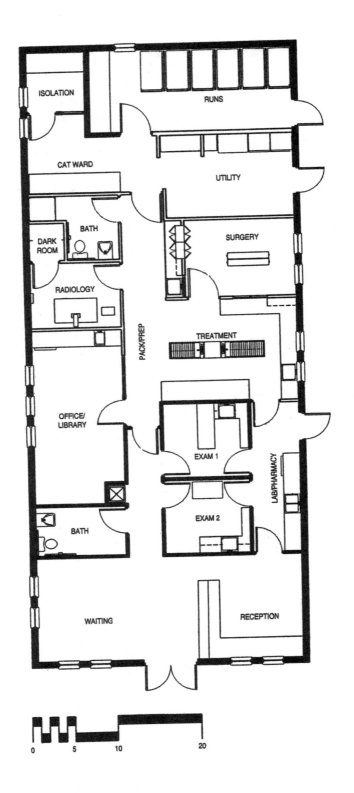

ISOLATION

RUNS

CAT WARD

UTILITY

DARK
ROOM

BATH

SURGERY

RADIOLOGY

PACK/PREP

TREATMENT

OFFICE/
LIBRARY

EXAM 1

LAB/PHARMACY

BATH

EXAM 2

WAITING

RECEPTION

0   5   10   20

Conclusion

THIS REFERENCE HAS attempted to provide the veterinary facility owner/planner a common language for hospital design, construction planning, programming, architecture, engineering, and construction. As such, there are alternative phrases and terms used throughout this reference, because there is *no* such common language except in the standard AIA forms and a few basic construction references (see glossary).

A complete veterinary facility project should be based upon a series of clear tasks and a straightforward schedule that is understood by the practice owner(s), project manager (clerk-of-the-works), consultant(s), architect, engineer, and contractor(s). During the past ten years it has often become a bidding game, where the contractor reviews the architect's plans, determines the shortfalls, bids on the plans as drawn, then adds to his or her income using change orders, because the veterinarian will *never* build something that does not fit his or her image of what he or she wants. In 2002, I discovered a reputable and noteworthy team (Fred and Joe) at SR Construction in Las Vegas, a pair of guys that not only did not charge for change orders but also spent an inordinate amount of their own time redrawing design defects that had been inserted by a less-than-aware architecture firm. As contractors, SR Construction set a new yardstick of client-service excellence in my mind.

The prices and estimates used in this reference are from 2001–2002 experiences and were averaged for standardization purposes, using the continental United States as a workplace. We all know that a standardized community does not exist anywhere in the world, much less within the free enterprise system of the United States. As time goes on and construction standards change in various locations, the estimated costs will likely escalate; in some cases, they are already higher due to the averaging used to provide general guidelines. This is where your trusted, construction-experienced, veterinary-specific consultant, or practice-specific project manager (clerk-of-the-works), will earn his or her paycheck many times over. The consultant or project manager is the check–and-balance for current construction, community, and veterinary-specific standards, any of which can greatly affect the construction costs.

Since even the plants in the reception area are seen as indicators of health-care delivery excellence, consider what a poorly planned, poorly constructed, or outdated facility conveys to the client. The veterinary practice of tomorrow must be client friendly, and the staff must be patient advocates. Programs, services, and procedures are delivered based on the effective design, construction, and use of the facility.

Appendix A

Knowing Your Value So They Can Know It Too

Robert W. Deegan, DVM

Learn that you need to speak the language of lenders
if you wish to have them play on your team.

THE NEED YOU HAVE is to grow or die. The accumulation of events and congestion of your medical facility have presented an absolute limit to quality medicine, a challenge to the very level that you and your clients deserve. You need another building or a radical reshaping of the one you are in. As you work your way through the design of the facility you need you are also working yourself through the question of "How much can the practice afford?"

Another way of asking that is "What is the value of my practice?" You need to know that because you have to decide which of two options you will use to finance. If you can do it on cash flow and accumulated assets you have no problem and you can move to chapter 4. If not, you will have to consider attracting capital from an outside source.

The problem with lenders is that while many bankers "kinda understand" service businesses, medical services seem to be from an alien planet. They understand assets and even cash flow. Most certainly the concept of net is as near and dear to their hearts as it is to yours. They have trouble identifying the actual nature of the net in a veterinary practice, given the widely varying reports to which they are subjected. And they are definitely unfamiliar with any method to measure the bonding of clients to the practice, which is the essential element in the practice's viability.

It is critical to make the connection between quality medical care and good business policies. Then the lenders will understand where the money comes from and the importance of the pride your staff has in the practice.

Business Plan

Your responsibility is to produce a business plan.

Here is where your vision is displayed, your procedure is spelled out, and your ability to deliver veterinary healthcare services and to operate a thriving business is demonstrated.

> **The Business Plan**
>
> Where you are.
> Where you need to be.
> What it will take to get there.
> How you will make it happen.

> **Assets**
>
> Net analysis of the historical business.
> Budget projections for three years.

The Tools

The tools you will apply to the lender's mind are fiscal at their root but based on community dynamics and acceptance of services provided, history of delivery, and projections using real analysis of services and ability to expand and alter existing practice.

The practice valuation shows what the practice has become in terms of the worth it can command by someone else who desires to buy it. The valuation, using historical documentation, shows where the practice was and how far it has come. The valuation identifies the tenor of the community that both drove and supported the growth of the practice. The valuation brings out the factors of the practice that made it stand out in the community. The valuation can also highlight the factors that encourage, or demand, additional services. Also note: Precision in results below 1 percent cannot be achieved, given the nature of the data. Do not pretend to more than that—round results to $1,000.

If this were only a building, the valuation would be the measure of the foundation. The valuation is not just a show piece for the triumphs and successes of the practice. It also identifies problem areas, those matters that you intend to rectify. It brings up issues that are needful of alteration and/or attention. Included in this is the matter of available documentation, and, hence, collection of management and medical data.

Given the variety and breadth of information garnered for the practice valuation it should not come as a surprise that there are more uses for the valuation than in a buy/sell situation. Which is why we have a fiscal audit! Just a rose by another name.

The Elements of the Fiscal Audit

The Major Elements	**The Factors**
Tangible assets	Present value of future earnings
Client records	Risk assessment
Net excess earnings	Retention

(See *Beyond the Successful Veterinary Practice: Succession Planning and Other Legal Issues.*)

The Tangible Assets

- Assets are the yesterday of the practice. Here we can see the capital investments of the practice: real estate, the equipment, the inventory, the accounts payable, and the accounts receivable. The cash on hand and any other instruments that can produce cash in the short term are included.
- Liabilities go along with the practice. The bulk of liabilities is attached to tangible assets. Note that overdue drug bills and snow removal charges are certainly a liability, but these types of debts get the more prosaic label of "expense."
- Cash on hand is also a readily understood asset. Any short-term investment easily redeemed is treated as cash. Accounts receivable can have a cash value. Accounts payable work like liabilities.

Client Records

All clients are not born equal. Most can end up being "favorite clients," but that comes later. Bonding can be measured as a function of return. Thusly, we have active clients who come in once a year, those who come in less than once a year, and those who come in more than once a year. "Inactive clients" have no fiscal value to the practice.

Determining Net

The net of the practice is what is left after all the legitimate expenses and liabilities of the practice are paid. Simple to say but frequently abused in practice. Beyond the cost of goods for sale, utilities, and continued education; past external lab services, uniforms, and advertising as well as salary for all clinicians, rent, and owner's draw; we arrive at the true net. This is the money for capital investment, debt reduction, and excessive continuing education on the Riviera.

Since the net is a static we need to see it as a dynamic. The experience of Veterinary Practice Consultants® is that the influence of the previous management can have a (decreasing) influence on the practice performance for three years. After that, the management of the current leadership team is fully functional. For this reason there is no justification to try to "sell" net or cash flow more than three years out. We do use the present value of future earnings to provide a value of promised returns "sometime soon."

The Factors

Present Value of Future Earnings

Consider the dilemma of your brother-in-law from whom you wish to borrow some money to buy a bass boat. He really wants you to get the boat so he can go fishing with you. But he has several options for his $4,000. Certificates of deposit, utility bonds, his bookie. So he needs to decide which option will give him the best return with the least risk. He decides to give it to you because he knows you will pay, he will have lots of fun with you out there molesting fish, and he is terrorized by his sister.

A commercial lender has a similar decision to make. How stable are you in the community? How well managed is your business? What will be the return to him in terms of fun, or interest? The lender considers this possible loan and attaches an interest rate to the deal.

The present value of future earnings is what the lender feels is the difference in value between a dollar from anybody today and a dollar from you next year. This concept is codified as a discount rate using the matrix of risk assessment.

Risk Assessment

This is close to being a capitalization rate but has more variance. The cap rate is denominated in whole numbers. For practices we see numbers from three to six. Meaning, for example, "I will let you have this money for three years but after that you give it back or I break your knees."

Risk is denominated as a percentage discount that is cumulative for each year out. A discount of 17 percent on one dollar for one year means you will get eighty-five cents now and you will pay one dollar in a year. If you want it for two years, you will get seventy-three cents.

Retention

The retention is the first measure of community stability and client bonding. Take the number of active clients at the end of this year minus new clients acquired this year divided by active clients last year and you have retention. For instance: 115 active clients this year, 16 new clients this year, 100 active clients last year.

115 − 16 = 99 ÷ 100 = .99, or 99%

Let's do it!

The Tangible Assets

Tangible assets are the hard, visible parts of the place where you do medicine. This may include building and ground if your corporate structure also owns the real estate. It includes the equipment inside and around the building. It includes the inventory, drugs and things that get used up in the rendering of care. It includes cash and near cash and anything that can be easily converted to cash and not taken away from the practice. It includes money that is due in soon.

Tangible assets also include the liabilities related to the assets. These are such things as mortgages on property, leases, and accounts payable. The actual list is only limited by the creativity of the owners. But the practice can only claim the stuff that is really part of the practice operations. The place to start looking is on the balance sheet that you get from your accountant every month or at least quarterly.

Cool Hand Kitties Veterinary Services
Balance Sheet
31 Dec 2000

Current assets	
Cash on hand	$ 500
Cash in bank	$ 7,673
Accounts receivables	$ 6,155
Inventory	$ 18,645
TOTAL CURRENT ASSETS	**$ 32,973**
Property and equipment	
Furniture and fixtures	$ 7,819
Leasehold improvements	$ 28,350
Machinery and equipment	$ 83,700
Office equipment	$ 17,628
Truck	$ 12,390
	$149,887
Less: accumulated depreciation	<$125,905>
Total property and equipment	**$ 23,982**
TOTAL ASSETS	**$ 56,955**
	(continued)

Liabilities	
Accounts payable	$ 18,988
Payroll taxes payable	$ 417
State withholding	$ 25
Unemployment	$ 47
FUTA	$ 164
Workmen's comp	$ 651
Sales tax	$ 316
TOTAL CURRENT LIABILITIES	<$ 20,608>
TOTAL TANGIBLE ASSETS LESS LIABILITIES	$ 36,347

There is more in the report but this is the crucial data.

Client Records

We are constantly measuring our intended quality of care against the response from our clients. We really want our clients to be as dedicated to their companions as we are. But we are worried that they do not take our recommendations as seriously as we do. So we call clients A or B or K and we strive to attract and keep the best for the niche we intend to occupy. Do not be deceived. Not all practices wish to be at the cutting edge of care. Many primary care practices serve their community well and fairly and refer cases in a timely and deliberate manner. Good for you all. Each evening when you go home you can say "I have done the best for my clients and myself and I have provided a quality place for my quality staff."

Now let us quantify the bonding Cool Hand Kitties Veterinary Services has with its clientele.

- Class 1 clients are those who came in more than once in the last twelve months.
- Class 2 clients came in once in the last twelve months.
- Class 3 clients came in less than once in the last twelve months.

All we need is numbers for each class. We will not attempt to put a personal value on any individual client. Statistics is the tool here.

For Cool Hand Kitties the numbers are	
Avg chg	= $62.59
Ret	= 77%
Risk	= 80%
ACT = $38.56	

Cool Hand Kitties data	
Class 1 =	1,200
Class 2 =	910
Class 3 =	1,680

The formulation is:

1. Average client transaction (ACT) is the previous year average charge times the retention rate (Ret) times the capitalization rate or risk assessment (Risk).

   Avg. chg. ($) $\times$ Ret (%) $\times$ Risk (%)= ACT ($)

2. Class size
   times class factor (f)
   times average client transaction.

   Class $\times$ f $\times$ ACT = $

3. The big calculation is thusly:

Class 1	1,200 times 1.5 times $38.56 =	$69,400
Class 2	910 times 1.0 times $38.56 =	$35,100
Class 3	1,680 times 0.5 times $38.56 =	$32,400
Total value of client records		$138,100

Net Excess Earnings

In a real profit and loss (P&L) or income and earnings statement there is a real *AAHA Chart of Accounts* that is designed for the edification of the practice owner. To wit:

Income		
Professional services	$326,800	53%
Vaccinations	$ 67,200	11%
Lab/diagnostic	$ 18,300	3%
Surg/dental	$ 49,000	8%
Hospital/nursing	$ 25,000	4%
Pharmaceuticals	$ 15,100	2%
Grooming/board	$ 93,700	15%
Food/OTC	$ 16,100	3%
TOTAL INCOME	$611,000	
Cost of services		
Drugs and med supply	$108,900	18.0%
Nutritional products	$ 24,400	4.0%
Lab/diagnostics	$ 6,700	1.0%
Nursing/boarding	$ 69,800	11.0%
Animal/waste disposal	$ 1,800	0.3%
Other	$ 3,000	0.5%
		(continued)

General and Administrative Expenses (partial)

DVM clinician salary	$152,700	25.0%
Staff wages	$ 42,800	7.0%
Technician wages	$ 73,300	12.0%
Admin dollars	$ 18,300	3.0%
Rent	$ 42,300	7.0%
Maint and repair	$ 6,100	1.0%
Cont ed	$ 4,200	0.7%
Advert/cl rel	$ 7,300	1.2%
Legal/accounting	$ 1,800	0.3%
Depreciation/amort	$ 11,000	1.8%
Consultants	$ 6,100	1.0%
All the rest . . .		
TOTAL EXPENSES	$550,000	
NET EXCESS EARNINGS	$ 61,000	10% of gross income

That $61,000 net converts into a conservative $55,000. That could be used to make monthly principal and interest payments of $4,600. For a capital improvement loan of fifteen years at 10.3 percent this will service a loan of $424,000.

Is that all there is? Don't give up yet. Now is the time to review the data and see if it is all it could be. Start over at the top and say "Whoa, back, mule. I have a whole lot more hard stuff in this practice than that shows!"

The Balance Sheet

You are right! The balance sheet and P&L (also called income and expense) documents are tax documents. They are created to convince the minions of the IRS that you do not owe any more money than you are required to pay out.

So take another look at your assets:

Current assets

Cash on Hand	$ 500
Cash in bank	$ 7,673
Accounts receivable	$ 6,155
Inventory	$18,645
TOTAL CURRENT ASSETS	$32,973

That equipment depreciated over a straight line does not actually wear out that fast. You must find the replacement value of your assets—that is, what it would cost you to go out and buy an identical replacement for–whatever it is. To do this you probably need a knowledgeable individual who is in the equipment (especially the used equipment) business to come through your practice and look at everything and put a value on it.

Property and Equipment	
Furniture and Fixtures	$ 7,819
Leasehold Improvements	$ 28,350
Machinery and Equipment	$ 83,700
Office Equipment	$ 17,628
Truck	$ 12,390
Total Property and Equipment	$ 49,887
Less:	
Accumulated Deprec.	<$125,905>
Equipment Value	$ 23,982
TOTAL ASSETS	$ 56,955

When the Cool Hand Kitties gets this "knowledgeable individual," they find out their equipment is worth $186,000.00.

Inventory

What we know about inventory is that resupply is a highly predictable response to ordering. Time elapsed is a few days to a week. Just-in-time ordering would have an inventory control officer working on a two-week cycle. Prudent management practices look more to a four-week supply on hand.

Last year Cool Hand Kitties spent $133,000 (remember you are rounding) on medical cost of goods sold (CoGS).

Cost of Services		
Drugs and med supply	$ 108,900	18%
Nutritional products	$ 24,400	4%

$133,000 ÷ 12 = $11,000

Cool Hand Kitties has $18,000 of supplies on hand.

On-hand inventory	$18,000
Calculated need	$11,000
Difference	$ 7,000

This is an excess of $7,000 over the reported needs of the practice. That should have been money in the net!

How interesting. Let's look at our overall inventory control. In the well-managed companion animal practice we expect to see CoGS at 13 percent of gross income. At Cool Hand Kitties that $611,000 gross income should require $80,000 per year. This is greater than a $50,000 reduction over the existing inventory control effort.

Reported CoGS	$133,000
Calculated CoGS	$ 80,000
Difference	$ 53,000

Let's be serious. Cool Hand Kitties is not going to obtain that level of inventory control in one year. Between the current 22 percent and the 13 percent goal is a 9 percent gap. Better control systems can easily effect a reduction to 17 percent. This gives us $104,000 for cost of goods sold, a savings of $30,000. This is half of the current net.

More on Client Records

There are three elements in client records:

- Average client transaction
- Retention
- Return rate (class balance)

Average client transaction is always open to review. In fact, quarterly reviews of charges are at the core of fiscal stability. A healthy attitude toward the "circle sheet" and staff involvement in the review process will avoid creeping income loss. A 10 percent increase in the ACT can be effected without a concurrent increase in fixed expenses or CoGS. Eighty percent of any increase goes to net.

The most medically significant element is in the distribution of the clients by class.

Class 1 clients are the driving force of the practice. These are people bonded and dedicated to their pets. They also follow the regime required to effect good health. They return for checkups and will work with you to provide the appropriate healthcare. This may involve spreading out treatments such as a class 3 dental this week and the spay next month.

Forty-four percent of the clients of Cool Hand Kitties came in less than once in the last twelve months. Ask yourself if you are providing the appropriate care for all those pets.

Move half of class 2 to class 1 and move half of class 3 to class 2.

Now class 1 is 44 percent, class 2 is 34 percent, and class 3 is 22 percent of the total client population.

And how do they effect this class migration?

(a) Full examinations of all consults, and identification of conditions that need action and/or monitoring—bring all to the attention of the client. (b) Develop a program to address all issues in a timely manner—you may need to offer information about pet insurance. (c) Recall, remind, recover.

(I refer you to *Building the Successful Veterinary Practice: Volume 2: Programs and Procedures.*)

With these changes, Cool Hand Kitties may expand their practice by half without increasing fees.

Remember that lender? This is how you show him you will be expanding services *if* you get into that new facility. It is part of the package.

Expenses

We looked at expenses when we examined inventory and cost of goods sold. Let's look at the expense form again.

Payroll: Don't try to cut the dollar amount. Increase the income and even as the dollar amount goes up the percentage of gross income goes down. Lenders understand this. If your staff doesn't, you need to pursue some remedial economics instruction. But I bet they understand already.

DVM clinician salary	$152,700	25%
Staff wages	$ 42,800	7%
Technician wages	$ 73,300	12%
Admin. dollars	$ 18,300	3%

Rent: Rent is aimed at hard assets. It is paid to keep a roof over the head. When the real estate is exteriorized $42,300 is currently available to pass thru old doc's LLC to support the mortgage. It also means that as the gross income increases so does the ability of the practice to take on more debt and pay it off faster. That, of course, is the intent of the business plan.

| $42,300 | 7% |

Maintenance and repair: Don't mess with maintenance. Even in a new building you have things going "critical" all the time.

$6,100	1%

Continuing education: As the income goes up so does this. This is an investment in services and staff motivation. Continuing education (CE) is not just for DVMs! Even the percentage is not written in stone. As Cool Hand Kitties develops their staff and their associates the overall attitude of the practice alters. Return on investment (ROI) in CE will increase.

$4,200	0.7%

Depreciation: Well, Cool Hand Kitties already knows that this is not expense. It was paid years ago. This is another $11,000 for the ROI.

Advert/cl rel	$ 7,300	1.2%
Legal/accounting	$ 1,800	0.3%
Depreciation/amort	$11,000	1.8%

Consultants: Consultants are good for when you are facing a meltdown or when you have identified a managerial issue in the operation. Consultants are also cool surgical specialists who come in and upgrade your orthopedic prowess. Consultants work with front staff, inpatient technicians, bookkeepers, owner/operators, and lawyers.

$6,100	1%

What do the Cool Hand Kitties have to offer the lender?

Tangible Assets	P&L Report $	Revised $	Adjust to Net
Inventory	18,600	17,600	<7,000>
Equipment	24,000	186,000	+162,000
Client Records	138,000	173,000	+35,000
Total Adjustment to Assets			+$190,000
			(continued)

Net Excess Earnings			
	P&L Report $	Revised $	Adjust to Net
Rent	42,300	-0-	+42,000
Depr/Amort	11,000	-0-	+11,000
CoGS	108,000	79,000	+29,000
Total Adjustment			+$ 82,000
Reported Net			$ 61,000
Revised Net Excess Earnings			$143,000

Note: Liquidity reality check: $12,000 payment per month on a loan at 10.3% for twenty years will service principle and interest on a loan of $1,218,000. But you don't have to blow it all on a mortgage loan.

The Pièce de Résistance: Numbers from the Business Plan

So far you have demonstrated that the practice is a going business concern. It is well run and profitable. It has good client bonding, increasing as programs for revitalizing the existing client base kick in. Now to directly respond to the question of why and how the new facility will be even better for the practice.

In a budget specifically tailored to the style and expertise of Cool Hand Kitties, the whole of it comes together (see table A.1). The practice is client and patient centered. The budget begins with income centers that state what procedures and concerns are the defining activities of the practice. Cool Hand Kitties also serves notice that they are beginning development of further medical procedures. The line is in the budget but there is no fiscal action. Yet.

What is available to the owner to finance the new project?

Rent	$ 25,200
Depreciation	$ 15,700
Net profit	$143,100
Net excess earnings	$184,000

Now you have it all. A strong tangible assets base. A historical and current net excess earnings that can justify securing funding. And a solid projection, based on medical procedures and community demand for services.

Go forth and do well by doing good.

Table A.1 Cool Hand Kitties Veterinary Hospital Budget for 2002

Projection for growth	Projected increase 12.0%	North America averages	Year 2001 actual $611,000	Year 2002 estimate $684,320
	% of income, not avg			
Income centers				
Outpatient professional	22.0	18.4		150,550
Emergency services	0.0	0.0		0
Vaccinations	11.2	11.1		76,644
Diagnostics lab	14.0	12.4		95,805
Diagnostics imaging	2.0	4.2		13,686
Hospital nursing	5.0	4.5		34,216
Boarding	5.0	6.4		34,216
Grooming	2.0	3.7		13,686
Alt therapy	0.0	0.0		0
Surgery w/o anesth	10.0	9.1		68,432
Dentistry	2.8	2.8		19,161
Anesthesia	5.9	3.4		40,375
Nutrition/OTC	4.8	6.5		32,847
Pharmacy/euth	15.3	17.5		104,702
Total income	100.0	100.0		$684,320
Cost of professional services				
Drugs/med supplies	18.0	12.5		123,178
Nutrition/OTC	4.0	4.4		27,373
Lab/diagnostics costs	1.9	1.5		13,002
Boarding expense	1.0	1.3		6,843
Animal waste/disposal	0.2	0.3		1,369
Other	0.5	0.7		3,422

(*continued*)

Table A.1 Cool Hand Kitties Veterinary Hospital Budget for 2002 (*continued*)

	Projected increase	North America	Year 2001	Year 2002
	% of income, not avg			
General and admin expenses				
DVM dollars	22.0	20.5		150,550
Staff dollars	19.0	19.5		130,021
Management/admin dollars	3.0	3.0		20,530
Payroll taxes	6.0	3.1		41,059
Insurance, health	1.0	1.1		6,843
NQA and uniforms	1.0	0.4		6,843
Rent	7.0	6.8		47,902
Office/computer supp	1.5	1.4		10,265
Service contracts	1.0	0.7		6,843
Maintenance and repair	1.0	1.3		6,843
Telephone	1.5	1.1		10,265
Utilities	3.0	1.2		20,530
Postage	1.0	0.7		6,843
Cont. education	0.8	0.8		5,475
Advertising	1.0	1.1		6,843
Charity and discounts	0.5	0.4		3,422
Sales tax	1.0	0.8		6,843
Property taxes	0.3	0.5		2,053
Dues/licenses	0.3	0.4		2,053
Legal/accounting	0.3	0.6		2,053
Bad debt	0.5	0.5		3,422
Bank charges and fees	0.3	0.3		2,053
Insurance, practice	1.0	1.1		6,843
Interest	0.5	1.3		3,422
Depreciation	2.3	0.9		15,739
Consultants	1.0	1.0		6,843
Other	1.0	0.7	100.0	6,843
Total expenses	78.8	71.2	100.0	$539,244

Appendix B

Pre-Architect Feasibility Review

Thomas E. Catanzaro, DVM, MHA, FACHE
Diplomate, American College of Healthcare Executives

When the *AAHA Design Starter Kit* was developed (it's now in third edition), I was very sincere about a practice needing to know what was needed before approaching an architect. These questionnaires were developed with a want-list in mind. Now it is becoming evident that "needs" must also be identified, to balance the "wants." In many cases, a full consultation is needed to get a practice ready for transition into a new facility, but that is *not* the intent of this review. This review is specifically a fast overview of feasibility matched to desires.

> **NOTE: There are no national or regional standards for these numbers; you must learn to measure progress against your own practice's commitment to change and your personal leadership effort.**

Income, Profitability, and Efficiency Trends

	2000	2001	2002	2003
Days open	____	____	____	____
New client visits	____	____	____	____
Total client visits	____	____	____	____
Total patient visits	____	____	____	____
xxxxxxxxxxxxxxxxxxxxxxxxxxxxxxxxxxxxxxxxxxxxxxxxxxxxxxxxxxxxxxxxxxxxxxxxx				
Total income from operations	____	____	____	____
Sales/FTV (doctor)	____	____	____	____
Sales/FTE (staff member)	____	____	____	____
Rent (as % of gross sales)	____	____	____	____
# Transactions	____	____	____	____
Average charge/client	____	____	____	____
Average charge/patient	____	____	____	____
xxxxxxxxxxxxxxxxxxxxxxxxxxxxxxxxxxxxxxxxxxxxxxxxxxxxxxxxxxxxxxxxxxxxxxxxx				
Profit (P&L net)/FTV (doctor)	____	____	____	____
Profit (P&L net)/FTE (staff)	____	____	____	____
xxxxxxxxxxxxxxxxxxxxxxxxxxxxxxxxxxxxxxxxxxxxxxxxxxxxxxxxxxxxxxxxxxxxxxxxx				

PROFILE THE PRACTICE BY USE OF A MEDICAL RECORD AUD

The audit of active medical records within the veterinary practice has traditionally been done by exception; that is, when we get a complaint or ask for help on a difficult case. We have developed an interesting set of tools to allow the medical record audit to become a management tool. The full set is available in the *Recovered Pet & Recovered Client Programs* Signature Series Monograph, available at www.v-p-c.com.

Determine a method to keep track of your progress as you sort through 100 client records. Note we said "client records." When you use 100, the data automatically converts to a percentage, which allows ready comparability to AAHA, AVMA, or other published data. Statistical sampling may indicate that you should pull records from the ----10 to ----19 terminal digits until you get 100, but we have found that 50 or 100 consecutive records work just as well for these instruments. Ensure all patients that belong to each of the 100 clients are included in the record pull.

"SNAPSHOT" CALIBRATION

Catanzaro & Associates, Inc., has evaluated off-site practice valuations and has come to a realization that all things are not always as they seem. The "snapshot valuation," described in *Beyond the Successful Veterinary Practice: Succession Planning and Other Legal Issues*, is based on a specific practice's data, often from the computer, and is based on the buyer-seller, partners, or principals agreeing on the data submitted. Since not all computers "count" the same, nor do all eyes perceive the same, we ask for one additional "litmus test" to assist your (and ours) feasibility review:

a)   Commit to reviewing *all* the "S" (last name) files in the client records.

b)   Smile . . . and get a cup of tea, coffee, or a Coke; you'll need it!

c)   Screen each record in the "S" client files, classify it as one of three categories, and fill in the total:

Clients who have not been in during the past twelve months: . . . . ____

(these are considered active by *your* definition).

Clients who have been in once during the past twelve months: . . . . . . ____

(these may have been in more than once but with each pet only once)

Clients who have been in two or more times during the past

twelve months: . . . .   ____

(pet has been in two or more times in the past twelve months)

d)   Celebrate completing the above task! Pat each other on the back!

e)   Make sure the total of the three numbers in c) above matches the total number of "S" clients (this ensures the data encompasses what you looked at).

COMMENTS:

By pulling 100 client records, you have a 100-percent client number for assessing the pets per household, pet mix, or similar parameters. The patient data comparisons will require a separate math assessment for internal comparisons.

QUICK CLIENT LOYALTY ASSESSMENT:

Count the total number of clients within the "S" file: _____(a)

Count those in "S" that haven't been in during the last FY: _____(b)

Subtract (b) from (a) to get active clients in FY: (a) − (b) = _____(c)

"S" is 10% of client base in USA, so multiply by 10: (c) x 10 = _____(d)

Count the rabies tags (certificates) for the last FY: _____(e)

Divide (e) by (d) to get client response rate to reminders: _____%

* If there are large amounts of new or walk-in clients, compute their percentage of the active client base (c) then subtract from above % to get an adjusted client loyalty impression.

CASELOAD MANAGEMENT PREFERENCES:

- Current number of client relations staff per shift . . . . ____
- Number of active client relations computer terminals . . . . ____
- Number of telephone receptionists . . . . ____
- Current number of exam/consultation/comfort rooms . . . . ____
- Current number of FTE doctors . . . . ____
- Number of exam rooms scheduled per doctor on outpatient . . . . ____
- Current number of outpatient nurses per shift . . . . ____
- Current number of aseptic surgery suites . . . . ____
- Current number of doctors who prefer to do surgery . . . . ____
- Current number of inpatient cages . . . . ____
- Current number of "drop-off" cases per day . . . . ____
- Current number inpatient nursing staff per shift . . . . ____
- Current number of doctors who have special interest in exotics . . . . ____
- Current number of boarding cages (not inpatient) . . . . ____
- Current number of boarding runs (not inpatient) . . . . ____
- Number of animal caretakers dedicated to boarding/wards . . . . ____

PRACTICE PROFILE INQUIRY

FILL IN THE BLANKS:	CHECK ONE:
Based on 168 Manhours/Month/Average	*Community Population Base*

Full-time equivalent DVM _____   Less than 10,000 _____   10,000 - 30,000 _____

Full-time equivalent VHT _____   30,001 - 70,000 _____   70,001 - 120,000 _____

FTE reception staff _____   120,001 - 190,000 _____   90,001 - 260,000 _____

FTE technician assistant staff _____   260,001 - 500,000 _____   500,001 or more _____

Practice manager _____

Grooming staff _____

Boarding staff _____

Other staff _____

Proprietorship __, Partnership __, Corporation (circle which: C, S, LLC) __, Number of years _____

PC-leased building _____   Third-party lease _____   Years in lease _____

Purchased facility _____   Year built _____   Square feet _____

Replacement value of: Facility $_____   Equipment $___

Services by appointment only _____,   Over 50% walk-in _____,   Combination _____

Average number of clients per month _____   Number of boarding cases _____

Record system used _____   Filing system used _____

Computer system type _____

Electric cash register type _____

Affiliations and Associations:	Doctor	Receptionists	Technicians	Manager
Local VMA	___	___	___	___
County VMA	___	___	___	___
State VMA	___	___	___	___
AVMA	___	___	___	___
AAHA	___	___	___	___
VHMA	___	___	___	___
ABKA	___	___	___	___

Specialty Board ___ list: _____

GENERAL VETERINARY PRACTICE INQUIRY

Please check or fill in as indicated:

1. The first 5 digits of my zip code are _____
2. Type of practice: Companion Animal _____ Mixed _____ Equine _____ Food Animal _____
3. Number of veterinarians: Full-time _____ Part-time _____
4. The practice is ___ years old and is: Freestanding _____ Mall _____ Shopping Center _____
5. My area is: Urban _____ Suburban _____ Rural _____
6. Number of receptionists: Full-time _____ Part-time _____
7. Number of technicians: Full-time _____ Part-time _____
8. Number of other nonprofessional staff (cleaning, etc.): _____
9. Our building is cleaned by outside services: Yes _____ No ___
10. Our hospital has _____ square feet and _____ exam rooms
11. We have point-of-purchase display(s): No ___; Yes ___ and it covers _____ square feet
12. We offer boarding: No __; Yes__ and we can accommodate: ___dogs, ___ cats, ___ birds
13. We accept credit cards: No___; Yes___ and our MC/VISA discount rate is _____%.
14. In the previous 12 months, the owner(s) averaged _____ weeks vacation (excluding C.E.)
15. We have a hospital administrator: No___; Yes___ at Full-time __ Part-time __ Salary $_____
16. We average _____ patients/transactions (circle one) per week
17. We have _____ transactions per month
18. In the previous 12 months, gross was: $_____
    Incorporated? Yes _____ No _____
    Our gross is: Up _____ Down _____ at _____% from last year
    Why do you think this occurred? _____
    _____
    _____
19. There are _____ owner(s); the net to owner(s) (combined) in previous 12 months: $_____
20. Our annual payroll (excluding veterinarians) is: $_____
21. Our highest paid non-doctor staff member is _____ at $_____
22. Our total W-2 payroll for veterinarians is: $_____
23. Veterinarian(s) salaries (including yours): #1 $_____ #2 $_____ #3 $_____
    #4 $_____ #5 $_____ #6 $_____ #7 $_____ #8 $_____
24. Cost of drugs and supplies for previous 12 months: $_____
25. Approximate resale inventory value on hand: $_____
26. Our land, building, and equipment today would sell for: $_____
27. Our building is: ___ Owned ___ Rented; our monthly rent is: $_____
28. Our legal fees in the previous 12 months were: $_____
29. Our accounting fees in the previous 12 months were: $_____
30. Our accounts receivable are: $_____
31. Computer: No ___ Yes _____ Software vendor name: _____
    We are on the net: VIN ___ @ _____ NOAH ___ @ _____ Other ___ @ _____
32. Computer investment: Hardware $_____ Software $_____
33. Advertising budget: Yellow Pages $_____ Newspaper $_____ Other ___ $ _____
34. The percentage of our clients using pet health insurance is: _____%

COMPUTER INQUIRY

_____ I plan to purchase a computer system within the next year.
_____ I use an in-house computer system.   Purchase date _____/_____/_____

Type of computer hardware system used: # terminals ____, # printers ____ & type _____

Hardware type: _____

Type of computer software:
_____ ALIS•VET (InformaVet)
_____ AviMark (Schein)
_____ Doty
_____ DVM Manager
_____ Idexx Cornerstone
_____ Idexx AVS
_____ Impromed Computer System
_____ Jade (Colgate)
_____ V-Boss
_____ Vet Tech
_____ Visionarian
_____ WinVet_____ Other_____

Operating system used:
_____ Windows ____ '95 ____ '98 ____ 32 bit ____ Earlier version
_____ NT_____
_____ Unix
_____ Xenix
_____ Other_____

Can your system perform the following functions:

_____ AAHA Chart of Accounts   ____ text for Improved Chart of Accounts (*Building the Successful Veterinary Practice: Volume 2: Programs and Procedures,* Iowa State Press)
_____ Reminders: _____ One   _____ Multiple   _____ Variable factors
_____ Recalls
_____ Billing: _____ Invoicing   _____ Fee compliance
_____ Accounting (maintain a general ledger)
_____ Inventory control
_____ Pharmacy labels
_____ Controlled substance accountability (with password, yes____, no ____)
_____ Word processing (which _____)
_____ Spread Sheet (which _____)

Would you use computer-assisted diagnostic assistance in your practice:
_____ Yes   _____ No   _____ Don't know

MARKETING INQUIRY

Please check the columns appropriate to your facility:
A = Active; I = Inactive; N = Never Used

Program status:

A	I	N	
___	___	___	Annual life-cycle consultation
___	___	___	Giardia screening
___	___	___	Travel with your pet safety program
___	___	___	Sympathy acknowledgment
___	___	___	Grief counseling
___	___	___	Donate to a memorial foundation (e.g., Delta Foundation)
___	___	___	Nutritional counseling — pet weight-loss program
___	___	___	Pet selection consultation
___	___	___	Puppy/kitten health wellness package
___	___	___	Puppy/kitten "first visit" packets
___	___	___	Behavior management assistance
___	___	___	Geriatric reminder, arthritis program
___	___	___	FeLV reminders
___	___	___	Lyme reminders
___	___	___	Rabies vaccination reminders
___	___	___	Multivalent vaccine reminders
___	___	___	Heartworm
___	___	___	Annual blood test
___	___	___	Annual physical
___	___	___	Program (flea) reminders
___	___	___	Six-month fecal reminders
___	___	___	Dental reminders
___	___	___	Newsletters
___	___	___	Video education
___	___	___	Practice-specific client handouts
___	___	___	Merchandising of pet products
___	___	___	Hospital tours
___	___	___	Open house for clients
___	___	___	School PR programs
___	___	___	Youth group support programs
___	___	___	Medical/surgical/treatment consent form
___	___	___	Euthanasia consent form
___	___	___	Financial (obligation to pay) consent form
___	___	___	Boarding agreement
___	___	___	Designated child-care areas in lobby
___	___	___	Brochure on your facility
___	___	___	All doctors' pictures/biographies displayed in hospital
___	___	___	Hospital pictures displayed in reception area or examination room scrapbook
___	___	___	Staff recognition displayed in the hospital
___	___	___	Nonhazardous parking areas with well-directed traffic patterns
___	___	___	Outside practice signage that clearly and professionally identifies the facility

HUMAN RESOURCE INQUIRY

_____ Number of animal technicians or trained hospital staff (full-time)
_____ a. Licensed/certified/registered   _____ b. Job trained
_____ Number of staff members assigned to reception area (full-time)
_____ Caretaker staff (if different from above)
_____ Groomer
_____ Bookkeeper
_____ Hospital administrator
_____ Marketing manager
_____ Number of support staff not specified/part-time

Proper training, education, evaluation, supervision, and benefits motivate personnel and encourage productivity. The hospital director should provide for the coverage of these responsibilities.

Please note if the following suggestions are used in your practice:
_____ Staff member benefit and responsibilities manual (employee personnel handbook)
_____ AAHA training tapes
_____ AVMA Client Link VCR tapes
_____ AVMA receptionist "Crisp" books
_____ Well-planned on-the-job training
_____ Written job descriptions, *with* or *without* performance standards - (circle one)
_____ Staff productivity data (sales per FTE, etc.)
_____ Hospital technical handbook for staff member
_____ Client information handbook
_____ Regular or periodic staff meetings
_____ Out-of-house training sessions (e.g., national meetings) for support staff
_____ Continuing para-veterinary training or administrative courses (local level)
_____ Distance learning programs
_____ Animal caretaker or technician assistant monthly training program
_____ Written performance review
_____ Verbal performance review
_____ Staff uniforms
_____ Paid vacations
_____ Sick time allowance
_____ Personal time
_____ Life insurance
_____ Medical insurance
_____ Pension or profit-sharing plans
_____ Paid holidays
_____ Bonus plans
_____ Cafeteria benefit package
_____ Pet care for employees
_____ Child care for employees
Other _____
_____
_____

FISCAL REALITIES - or - THE OWNER'S COMPENSATION FORMULA!

There are three "salaries" (besides rental payments) which every veterinarian who is a practice owner should be drawing on a monthly or quarterly basis . . . are you?

PART 1. Clinical duties salary at current rate of training, hours worked and years of experience (+/- $45,000 first year, $4,000/yr raise for 5 yrs)(maximum compensation is 23% of production). . . . .$ _____

PART 2. Salary for management duties, hospital administration functions, and overall business responsibilities according to hours worked and pay scale of region (+/- administration/management is 10% of gross, including CPA, lawyer, personnel, bookkeeping, job replacement cycles, inventory management, etc., with 2.5-3.25% of gross for hospital manager) . . . . $ _____

PART 3. Return on investment, taking into consideration proper investment rate for high competency, small business, investment risk situations (+/- occupancy cost @ 6-11%, ROI @ medical CPI plus 6% - or - about 11-16% in the new millennium) . . . .$ _____

COMPENSATION FROM ABOVE . . . . . $ _____

There is more to the owner's compensation than what the W-2 reports to the IRS each year, so look at the total compensation in this formula for your "fiscal reality."

Adjusted Owner's Income (AOI)

All salaries/draw to owner veterinarians	$_____
+ all owner fringe benefits	$_____
+ all profit sharing to owner	$_____
+ depreciation	$_____
+ excess auto expense	$_____
+ excess continuing education	$_____
+ excess rent (above fair level)	$_____
+ any hidden income or draws	$_____

* SUBTOTAL OF AOI DATA . . . . $ _____

* Excess CE defined as greater than 0.8% gross or in excess of $1,800 per veterinarian.
* Excess rent is usually that over 10% of gross revenues.
* Excess auto is generally amounts over 30% of vehicle value.

Owner's Average Income Computation: Adjusted owners income subtotal
                                                              Number of owners

HINT: The difference between the compensation total from above and the AOI (which is a form of ROI) is what needs to be addressed in the annual cash budget (programmed-based) planning process.

PROGRAM PROCEDURES - AN "IN DETAIL" ASSESSMENT OF TRENDS

CONDITION MO	J	F	M	A	M	J	J	A	S	O							
Anaerobic culture																	
ATCH stimulation																	
Autoimmune profile																	
Blood pressure check																	
CBC																	
Cerebral spinal tap																	
Conjunctival cytology																	
Cruciate diagnosis																	
Cytology, general																	
Direct stool smear																	
Echocardiography																	
Endoscopic exam																	
Erhlichia exam																	
Eyelid disticaisis exam																	
Fecal flotations																	
FeLV tests																	
Glaucoma exam																	
Glucose tolerance																	
Kidney biopsy																	
Liver biopsy																	
Lymph node biopsy																	
Lecroix-Zepp surgery																	
Necropsy																	
Shirmer tear test																	
Skin biopsy																	
Skin scrape/culture																	
Transtracheal wash																	
Urine cytology																	

FACILITY "DREAM" RESOURCE INQUIRY

PLAN:

Remodel owned facility ____, Remodel leasehold ____, Storefront build-out ____,
Build at same site ____, Build on other owned property ____, Build at new site ____,
General practice ____, Specialty practice ____, Urgent care (emergency) practice ____.

CAPTIALIZATION:

Bank ready to loan money ____, Other: _____
Equity leverage available: $_____,___% down payment available, Other:
_____
Desire to cash flow finance ____, Other: _____

CLIENT ACCESS DESIRES:

Morning drop-off ____, Evening____, Saturday only weekend, Sunday weekend ____,
24/7 access ____, Walk-ins welcomed ____, Mixed ____, Cat & dog ____, Exotics ____,

DELIVERY CHANGES PLANNED:

High-density scheduling: _____,
Outpatient nurses: _____,
Zoning of the hospital operations (inpatient, outpatient): _____,
Drop-off increases: _____,
Boarding vs guest resort: _____,
Urgent care vs appointments only: _____,
Hours of operation: _____,
House call/ambulatory: _____,
Community affiliation with other providers: _____,
Other: _____,

_____
_____
_____
_____

Appendix C

2002 Building Costs
(National Building Cost Manual)

NOT MANY VETERINARY practices have access to the *National Building Cost Manual,* simply because they do not know it exists. We have included an extract of the 2002 *National Building Cost Manual* in this book, not as a yardstick, but as an example of what veterinary practices "should cost." The web site with the most current construction cost data can be found at www.building-cost.net.

In veterinary medicine, we have always had rules of thumb to estimate construction costs; they have been provided by experienced veterinary facility architects and thumbnail reports in our journals. This is not the best yardstick for computing costs for your new facility, since even the number of outside corners changes the cost, as do geographic variances. We have usually planned on the second floor offices and meeting space in a veterinary hospital to cost between fifty-five dollars and seventy-five dollars a square foot (about 50 percent of the main floor), while basements are only 25–35 percent of the cost of the main floor. Boarding facilities should be less than half the main floor, but with the abundance of VIP resorts, exploration zones, and boutique plans we are seeing, even those factors have become highly variable. Even these basic factors change with the amount of finish and detailing that is required for occupancy.

When we negotiate for a building loan, we have three components that we ask for in the term sheet (the bank bid of the loan). First is the building loan itself, usually within a couple of points of the Treasury Note rate. Second is an unsecured line of credit for the equipment, which will self-collateralize as equipment is procured, thereby keeping the interest rates down. The third component is the contingency line of credit, usually about two months' operating capital, and hopefully it will never be used. As we assist our clients in negotiating for a loan package, other elements come onto the table: interest on bank card rates, cost and/or combining of sweep accounts, interest on daily sweeps, banking services for staff, and a host of other bank offerings. These banking elements are usually very negotiable for "best rates" when an established practice is expanding, and less negotiable for a new practitioner entering the area. We have also negotiated a D&B (Dun & Bradstreet) review in lieu of a Class I Environmental Review when the property has a "community known" history, a savings of more than $6,000.

Veterinary design has many factors, and experience does not always equate with logic. In one case we had a call from an old client who had gone off and negotiated with an architect for new facility design without using our assistance. He called us when it "did not feel right." He had been caught up in the "increased capacity" mentality and was doubling the number of consultation rooms as well as building a mega-design with curved walls and an abundance of glass block to "let the light in." Because he was in a location with geographic boundaries on every side, and he was staying in same area, we questioned his current "fill rate" of consultation rooms; he had never even looked at his own history. When we assessed his fill rates, he was at only 55 percent capacity at his existing facility. He was even considering leasing his current facility out to another veterinarian when the new building was complete, which would have diluted his demographic market further, considering the severe geographic limitations of the area. Needless to say, he then considered the $80,000 already spent with the architect as a great learning experience, downscaled his plans, using the same architect but now with knowledge of what was needed for a practice-specific twenty-year growth plan, and sublet the old practice facility to a grooming and boarding operation.

In another case, a four-million-dollar bid was offered on a design-build veterinary hospital, we got the quote, ran the numbers, and challenged the cost estimate. We could only find about $2.26 million in costs using the national factors, and the design-build group stated within twenty-four hours that they had miscalculated, and it was in fact about $2.5 million. Concurrently, their architect fees dropped from $400,000 to $226,000 in itemized bidding (showing how easy the 10 percent computation really can be). A savings of $174,000 for less than one day of consulting support repaid our client many times over for having a skilled second opinion in their corner.

In a third case, the architects had designed a flat roof on a Colorado veterinary practice building, although the veterinarian wanted a pitched roof. In a joint conference, the architects stated that it was for a cost savings, and when confronted with the cost difference, stated they did not know unless they contacted the contractor. We knew from experience that the cost was about three dollars a square foot to go from a flat to a pitched roof (which is very desirable in snow country), confronted the architects right then and there, and they agreed that was about right. We had the architects inform the client, who was also sitting at the table, that the cost was about $15,000, on a building already estimated at costing $750,000. Needless to say, today she has a pitched roof on a wonderful veterinary facility.

In a final example, a mixed animal practice was building a new companion animal facility with a veterinary-specific architect, and when we reviewed the plans, we saw immediately that the companion animal practice had been built with a chute system called "too many hallways." We reduced the circulation space by 20 percent, keeping most every other feature as originally drawn. Since this was a "percentage of cost" based architect, that circulation space reduction of more than 1,000 sq. ft. cost the architect more than $140,000 in design fees. The architect told me directly that if I was going to do architecture, he was going to start doing consulting. I responded that designing a poor-flowing hospital was consulting of the worst kind; it was an overhead expense without a return on investment. He has seldom tried to add excess hallways for a client of ours ever since, although we do have to remind him occasionally that veterinary teaching hospital hallways are for students, and specialty hospitals do not require a hallway system to divide fiefdoms if there is good facility governance (chapter 2 of *Veterinary Management in Transition: Preparing for the Twenty-First Century*).

Studies of the Myers-Briggs personality factors of most architects show many are introverts by nature and do not negotiate very well. In most cases, a well-informed practice owner (or practice owner-to-be) can negotiate a very equitable design deal when he or she comes armed with knowledge and a clear picture of what he or she wants. This appendix is designed to give readers some information and costs that they can use when interviewing architects to decide with whom they will be discussing their plans for the next twelve months (the minimum design-build time with zoning and permit cycles in most communities).

Explanation of Cost Tables

This manual provides construction or replacement costs for a wide variety of residential, commercial, industrial, agricultural, and military buildings. For your convenience and to avoid possible errors, all the cost and reference information you need for each building type is listed with the primary cost figures for that building. After reading this and the following pages you should be able to turn directly to any building type and make an error-free estimate or appraisal.

The costs are per square foot of floor area for the basic building and additional costs for optional or extra components that differ from building to building. Building shape, floor area, design elements, materials used, and overall quality influence the basic structure cost. These and other cost variables are isolated for the building types. Components included in the basic square foot cost are listed with each building type. Instructions for using the basic building costs are included above the cost tables. These instructions include a list of components that may have to be added to the basic cost to find the total cost for your structure.

The figures in this manual are intended to reflect the amount that would be paid by the end user of a building as of mid 2002.

They show the total construction cost including all design fees, permits, and the builder's supervision, overhead, and profit. These figures do not include land value, site development costs, or the cost of modifying unusual soil conditions or grades.

Building Quality

Structures vary widely in quality and the quality of construction is the most significant variable in the finished cost. For estimating purposes the structure should be placed in one or more quality classes. These classes are numbered from 1 which is the highest quality generally encountered. Each section of this manual has a page describing typical specifications which define the quality class. Each number class has been assigned a word description (such as best, good, average, or low) for convenience and to help avoid possible errors.

The quality specifications do not reflect some design features and construction details that can make building both more desirable and more costly. When substantially more than basic design elements are present, and when these elements add significantly to the cost, it is appropriate to classify the quality of the building as higher than would be warranted by the materials used in construction. Thanks to the Internet, "built-in" components, e.g., cabinets and counters, can be found very economically, such as at www.BuyNewKitchen.com and similar sites; ensure you review these Internet resources with your contractor to ensure the highest quality at the best cost.

Many structures do not fall into a single class and have features of two quality classes. The tables have "half classes" which apply to structures which have some features of one class and some features of a higher or lower class. Classify a building into a "half class" when the quality elements are fairly evenly divided between two classes. Generally quality elements do not vary widely in a single building. For example, it would be unusual to find a top quality single family residence with minimum quality roof cover. The most weight should be given to the quality elements that have the greatest cost. For example, the type of wall and roof framing or the quality of interior finish are more significant than the roof cover or bathroom wall finish. Careful evaluation may determine that certain structures fall into two distinct classes. In this case the cost of each part of the building should be evaluated separately.

Building Shapes

Shape classification considers any cost differences that arise from variations in building outline. Shape classification considerations vary somewhat with different building types. Where the building shape often varies widely between buildings and shape has a significant effect on the building cost, basic building costs are given for several shapes. Use the table that most closely matches the shape of the building you are evaluating. If the shape falls near the division between two basic building cost tables, it is appropriate to average the square foot cost from those two tables.

Area of Buildings

The basic building cost tables reflect the fact that larger buildings generally cost less per square foot than smaller buildings. The cost tables are based on square foot areas which include the following:

1. All floor area within and including the exterior walls of the main building.
2. Inset areas such as vestibules, entrances or porches outside of the exterior wall but under the main roof.
3. Any enclosed additions, annexes or lean-tos with a square foot cost greater than three-fourths of the square foot cost of the main building.

Select the basic building cost listed below the area which falls closest to the actual area of your building. If the area of your building falls nearly mid-way between two listed building areas, it is appropriate to average the square foot costs for the listed areas.

Wall Heights

Building costs are based on the wall heights given in the instructions for each building cost table. Wall height for the various floors of a building are computed as follows: The basement is measured from the bottom of floor slab to the bottom of the first floor slab or joist. The main floor or first floor extends from the bottom of the first floor slab or joist to the top of the roof slab or ceiling joist. Upper floors are measured from the top of the floor slab or floor joist to the top of the roof slab or ceiling joist. These measurements may be illustrated as follows:

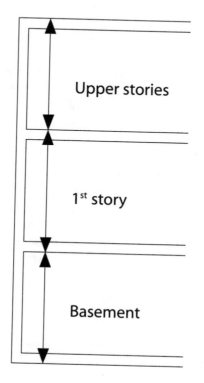

Square foot costs of most building design types must be adjusted if the actual wall height differs from the listed wall height. Wall height adjustment tables are included for buildings requiring this adjustment. Wall height adjustment tables list square foot costs for a foot of difference in perimeter wall height of buildings of various areas. The amount applicable to the actual building area is added or deducted for each foot of difference from the basic wall height.

Buildings such as residences, medical-dental buildings, funeral homes and convalescent hospitals usually have a standard 8-foot ceiling except in chapels or day room areas. If a significant cost difference exists due to a wall height variation, this factor should be considered in establishing the quality class.

Other Adjustments

A common wall exists when two buildings share one wall. Common wall adjustments are made by deducting the in-place cost of the exterior wall finish plus one-half of the in-place cost of the structural portion of the common wall area.

If an owner has no ownership in a wall, the in-place cost of the exterior wall finish plus the in-place cost of the structural portion of the wall should be deducted from the total building costs. Suggested common wall and no wall ownership costs are included for many of the building types.

Some square foot costs include the cost of expensive veneer finishes on the entire perimeter wall. When these buildings butt against other buildings, adjustments should be made for the lack of this finish. Where applicable, linear foot cost deductions are provided.

The square foot costs in this manual are based on composite costs of total buildings including usual work room or storage areas. They are intended to be applied on a 100% basis to the total building area even though certain areas may or may not have interior finish. Only in rare instances will it be necessary to modify the square foot cost of a portion of a building.

Multiple story buildings usually share a common roof structure and cover, a common foundation and common floor or ceiling structures. The costs of these components are included in the various floor levels as follows:

The first or main floor includes the cost of a floor structure built at ground level, foundation costs for a one-story building, a complete ceiling and roof structure, and a roof cover. The basement includes the basement floor structure and the difference between the cost of the first floor structure built at ground level and its cost built over a basement. The second floor includes the difference between the cost of a foundation for a one-story building and the cost of a foundation for a two-story building and the cost of the second story floor structure.

Location Adjustments

The figures in this manual are intended as national averages for metropolitan areas of the United States. Use the information starting on page 207 to adapt the basic building costs to any area listed. Frequently building costs outside metro-politan areas are 2% to 6% lower if skilled, productive, lower cost labor is avail-able in the area. The factors on pages 207–115 can be applied to nearly all the square foot costs and some of the "additional" costs in this book.

Depreciation

Depreciation is the loss in value of a structure from all causes and is caused primarily by three forms of obsolescence: (1) physical, (2) functional, and (3) economic.

Physical obsolescence is the deterioration of building components such as paint, carpets or roofing. This deterioration may be partially curable. Several tables in the *Building Cost Manual* consider only typical physical obsolescence. Individual adjustments will have to be made for functional and economic obsolescence.

Functional obsolescence is due to a deficiency or inadequacy in some char-acteristic of the building, such as too few bathrooms for the number of bed-rooms, or some excess, such as a 10 foot ceiling in a residence. This obso-lescence may be curable. The tables do not include functional obsolescence considerations.

Economic obsolescence is caused by factors not directly concerning the structure, but rather, by adverse environmental factors, resulting in loss of desirability. Examples include the obsolescence of a store in an area of declin-ing economic activity, or obsolescence resulting from governmental regulation changing the zone of an area. Because this kind of obsolescence is particular-ly difficult to measure, it is not included in the tables.

"Effective age" considers all forms of depreciation. It may be less than chronological age, if recently remodeled or improved, or more than the actual age, if deterioration is particularly bad. Though effective age is not considered in the physical life tables, it may yield a better picture of a structure's life than the actual physical age. Once the effective age is determined, considering phys-ical, functional and economic deterioration, use the percent good tables on page 40 or 200 of the *Building Cost Manual* to determine the present value of a depreciated building. Present value is the result of multiplying the replace-ment cost (found by using the cost tables) by the appropriate percent good.

Limitations

This manual will be a useful reference for anyone who has to develop budg-et estimates or replacement costs for buildings. Anyone familiar with construc-tion estimating understands that even very competent estimators with complete working drawings, full specifications and precise labor and material costs can disagree on the cost of a building. Frequently exhaustive estimates for even rel-atively simple structures can vary 5% or more. The range of competitive bids on some building projects is as much as 10%. Estimating costs is not an exact science and there is room for legitimate disagreement on what the "right" cost is. This manual can not help you do in a few minutes what skilled estimators may not be able to do in several hours. This manual will help you determine a reasonable replacement or construction cost for most buildings. It is not intended as a substitute for judgement or as a replacement for sound professional practice, but should prove a valuable aid to developing an informed opinion of value.

Area Modification Factors

Construction costs are higher in some cities than in other cities. Add or deduct the percentage shown in the table that starts on page 207 in this book to adapt the costs to your job site. Adjust your estimated total project cost by the percentage shown for the appropriate city in this table to find your total estimated cost. Where no percentage is shown it means no modification is required. Factors for Canada adjust to Canadian dollars.

These percentages were compiled by comparing the construction cost of buildings in nearly 600 communities throughout North America. Because these percentages are based on completed projects, they consider all construction cost variables, including labor, equipment and material cost, labor productivity, climate, job conditions and markup.

Modification factors are listed alphabetically by state. Areas within each state are listed by the first three digits of the postal zip code. For convenience, one representative city is identified in each zip code or range of zip codes.

These percentages are composites of many costs and will not necessarily be accurate when estimating the cost of any particular part of a building. But when used to modify costs for an entire structure, they should improve the accuracy of your estimates.

Building Cost Historical Index

Use this table to find the approximate current dollar building cost when the actual cost is known for any year since 1935. Multiply the figure listed below for the building type and year of construction by the known cost. The result is the estimated 2002 construction cost.

Square foot costs include the following components: Foundations as required for normal soil conditions. Floor, wall and roof structures. Interior floor, wall and ceiling finishes. Exterior wall finish and roof cover. Interior partitions. Cabinets, doors and windows. Basic electrical systems and lighting fixtures. Rough plumbing and fixtures. Permits and fees. Contractors' mark-up. In addition to the above components, costs for buildings with more than 10,000 feet include the cost of lead shielding for typical X-ray rooms.

Medical-Dental Buildings—Masonry or Concrete—Exterior Suite Entrances, Length Less Than 2 Times Width

Estimating Procedure

1. Use these figures to estimate medical, dental, surgical, and similar professional buildings in which access to each office suite is through an exterior entrance. Buildings in this section have more plumbing fixtures per square

Area modification factors: percentages added or subtracted to modify construction costs, listed by state

Alabama Average		**-14**
350-352	Birmingham	-13
354	Tuscaloosa	-13
355	Jasper	-13
356	Sheffield	-16
357	Scottsboro	-16
358	Huntsville	-13
359	Gadsden	-13
360-361	Montgomery	-13
362	Anniston	-13
363	Dothan	-16
364	Evergreen	-16
365-366	Mobile	-11
367	Selma	-13
368	Auburn	-13
369	Bellamy	-13

Alaska Average		**43**
995	Anchorage	30
996	King Salmon	51
997	Fairbanks	45
998	Juneau	44
999	Ketchikan	46

Arizona Average		**1**
850	Phoenix	-1
852-853	Mesa	-1
855	Douglas	-1
856-857	Tucson	-2
859	Show Low	4
860	Flagstaff	-1
863	Prescott	3
864	Kingman	3
865	Chambers	3

Arkansas Average		**-12**
716	Pine Bluff	-11
717	Camden	-12
718	Hope	-12
719	Hot Springs	-12
720-722	Little Rock	-12
723	West Memphis	-12
724	Jonesboro	-12
725	Batesville	-12
726	Harrison	-12
727	Fayetteville	-11
728	Russellville	-9
729	Fort Smith	-9

California Average		**14**
900-901	Los Angeles	14
902-905	Inglewood	13
906	Whittier	13
907-908	Long Beach	14
910-912	Pasadena	13
913-916	Van Nuys	13
917-918	Alhambra	13
919-921	San Diego	10
922	El Centro	10
923-925	San Bernardino	13
926-928	Anaheim	13
930	Oxnard	11
931	Santa Barbara	11
932-933	Bakersfield	13
934	Lompoc	11
935	Mojave	10
936-938	Fresno	13
939	Salinas	14
940	Sunnyvale	17
941	San Francisco	24
942	Sacramento	10
943-944	San Mateo	16
945-947	Oakland	16
948	Richmond	22
949	Novato	22
950-951	San Jose	17
952-953	Stockton	11
954	Santa Rosa	22
955	Eureka	16
956-958	Rancho Cordova	11
959	Marysville	11
960	Redding	12
961	Herlong	18

Colorado Average		**-1**
800-801	Aurora	-3
802-804	Denver	0
805	Longmont	-3
806	Greeley	-3
807	Fort Morgan	-3
808-809	Colorado Springs	1
810	Pueblo	-4
811	Pagosa Springs	-3
812	Salida	-3
813	Durango	-3
814-815	Grand Junction	-3

(*continued*)

207

816	Glenwood Spgs	-3		303	Atlanta	-1
	Ski Resorts	13		304	Statesboro	-11
				305	Buford	-11
Connecticut Average		**9**		306	Athens	-11
060-061	Hartford	9		307	Calhoun	-11
062	West Hartford	9		308-309	Augusta	-17
063	Norwich	8		310	Dublin	-11
064	Fairfield	10		311	Fort Valley	-11
065	New Haven	10		312	Macon	-11
066	Bridgeport	8		313	Hinesville	-13
067	Waterbury	11		314	Savannah	-13
068-069	Stamford	11		315	Kings Bay	-12
				316	Valdosta	-11
Delaware Average		**3**		317	Albany	-13
197	Newark	3		318-319	Columbus	-16
198	Wilmington	4				
199	Dover	3		**Hawaii Average**		**34**
				967	Ewa	34
District of Columbia		**2**		967	Halawa Heights	34
200-201	Washington	2		967	Hilo	34
202-205	Washington	2		967	Lualualei	34
				967	Mililani Town	34
Florida Average		**-8**		967	Pearl City	34
320	Saint Augustine	-10		967	Wahiawa	34
321	Daytona Beach	-10		967	Waianae	34
322	Jacksonville	-3		967	Wailuku	34
323	Tallahassee	-14		968	Alimanu	34
324	Panama City	-13		968	Honolulu	34
325	Pensacola	-13		968	Kailua	35
326	Gainesville	-10				
327	Altamonte Spgs	-1		**Idaho Average**		**-6**
328	Orlando	-1		832	Pocatello	-6
329	Melbourne	-1		833	Sun Valley	-5
330-332	Miami	-6		834	Idaho Falls	-6
333	Fort Lauderdale	-1		835	Lewiston	-8
334	W Palm Beach	-1		836	Meridian	-8
335-336	Tampa	-11		837	Boise	-6
337	St Petersburg	-11		838	Coeur d'Alene	-2
338	Lakeland	-10				
339	Fort Myers	-10		**Illinois Average**		**6**
342	Bradenton	-10		600	Arlington Hts	6
344	Ocala	-10		601	Carol Stream	10
346	Brooksville	-10		602	Quincy	6
347	Saint Cloud	-10		603	Oak Park	6
349	Fort Pierce	-10		604	Joliet	6
				605	Aurora	6
Georgia Average		**-11**		606-608	Chicago	10
300-302	Marietta	-1		609	Kankakee	5

Area modification factors: percentages to be added or subtracted (*continued*)

610-611	Rockford	2		526	Burlington	-5
612	Green River	5		527-528	Davenport	-2
613	Peru	6				
614	Galesburg	5		**Kansas Average**		**-5**
615-616	Peoria	6		660-662	Kansas City	-5
617	Bloomington	5		664-666	Topeka	-5
618-619	Urbana	6		667	Fort Scott	-5
620	Granite City	5		668	Emporia	-6
622	Belleville	3		669	Concordia	-5
623	Decatur	5		670-672	Wichita	-4
624	Lawrenceville	6		673	Independence	-5
625-627	Springfield	6		674	Salina	-5
628	Centralia	5		675	Hutchinson	-6
629	Carbondale	5		676	Hays	-5
				677	Colby	-5
Indiana Average		**3**		678	Dodge City	-5
460-462	Indianapolis	3		679	Liberal	-5
463-464	Gary	4				
465-466	South Bend	4		**Kentucky Average**		**-4**
467-468	Fort Wayne	4		400-402	Louisville	-5
469	Kokomo	3		403-406	Lexington	-5
470	Aurora	3		407-409	London	-7
471	Jeffersonville	3		410	Covington	-5
472	Columbus	4		411-412	Ashland	-5
473	Muncie	4		413-414	Campton	-5
474	Bloomington	4		415-416	Pikeville	-5
475	Jasper	1		417-418	Hazard	-5
476-477	Evansville	1		420	Paducah	-5
478	Terre Haute	4		421	Bowling Green	-5
479	Lafayette	4		422	Hopkinsville	-4
				423	Owensboro	-5
Iowa Average		**-4**		424	White Plains	-3
500-503	Des Moines	1		425-426	Somerset	-3
504	Mason City	-4		427	Elizabethtown	-3
505	Fort Dodge	-4				
506-507	Waterloo	-4		**Louisiana Average**		**-4**
508	Creston	-4		700-701	New Orleans	1
510	Cherokee	-4		703	Houma	1
511	Sioux City	-4		704	Mandeville	-6
512	Sheldon	-4		705	Lafayette	-5
513	Spencer	-4		706	Lake Charles	-5
514	Carroll	-5		707-708	Baton Rouge	-5
515	Council Bluffs	-4		710	Minden	-8
516	Shenandoah	-5		711	Shreveport	-6
520	Dubuque	-4		712	Monroe	-6
522-524	Cedar Rapids	-4		713-714	Alexandria	-6
521	Decorah	-4				
525	Ottumwa	-4				

(*continued*)

Maine Average		**-4**
039-040	Brunswick	-2
041	Portland	-2
042	Auburn	-4
043	Augusta	-4
044	Bangor	-6
045	Bath	-4
046	Cutler	-4
047	Northern Area	-4
048	Camden	-5
049	Dexter	-4
Maryland Average		**0**
206-207	Laurel	2
208-209	Bethesda	0
210-212	Baltimore	0
214	Annapolis	1
215	Cumberland	0
216	Church Hill	0
217	Frederick	0
218	Salisbury	0
219	Elkton	0
Massachusetts Average		**15**
015-016	Ayer	15
010	Chicopee	15
011	Springfield	15
012	Pittsfield	15
013	Northfield	15
014	Fitchburg	14
017	Bedford	15
018	Lawrence	15
019	Dedham	15
020	Hingham	16
021-022	Boston	16
023-024	Brockton	15
025	Nantucket	15
026	Centerville	15
027	New Bedford	15
Michigan Average		**6**
480	Royal Oak	7
481-482	Detroit	6
483	Pontiac	6
484-485	Flint	6
486-487	Saginaw	1
488-489	Lansing	6
490-491	Battle Creek	7

492	Jackson	6
493-495	Grand Rapids	7
496	Traverse City	6
497	Grayling	6
498-499	Marquette	1
Minnesota Average		**5**
550-551	St Paul	9
553-555	Minneapolis	9
556-558	Duluth	3
559	Rochester	5
560	Mankato	5
561	Magnolia	5
562	Wilmar	5
563	St Cloud	5
564	Brainerd	5
565	Fergus Falls	5
566	Bemidji	5
567	Thief River Falls	5
Mississippi Average		**-13**
386	Clarksdale	-14
387	Greenville	-5
388	Tupelo	-14
389	Greenwood	-14
390-392	Jackson	-14
393	Meridian	-14
394	Laurel	-14
395	Gulfport	-12
396	McComb	-12
397	Columbus	-16
Missouri Average		**1**
630-631	St Louis	5
633	Saint Charles	5
634	Hannibal	1
635	Kirksville	1
636	Farmington	1
637	Cape Girardeau	1
638	Caruthersville	1
639	Poplar Bluff	0
640-641	Independence	1
644-645	Saint Joseph	1
646	Chillicothe	1
647	East Lynne	1
648	Joplin	1
650-651	Jefferson City	-1
652	Columbia	0

653	Knob Noster	-1	077	Monmouth	8
654-655	Lebanon	2	078	Dover	9
656-658	Springfield	1	079	Summit	9
			080-084	Atlantic City	9
Montana Average		**1**	085	Princeton	9
590-591	Billings	1	086	Trenton	8
592	Fairview	1	087	Brick	9
593	Miles City	1	088-089	Edison	9
594	Great Falls	2			
595	Havre	1	**New Mexico Average**		**-5**
596	Helena	1	870-871	Albuquerque	-4
597	Butte	1	873	Gallup	-4
598	Missoula	1	874	Farmington	-4
599	Kalispell	1	875	Sante Fe	-4
			877	Holman	-4
Nebraska Average		**-11**	878	Socorro	-5
680-681	Omaha	-8	879	Truth or Con.	-5
683-685	Lincoln	-11	880	Las Cruces	-5
686	Columbus	-11	881	Clovis	-6
687	Norfolk	-11	882	Fort Sumner	-4
688	Grand Island	-11	883	Alamogordo	-5
689	Hastings	-11	884	Tucumcari	-4
690	McCook	-11			
691	North Platte	-11	**New York Average**		**9**
692	Valentine	-11	100	NYC (Manhattan)	26
693	Alliance	-11	100	New York City	13
			103	Staten Island	9
Nevada Average		**5**	104	Bronx	9
889-891	Las Vegas	4	105-108	White Plains	9
893	Ely	4	109	West Point	9
894	Fallon	7	110	Queens	16
895	Reno	4	111	Long Island	16
897	Carson City	6	112	Brooklyn	9
898	Elko	6	113	Flushing	9
			114	Jamaica	9
New Hampshire Average		**2**	115	Garden City	9
030-031	New Boston	3	116	Rockaway	9
032-033	Manchester	2	117	Amityville	9
034	Concord	3	118	Hicksville	9
035	Littleton	2	119	Montauk	9
036	Charlestown	2	120-123	Albany	6
037	Lebanon	2	124	Kingston	7
038	Dover	2	125-126	Poughkeepsie	7
			127	Stewart	7
New Jersey Average		**9**	128	Newcomb	6
070-073	Newark	9	129	Plattsburgh	7
074-075	Paterson	9	130-132	Syracuse	8
076	Hackensack	9			

(*continued*)

Area modification factors: percentages to be added or subtracted (*continued*)

133-135	Utica	8	457	Marietta	1
136	Watertown	6	458	Lima	2
137-139	Binghampton	8			
140	Batvia	8	**Oklahoma Average**		**-8**
141	Tonawanda	8	730-731	Oklahoma City	-7
142	Buffalo	8	734	Ardmore	-8
143	Niagara Falls	8	735	Lawton	-8
144-146	Rochester	7	736	Clinton	-8
147	Jamestown	5	737	Enid	-8
148-149	Ithaca	5	738	Woodward	-8
			739	Adams	-8
North Carolina Average		**-16**	740-741	Tulsa	-8
270-274	Winston-Salem	-17	743	Pryor	-8
275-277	Raleigh	-17	744	Muskogee	-6
278	Rocky Mount	-17	745	McAlester	-12
279	Elizabeth City	-17	746	Ponca City	-8
280-282	Charlotte	-17	747	Durant	-8
283	Fayetteville	-11	748	Shawnee	-8
284	Wilmington	-11	749	Poteau	-8
285	Kinston	-17			
286	Hickory	-17	**Oregon Average**		**6**
287-289	Asheville	-17	970-972	Portland	
			973	Salem	
North Dakota Average		**-4**	974	Eugene	
580-581	Fargo	-4	975	Grants Pass	
582	Grand Forks	-4	976	Klamath Falls	
583	Nekoma	-4	977	Bend	
584	Jamestown	-4	978	Pendleton	
585	Bismarck	-4	979	Adrian	
586	Dickinson	-4			
587	Minot	-3	**Pennsylvania Average**		**5**
588	Williston	-4	150-151	Warrendale	2
			152	Pittsburgh	2
Ohio Average		**1**	153	Washington	2
430-431	Newark	1	154	Uniontown	2
432	Columbus	1	155	Somerset	2
433	Marion	0	156	Greensburg	2
434-436	Toledo	2	157	Punxsutawney	5
437-438	Zanesville	0	158	DuBois	5
439	Stubenville	1	159	Johnstown	5
440-441	Cleveland	3	160	Butler	5
442-443	Akron	1	161	New Castle	5
444-445	Youngstown	1	162	Kittanning	5
446-447	Canton	1	163	Meadville	5
448-449	Sandusky	0	164-165	Erie	5
450-452	Cincinnati	0	166	Altoona	5
453-455	Dayton	0	167	Bradford	5
456	Chillicothe	0	168	Clearfield	5

169	Genesee	5	**Tennessee Average**		**-8**	
170-171	Harrisburg	5	370-372	Nashville	-9	
172	Chambersburg	2	373	Cleveland	-9	
173-174	York	5	374	Chattanooga	-8	
175-176	Lancaster	5	376	Kingsport	-8	
177	Williamsport	5	377-379	Knoxville	-8	
178	Beaver Springs	5	380-381	Memphis	-7	
179	Pottsville	5	382	McKenzie	-8	
180-181	Allentown	5	383	Jackson	-8	
182	Hazleton	5	384	Columbia	-8	
183	East Stroudsburg	5	385	Cookeville	-8	
184-185	Scranton	4				
186-187	Wilkes Barre	5	**Texas Average**		**-9**	
188	Montrose	5	750	Plano	-5	
189	Warminster	8	751-753	Dallas	-5	
190-191	Philadelphia	9	754	Greenville	-11	
195-196	Reading	5	755	Texarkana	-8	
193	Southeastern	5	756	Longview	-11	
194	Valley Forge	5	757	Tyler	-11	
			758	Palestine	-11	
Rhode Island Average		**10**	759	Lufkin	-11	
028	Bristol	9	760	Arlington	-11	
028	Coventry	9	761-762	Ft Worth	-5	
028	Davisville	9	763	Wichita Falls	-11	
028	Narragansett	9	764	Woodson	-11	
028	Newport	10	765-767	Waco	-11	
028	Warwick	10	768	Brownwood	-12	
029	Cranston	10	769	San Angelo	-12	
029	Providence	10	770-772	Houston	-10	
			773	Huntsville	-9	
South Carolina Avg		**-13**	774	Bay City	-10	
290-292	Columbia	-15	775	Galveston	-11	
293	Spartanburg	-15	776-777	Beaumont	-11	
294`	Charleston	-13	778	Bryan	-11	
295	Myrtle Beach	-13	779	Victoria	-10	
296	Greenville	-15	780-782	San Antonio	-8	
297	Rock Hill	-15	783-784	Corpus Christi	-11	
298	Aiken	-9	785	McAllen	-11	
299	Beaufort	-9	786-787	Austin	-11	
			788	Del Rio	-2	
South Dakota Average		**-8**	789	Giddings	-2	
570-571	Sioux Falls	-10	790-791	Amarillo	-11	
572	Watertown	-8	792	Childress	-9	
573	Mitchell	-8	793-794	Lubbock	-8	
574	Aberdeen	-7	795-796	Abilene	-11	
575	Pierre	-7	797	Midland	-10	
576	Mobridge	-8	798-799	El Paso	-11	
577	Rapid City	-8				

(continued)

Utah Average		**-7**
840	Clearfield	-7
841	Salt Lake City	-8
843-844	Ogden	-6
845	Green River	-7
846-847	Provo	-8

Vermont Average		**-4**
050	White Rv. Junct.	-4
051	Springfield	-4
052	Bennington	-4
053	Battleboro	-4
054	Burlington	-3
056	Montpelier	-5
057	Rutland	-4
058	Albany	-4
059	Beecher Falls	-5

Virginia Average		**-10**
220-223	Alexandria	-11
224-225	Fredericksburg	-15
226	Winchester	-10
227	Culpeper	-10
228	Harrisonburg	-10
229	Charlottesville	-10
230-231	Williamsburg	-7
232	Richmond	-10
233-237	Norfolk	-7
238	Petersburg	-9
239	Farmville	-8
240-241	Radford	-10
242	Abingdon	-10
243	Galax	-10
244	Staunton	-10
245	Lynchburg	-10
246	Tazewell	-10

Washington Average		**8**
980-981	Seattle	8
982	Everett	8
983-984	Tacoma	8
985	Olympia	8
986	Vancouver	8
988	Wenatchee	7
989	Yakima	6
990-992	Spokane	10
993	Pasco	8
994	Clarkston	8

West Virginia Average		**-1**
247-248	Bluefield	-3
249	Lewisburg	-1
250-253	Charleston	-1
254	Martinsburg	-1
255-257	Huntington	-1
258-259	Beckley	-1
260	Wheeling	-1
261	Parkersburg	-1
262	New Martinsville	-1
263-264	Clarksburg	-1
265	Morgantown	-1
266	Fairmont	-1
267	Romney	-1
268	Sugar Grove	-3

Wisconsin Average		**-2**
530-534	Milwaukee	4
535	Beloit	-2
537	Madison	-6
538	Prairie du Chien	-6
539	Portage	-7
540	Amery	-2
541-543	Green Bay	-1
544	Wausau	-2
545	Clam Lake	-2
546	La Crosse	-2
547	Eau Claire	-2
548	Ladysmith	-2
549	Oshkosh	-2

Wyoming Average		**-11**
820	Cheyenne	-10
821	Laramie	-11
822	Wheatland	-11
823	Rawlins	-10
824	Powell	-11
825	Riverton	-11
826	Casper	-11
827	Gillette	-11
828	Sheridan	-11
829-831	Rock Springs	-10

Canada		
Alberta Average		**53.0**
Calgary		49.3
Edmonton		54.1
Ft. McMurray		55.7

Area modification factors: percentages to be added or subtracted (*continued*)

British Columbia Avg	51.6		Newfoundland Avg	49.8
Fraser Valley	50.9		Newfoundland & Labrador	49.8
Okanagan HRCC	45.6			
Vancouver 62.5			**Ontario Average**	**51.1**
			London	59.1
Manitoba Average	**57.3**		Thunder Bay	48.3
North Manitoba	67.7		Toronto	59.1
South Manitoba	57.0			
Selkirk	49.7		**Quebec Average**	**59.5**
Winnipeg	54.6		Montreal	63.4
			Quebec	55.4
New Brunswick Avg	**49.1**			
Moncton	49.1		**Saskatchewan Avg**	**58.6**
			La Ronge	62.3
Nova Scotia Average	**57.8**		Prince Albert	57.7
Amherst	56.9		Saskatoon	55.7
Nova Scotia	52.7			
Sydney	63.9			

Building costs: historical index

Year	Masonry Buildings	Concrete Buildings	Steel Buildings	Wood-Frame Buildings	Agricultural Buildings	Year of Construction
1935	24.41	24.70	24.86	22.02	22.35	1935
1936	23.95	24.49	24.86	21.26	21.00	1936
1937	21.41	22.49	21.55	19.28	19.11	1937
1938	20.76	22.42	21.42	19.28	18.91	1938
1939	20.55	22.25	21.15	18.72	18.88	1939
1940	20.31	22.03	20.62	18.48	18.34	1940
1941	19.00	20.39	19.72	18.16	17.01	1941
1942	17.33	18.98	18.55	15.56	16.01	1942
1943	17.10	18.17	17.73	14.83	14.35	1943
1944	16.18	17.62	17.06	13.57	13.70	1944
1945	15.29	16.94	16.53	12.86	12.89	1945
1946	13.12	14.87	14.70	11.51	11.15	1946
1947	11.20	12.28	12.85	9.25	9.03	1947
1948	9.81	10.52	11.47	8.47	8.26	1948
1949	9.88	10.41	11.40	8.58	8.51	1949
1950	9.39	9.94	11.19	8.19	7.92	1950
1951	8.78	9.37	10.16	7.66	7.35	1951
1952	8.48	9.16	9.93	7.53	7.28	1952
1953	8.36	8.85	9.49	7.35	7.12	1953
1954	8.21	8.54	9.49	7.35	7.12	1954
1955	7.86	8.14	8.99	6.96	6.80	1955
1956	7.47	7.77	8.28	6.67	6.53	1956
1957	7.25	7.49	7.95	6.61	6.38	1957

(*continued*)

Building costs: historical index (*continued*)

Year	Masonry Buildings	Concrete Buildings	Steel Buildings	Wood-Frame Buildings	Agricultural Buildings	Year of Construction
1958	7.05	7.20	7.57	6.60	7.60	1958
1959	6.83	6.97	7.38	6.32	6.09	1959
1960	6.67	6.85	7.25	6.22	5.97	1960
1961	6.52	6.82	7.14	6.11	5.95	1961
1962	6.38	6.62	6.98	6.04	5.85	1962
1963	6.28	6.45	6.89	5.92	5.32	1963
1964	6.11	6.36	6.79	5.71	5.59	1964
1965	5.91	6.21	6.56	5.60	5.43	1965
1966	5.64	6.04	6.31	5.36	5.28	1966
1967	5.51	5.74	5.90	5.10	5.07	1967
1968	5.28	5.43	5.63	4.81	4.85	1968
1969	4.99	5.19	5.44	4.63	4.57	1969
1970	4.80	4.95	5.17	4.41	4.35	1970
1971	4.50	4.55	4.80	3.80	4.05	1971
1972	4.18	4.20	4.47	3.81	3.76	1972
1973	3.81	3.99	3.97	3.51	3.53	1973
1974	3.39	3.65	3.72	3.28	3.29	1974
1975	3.10	3.23	3.37	3.09	2.92	1975
1976	2.89	3.08	3.19	2.97	2.77	1976
1977	2.69	2.88	3.02	2.76	2.60	1977
1978	2.52	2.69	2.79	2.53	2.37	1978
1979	2.31	2.40	2.49	2.33	2.25	1979
1980	2.09	2.18	2.22	2.09	2.03	1980
1981	1.96	2.05	2.04	2.00	1.89	1981
1982	1.89	1.96	1.98	1.93	1.81	1982
1983	1.82	1.89	1.93	1.83	1.72	1983
1984	1.71	1.79	1.85	1.70	1.66	1984
1985	1.66	1.71	1.79	1.64	1.63	1985
1986	1.62	1.69	1.77	1.61	1.61	1986
1987	1.61	1.66	1.75	1.59	1.59	1987
1988	1.57	1.59	1.70	1.57	1.56	1988
1989	1.53	1.56	1.64	1.53	1.52	1989
1990	1.44	1.51	1.54	1.44	1.45	1990
1991	1.56	1.48	1.48	1.36	1.37	1991
1992	1.39	1.46	1.45	1.35	1.36	1992
1993	1.35	1.44	1.40	1.33	1.33	1993
1994	1.32	1.34	1.35	1.29	1.25	1994
1995	1.25	1.22	1.26	1.21	1.18	1995
1996	1.21	1.20	1.21	1.19	1.16	1996
1997	1.17	1.17	1.16	1.16	1.13	1997
1998	1.12	1.12	1.12	1.11	1.11	1998
1999	1.09	1.09	1.09	1.09	1.09	1999
2000	1.06	1.06	1.06	1.05	1.05	2000
2001	1.03	1.03	1.03	1.02	1.02	2001
2002	1.00	1.00	1.00	1.00	1.00	2002
(estimated)						

Medical-Dental Buildings—Masonry or Concrete

	Class 1 Best Quality	Class 2 Good Quality	Class 3 Average Quality	Class 4 Low Quality
First Floor Structure (10% of total cost)	Reinforced concrete slab on grade or standard wood frame.	Reinforced concrete slab on grade or standard wood frame.	Reinforced concrete slab on grade.	Reinforced concrete slab on grade.
Upper Floor Structure (8% of total cost)	Standard wood frame, plywood and 1-1/2" lightweight concrete subfloor.	Standard wood frame, plywood and 1-1/2" lightweight concrete subfloor.	Standard wood frame. 5/8" plywood subfloor.	Standard wood frame. 5/8" plywood subfloor.
Walls (9% of total cost)	8" decorative concrete block or 6" concrete tilt-up.	8" decorative concrete block or 6" concrete tilt-up.	8" reinforced concrete block or 8" reinforced brick.	8" reinforced concrete block or clay tile.
Roof Structure (6% of total cost)	Standard wood frame, flat or low pitch.	Standard wood frame, flat or low pitch.	Standard wood frame, flat or low pitch.	Standard wood frame, flat or low pitch.
Exterior Wall Finish (8% of total cost)	Decorative block or large rock imbedded in tilt-up panels with 10 to 20% brick or stone veneer.	Decorative block or exposed aggregate and 10 to 20% brick or stone veneer.	Stucco or colored concrete block.	Painted.
Windows (5% of total cost)	Average number in good aluminum frame. Fixed float glass in good frame on front.	Average number in good aluminum frame. Some fixed float glass in front.	Average number of average aluminum sliding type.	Average number of low cost aluminum sliding type.
Roof Cover (5% of total cost)	5 ply built-up roofing on flat roofs/Heavy shake or tile on sloping roofs.	5 ply built-up roofing on flat roofs. Average shake or composition, tar and large rock on sloping roofs.	4 ply built-up roofing on flat roofs. Wood shingle or composition, tar and pea gravel on sloping roofs.	3 ply built-up roofing on flat roofs. Composition shingle on sloping roofs.

(continued)

Medical-Dental Buildings—Masonry or Concrete (*continued*)

	Class 1 Best Quality	Class 2 Good Quality	Class 3 Average Quality	Class 4 Low Quality
Overhang (3% of total cost)	3" closed overhang, fully guttered.	2" closed overhang, fully guttered.	None on flat roofs. 18" open on sloping roofs, fully guttered.	None on flat roofs. 12" to 16" open on sloping roofs, gutters over entrances.
Business Offices (3% of total cost)	Good hardwood veneer paneling. Solid vinyl or carpet.	Hardwood paneling or vinyl wall cover. Resilient tile or carpet.	Gypsum wallboard, texture and paint. Composition tile.	Gypsum wallboard, texture and paint. Minimum grade tile.
Corridors (6% of total cost)	Good hardwood veneer paneling. Solid vinyl or carpet.	Gypsum wallboard and vinyl wall cover. Resilient tile.	Gypsum wallboard, some paneling. Composition tile.	Gypsum wallboard, texture and paint. Minimum grade tile.
Waiting Rooms (7% of total cost)	Good hardwood veneer paneling. Carpet.	Hardwood paneling. Carpet.	Gypsum wallboard, some paneling. Resilient tile or carpet.	Gypsum wallboard, texture and paint. Minimum grade tile.
Private Offices (2% of total cost)	Good hardwood veneer paneling. Carpet.	Textured wall cover and hardwood paneling. Carpet.	Gypsum wallboard and paper, wood paneling. Resilient tile or carpet.	Gypsum wallboard, texture and paint. Minimum grade tile.
Treatment Rooms (5% of total cost)	Gypsum wallboard and vinyl wall covering. Sheet vinyl or carpet.	Gypsum wallboard and enamel. Sheet vinyl.	Gypsum wallboard and enamel. Resilient tile.	Gypsum wallboard, texture and paint. Minimum grade tile.
Bathrooms (3% of total cost)	Gypsum wallboard and enamel with ceramic tile wainscot. Sheet vinyl or ceramic tile.	Gypsum wallboard and enamel or vinyl wall covering. Sheet vinyl or ceramic tile.	Gypsum wallboard and enamel. Resilient tile.	Gypsum wallboard, texture and paint. Minimum grade tile.
Ceiling Finish (4% of total cost)	Suspended "T" bar and acoustical tile.	Gypsum wallboard and acoustical tile.	Gypsum wallboard and acoustical tile.	Gypsum wallboard and paint.

Medical-Dental Buildings—Masonry or Concrete (*continued*)

	Class 1 Best Quality	Class 2 Good Quality	Class 3 Average Quality	Class 4 Low Quality
Utilities				
Plumbing (6% of total cost)	Copper tubing, good fixtures.	Copper tubing, good fixtures.	Copper tubing, average fixtures.	Copper tubing, economy fixtures.
Lighting (6% of total cost)	Conduit wiring, good fixtures.	Conduit wiring, good fixtures.	Romex or conduit wiring, average fixtures.	Romex wiring, economy fixtures.
Cabinets (4% of total cost)	Formica faced with formica tops.	Good grade of hardwood with formica tops.	Average amount of painted wood or low grade hardwood with formica top.	Minimum amount of painted wood with formica top.

Note: Use the percent of total cost to help identify the correct quality classification.

foot of floor and smaller room sizes than general office buildings. Note also that buildings with more than 10,000 square feet are assumed to have lead-shielded X-ray rooms.

2. Establish the building-quality class by applying the information on pages 217–219.

3. Compute the first floor area. This should include everything within the exterior walls and all insets outside the main walls but under the main roof.

4. If the first floor wall height is more or less than 10 feet, add to or subtract from the first floor square foot cost below the appropriate amount from the wall height adjustment table on page 232.

5. Multiply the adjusted square foot cost by the first floor area.

6. Deduct, if appropriate, for common walls or no wall finish. Use the figures on page 231.

7. If there are second or higher floors, compute the square foot area on each floor. Locate the appropriate square foot cost from the table on page 221. Adjust this figure for a wall height more or less than 9 feet, using the figures on page 232. Multiply the adjusted cost by the square foot area on each floor. Use the figures on page 231 to deduct for common walls or no wall finish. Add the result to the cost from step 6 above.

8. Multiply the total cost by the location factor listed on pages 207–215.

9. Add the cost of heating and air conditioning systems, elevators, fire sprinklers, exterior signs, paving and curbing, miscellaneous yard improvements, covered porches and garages.

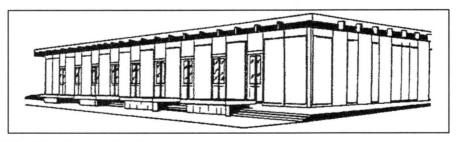

Medical–Dental building, Class 2

Medical-Dental Buildings—Masonry or Concrete—Exterior Suite Entrances, Length Between 2 and 4 Times Width

Estimating Procedure

1. Use these figures to estimate medical, dental, surgical, and similar professional buildings in which access to each office suite is through an exterior entrance. Buildings in this section have more plumbing fixtures per square foot of floor and smaller room sizes than general office buildings. Note also that buildings with more than 10,000 square feet are assumed to have lead shielded X-ray rooms.

2. Establish the building-quality class by applying the information on pages 217–219.

Masonry or Concrete—Exterior Suite Entrances, Length Less Than 2 Times Width

First Story—Square Foot Area

Quality Class	1,000	1,500	2,000	2,500	3,000	4,000	5,000	7,500	10,000	15,000	20,000
Exceptional	177.87	167.38	161.27	157.20	154.19	150.06	147.25	413.00	140.47	137.50	135.77
1, Best	164.64	154.91	149.27	145.47	142.72	138.90	136.30	132.36	130.01	127.27	125.67
1 & 2	156.10	146.85	141.53	137.94	135.32	131.69	129.24	125.49	123.27	120.68	119.14
2, Good	149.08	140.29	135.18	131.76	129.24	125.78	123.45	119.85	117.75	115.27	113.79
2 & 3	137.82	129.66	124.94	121.76	119.45	116.25	114.11	110.78	108.81	106.53	105.18
3, Average	129.23	121.77	117.25	114.30	112.12	108.00	107.07	103.97	102.13	99.98	98.72
3 & 4	121.82	114.64	110.47	107.65	105.63	102.79	100.85	97.93	96.21	94.19	92.98
4, Low	113.46	106.79	102.89	100.29	98.35	95.74	93.96	91.23	89.62	87.72	86.59

Second and Higher Stories—Square Foot Area

Quality Class	1,000	1,500	2,000	2,500	3,000	4,000	5,000	7,500	10,000	15,000	20,000
Exceptional	159.25	148.60	142.84	139.15	136.59	133.15	130.91	127.70	125.87	123.83	122.66
1, Best	155.49	145.10	139.50	135.89	133.38	130.04	127.85	124.67	122.90	120.93	119.77
1 & 2	147.74	137.85	132.53	129.11	126.72	123.53	121.45	118.46	116.77	114.87	113.80
2, Good	142.57	133.05	127.89	124.61	122.30	119.21	117.24	114.32	112.67	110.86	109.82
2 & 3	131.65	122.86	118.09	115.03	112.89	110.10	108.24	105.55	104.06	102.38	101.39
3, Average	123.58	115.33	110.86	107.99	106.04	103.34	101.62	99.09	97.68	96.09	95.21
3 & 4	116.37	108.59	104.39	101.68	99.81	97.31	95.66	93.29	91.79	90.47	89.62
4, Low	108.47	101.24	97.29	94.80	93.05	90.69	89.18	86.97	85.72	84.37	83.57

3. Compute the first floor area. This should include everything within the exterior walls and all insets outside the main walls but under the main roof.
4. If the first floor wall height is more or less than 10 feet, add to or subtract from the first floor square foot cost below the appropriate amount from the wall height adjustment table on page 232.
5. Multiply the adjusted square foot cost by the first floor area.
6. Deduct, if appropriate, for common walls or no wall finish. Use the figures on page 231.
7. If there are second or higher floors, compute the square foot area on each floor. Locate the appropriate square foot cost from the table on page 223. Adjust this figure for a wall height more or less than 9 feet, using the figures on page 232. Multiply the adjusted cost by the square foot area on each floor. Use the figures on page 231 to deduct for common walls or no wall finish. Add the result to the cost from step 6 above.
8. Multiply the total cost by the location factor listed on pages 207–215.
9. Add the cost of heating and air conditioning systems, elevators, fire sprinklers, exterior signs, paving and curbing, miscellaneous yard improvements, covered porches and garages.

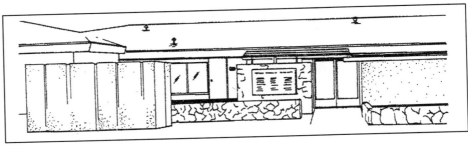

Medical–Dental building, Classes 3 and 4

Medical-Dental Building—Masonry or Concrete—Exterior Suite Entrances, Length More Than 4 Times Width

Estimating Procedure

1. Use these figures to estimate medical, dental, surgical, and similar professional buildings in which access to each office suite is through an exterior entrance. Buildings in this section have more plumbing fixtures per square foot of floor and smaller room sizes than general office buildings. Note also that buildings with more than 10,000 square feet are assumed to have lead shielded X-ray rooms.
2. Establish the building-quality class by applying the information on pages 217–219.
3. Compute the first floor area. This should include everything within the exterior walls and all insets outside the main walls but under the main roof.
4. If the first floor wall height is more or less than 10 feet, add to or subtract from the first floor square foot cost below the appropriate amount from the wall height adjustment table on page 232

Masonry or Concrete—Exterior Suite Entrances, Length Between 2 and 4 Times Width

First Story—Square Foot Area

Quality Class	1,000	1,500	2,000	2,500	3,000	4,000	5,000	7,500	10,000	15,000	20,000
Exceptional	191.74	177.53	169.55	164.26	160.48	155.28	151.87	146.70	143.68	140.22	138.18
1, Best	177.77	164.62	157.19	152.29	148.79	143.99	140.79	135.99	133.23	130.01	128.13
1 & 2	167.18	154.83	147.86	143.25	139.96	135.44	132.44	127.94	125.31	122.27	120.54
2, Good	159.53	147.75	141.06	136.69	133.53	129.23	126.40	122.08	119.58	116.70	115.01
2 & 3	147.44	136.55	130.36	126.33	123.41	119.42	116.79	112.81	110.52	107.82	106.27
3, Average	138.44	128.19	122.41	118.61	115.87	112.14	109.68	105.90	103.74	101.23	99.78
3 & 4	130.33	120.68	115.23	111.64	109.08	105.58	103.22	99.71	97.67	95.31	93.94
4, Low	121.37	112.38	107.32	104.02	101.59	98.32	96.12	92.84	90.98	88.75	87.46

Second and Higher Stories—Square Foot Area

Quality Class	1,000	1,500	2,000	2,500	3,000	4,000	5,000	7,500	10,000	15,000	20,000
Exceptional	176.72	164.29	157.29	152.66	149.33	144.79	141.80	137.27	134.61	131.57	129.78
1, Best	163.84	152.45	145.82	141.50	138.44	134.20	131.46	127.24	124.78	121.94	120.31
1 & 2	155.61	144.66	138.46	134.42	131.50	127.48	124.83	120.83	118.52	115.84	114.25
2, Good	150.11	139.52	133.59	129.66	126.84	122.97	120.43	116.57	114.32	111.76	110.22
2 & 3	138.56	128.84	123.34	119.71	117.11	113.57	111.18	107.63	105.56	103.18	101.77
3, Average	130.07	120.93	115.76	112.36	109.90	106.58	104.39	101.01	99.08	96.85	95.55
3 & 4	122.52	113.93	109.07	105.87	103.57	100.40	98.32	95.17	93.36	91.21	89.98
4, Low	114.29	106.26	101.71	98.74	96.58	93.65	91.71	88.75	87.03	85.10	83.96

223

5. Multiply the adjusted square foot cost by the first floor area.
6. Deduct, if appropriate, for common walls or no wall finish. Use the figures on page 231.
7. If there are second or higher floors, compute the square foot area on each floor. Locate the appropriate square foot cost from the table on page 225. Adjust this figure for a wall height more or less than 9 feet, using the figures on page 232. Multiply the adjusted cost by the square foot area on each floor. Use the figures on page 231 to deduct for common walls or no wall finish. Add the result to the cost from step 6 above.
8. Multiply the total cost by the location factor listed on pages 207–215.
9. Add the cost of heating and air conditioning systems, elevators, fire sprinklers, exterior signs, paving and curbing, miscellaneous yard improvements, covered porches and garages.

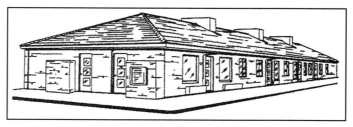

Medical–Dental building, Classes 2 and 3

Medical-Dental Building—Masonry or Concrete—Interior Suite Entrance, Length Less Than 2 Times Width

Estimating Procedure

1. Use these figures to estimate medical, dental, surgical, and similar professional buildings in which access to each office suite is through an interior entrance. Buildings in this section have more plumbing fixtures per square foot of floor and smaller room sizes than general office buildings. Note also that buildings with more than 10,000 square feet are assumed to have lead shielded X-ray rooms.
2. Establish the building quality class by applying the information on pages 217–219.
3. Compute the first floor area. This should include everything within the exterior walls and all insets outside the main walls but under the main roof.
4. If the first floor wall height is more or less than 10 feet, add to or subtract from the first floor square foot cost below the appropriate amount from the wall height adjustment table on page 232.
5. Multiply the adjusted square foot cost by the first floor area.
6. Deduct, if appropriate, for common walls or no wall finish. Use the figures on page 231.
7. If there are second or higher floors, compute the square foot area on each floor. Locate the appropriate square foot cost from the table on page 227.

Masonry or Concrete—Exterior Suite Entrances, Length More Than 4 Times Width

First Story—Square Foot Area

Quality Class	1,000	1,500	2,000	2,500	3,000	4,000	5,000	7,500	10,000	15,000	20,000
Exceptional	206.66	188.75	178.76	172.22	167.54	161.22	157.05	150.81	147.20	143.10	140.70
1, Best	191.58	175.00	165.71	159.66	155.34	149.46	145.60	139.79	136.48	132.66	130.43
1 & 2	179.89	164.28	155.56	149.88	145.85	140.30	136.66	131.24	128.11	124.55	122.44
2, Good	172.14	157.21	148.89	143.44	139.57	134.29	130.82	125.60	122.59	119.18	117.21
2 & 3	158.41	144.68	137.02	131.99	128.43	123.55	120.39	115.58	112.83	109.69	107.82
3, Average	148.56	135.67	128.47	123.80	120.43	115.88	112.88	108.38	105.81	102.83	101.13
3 & 4	139.83	127.68	120.94	116.50	113.37	109.08	106.26	102.41	99.57	96.80	95.18
4, Low	130.20	118.89	112.60	108.48	105.54	101.57	98.90	94.98	92.72	90.12	88.60

Second and Higher Stories—Square Foot Area

Quality Class	1,000	1,500	2,000	2,500	3,000	4,000	5,000	7,500	10,000	15,000	20,000
Exceptional	189.01	173.76	165.15	159.51	155.43	149.88	146.17	140.63	137.38	133.66	131.50
1, Best	174.50	160.42	152.49	147.24	143.50	138.36	134.94	129.82	126.84	123.41	121.41
1 & 2	166.32	152.92	145.35	140.37	136.77	131.89	128.65	123.73	120.92	117.63	115.70
2, Good	160.40	147.47	140.16	135.33	131.90	127.19	124.07	119.33	116.59	113.43	111.60
2 & 3	148.12	136.18	129.43	124.97	121.78	117.41	114.52	110.18	107.65	104.74	103.02
3, Average	138.98	127.79	121.44	117.30	114.31	110.22	107.50	103.40	101.03	98.29	96.70
3 & 4	131.12	120.51	114.57	110.63	107.81	103.95	101.41	97.53	95.30	92.71	91.19
4, Low	122.10	112.25	106.69	103.03	100.40	96.80	94.40	90.84	88.75	86.36	84.92

Adjust this figure for a wall height more or less than 9 feet, using the figures on page 232. Multiply the adjusted cost by the square foot area on each floor. Use the figures on page 231 to deduct for common walls or no wall finish. Add the result to the cost from step 6 above.

8. Multiply the total cost by the location factor listed on pages 207–215.
9. Add the cost of heating and air conditioning systems, elevators, fire sprinklers, exterior signs, paving and curbing, miscellaneous yard improvements, covered porches and garages.

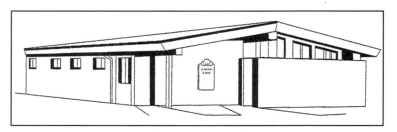

Medical–Dental building, Classes 3 and 4

Medical-Dental Building—Masonry or Concrete—Interior Suite Entrances, Length Between 2 and 4 Times Width

Estimating Procedure

1. Use these figures to estimate medical, dental, surgical, and similar professional buildings in which access to each office suite is through an interior entrance. Buildings in this section have more plumbing fixtures per square foot of floor and smaller room sizes than general office buildings. Note also that buildings with more than 10,000 square feet are assumed to have lead shielded X-ray rooms.
2. Establish the building quality class by applying the information on pages 217–219.
3. Compute the first floor area. This should include everything within the exterior walls and all insets outside the main walls but under the main roof.
4. If the first floor wall height is more or less than 10 feet, add to or subtract from the first floor square foot cost below the appropriate amount from the wall height adjustment table on page 232.
5. Multiply the adjusted square foot cost by the first floor area.
6. Deduct, if appropriate, for common walls or no wall finish. Use the figures on page 231.
7. If there are second or higher floors, compute the square foot area on each floor. Locate the appropriate square foot cost from the table on page 229. Adjust this figure for a wall height more or less than 9 feet, using the figures on page 232. Multiply the adjusted cost by the square foot area on each floor. Use the figures on page 231 to deduct for common walls or no wall finish. Add the result to the cost from step 6 above.
8. Multiply the total cost by the location factor listed on pages 207–215.

Masonry or Concrete—Interior Suite Entrances, Length Less Than 2 Times Width

First Story—Square Foot Area

Quality Class	2,000	2,500	3,000	4,000	5,000	7,500	10,000	15,000	20,000	30,000	40,000
Exceptional	150.36	146.29	143.44	139.94	136.54	132.38	129.93	127.08	125.42	123.48	122.32
1, Best	143.27	139.42	136.59	132.74	130.12	126.17	123.85	121.11	119.55	117.68	116.57
1 & 2	135.18	131.52	128.83	125.19	122.77	118.99	116.81	114.24	112.76	111.00	109.98
2, Good	129.36	125.86	123.32	119.84	117.47	113.88	111.80	109.36	107.93	106.23	105.24
2 & 3	119.90	116.67	114.30	111.06	108.89	105.56	103.65	101.35	100.03	98.45	97.54
3, Average	111.87	108.83	106.63	103.63	101.59	98.50	96.67	94.56	93.32	91.87	91.00
3 & 4	105.87	103.00	100.93	98.07	96.12	93.21	91.50	89.50	88.32	86.94	86.13
4, Low	99.25	96.54	94.60	91.91	90.12	87.37	85.76	83.92	82.78	81.51	80.74

Second and Higher Stories—Square Foot Area

Quality Class	2,000	2,500	3,000	4,000	5,000	7,500	10,000	15,000	20,000	30,000	40,000
Exceptional	142.15	138.51	135.88	132.26	129.82	126.11	123.94	121.43	119.96	118.21	117.19
1, Best	135.56	132.09	129.60	126.14	123.83	120.28	118.23	115.85	114.41	112.74	111.80
1 & 2	128.66	125.38	122.97	119.72	117.53	114.15	112.22	109.95	108.59	107.00	106.08
2, Good	123.95	120.80	118.51	115.33	113.20	110.00	108.11	105.90	104.60	103.10	102.19
2 & 3	114.60	111.66	109.54	106.65	104.66	101.69	99.97	97.91	96.72	95.31	94.49
3, Average	107.58	104.85	102.84	100.08	98.25	95.46	93.83	91.93	90.80	89.47	88.70
3 & 4	101.20	98.59	96.74	94.17	92.46	89.83	88.24	86.51	85.42	84.17	83.46
4, Low	95.29	92.84	91.08	88.65	87.01	84.54	83.12	81.43	80.43	79.25	78.57

9. Add the cost of heating and air conditioning systems, elevators, fire sprinklers, exterior signs, paving and curbing, miscellaneous yard improvements, covered porches and garages.

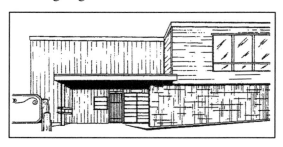

Medical–Dental building, Class 3

Medical-Dental Building—Masonry or Concrete—Interior Suite Entrances, Length More Than 4 Times Width

Estimating Procedure

1. Establish the building quality class by applying the information on pages 217–219.
2. Compute the first floor area. This should include everything within the exterior walls and all insets outside the main walls but under the main roof.
3. If the first floor wall height is more or less than 10 feet, add to or subtract from the first floor square foot cost below the appropriate amount from the wall height adjustment table on page 232.
4. Multiply the adjusted square foot cost by the first floor area.
5. Deduct, if appropriate, for common walls or no wall finish. Use the figures on page 231.
6. If there are second or higher floors, compute the square foot area on each floor. Locate the appropriate square foot cost from the table on page 230. Adjust this figure for a wall height more or less than 9 feet, using the figures on page 232. Multiply the adjusted cost by the square foot area on each floor. Use the figures on page 231 to deduct for common walls or no wall finish. Add the result to the cost from step 6 above.
7. Multiply the total cost by the location factor listed on pages 207–215.
8. Add the cost of heating and air conditioning systems, elevators, fire sprinklers, exterior signs, paving and curbing, miscellaneous yard improvements, covered porches and garages.

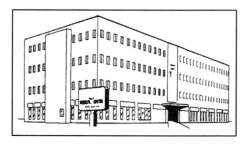

Medical–Dental building, Classes 2 and 3

Masonry or Concrete—Interior Suite Entrances, Length Less Than 2 and 4 Times Width

First Story—Square Foot Area

Quality Class	2,000	2,500	3,000	4,000	5,000	7,500	10,000	15,000	20,000	30,000	40,000
Exceptional	157.39	152.38	148.75	143.79	140.49	135.48	132.58	129.19	127.20	124.90	123.52
1, Best	150.02	145.25	141.80	137.06	133.92	129.13	126.36	123.12	121.23	119.01	117.73
1 & 2	141.38	136.90	133.65	129.17	126.20	121.70	119.08	116.06	114.25	112.21	110.97
2, Good	135.18	130.90	127.80	123.52	120.69	116.39	113.88	110.97	109.28	107.28	106.13
2 & 3	125.21	121.23	118.33	114.42	111.79	107.76	105.45	102.78	101.21	99.35	98.28
3, Average	116.73	113.01	110.33	106.63	104.19	100.48	98.30	95.79	94.33	92.62	91.59
3 & 4	110.58	107.05	104.54	101.03	98.69	95.20	93.14	90.73	89.37	87.73	86.81
4, Low	103.49	100.20	97.82	94.55	92.38	89.10	87.21	84.92	83.65	82.12	81.22

Second and Higher Stories—Square Foot Area

Quality Class	2,000	2,500	3,000	4,000	5,000	7,500	10,000	15,000	20,000	30,000	40,000
Exceptional	148.36	143.87	140.68	136.24	133.29	128.83	126.24	123.23	121.45	119.44	118.19
1, Best	141.40	137.12	134.06	129.85	127.01	122.81	120.29	117.44	115.74	113.82	112.65
1 & 2	134.14	130.10	127.18	123.18	120.54	116.46	114.13	111.42	109.81	107.97	106.88
2, Good	129.26	125.38	122.54	118.68	116.14	112.27	110.02	107.39	105.83	104.05	102.99
2 & 3	119.34	115.74	113.16	109.60	107.23	103.67	101.56	99.13	97.73	96.04	95.11
3, Average	111.95	108.61	106.13	102.81	100.59	97.21	95.24	92.98	91.67	90.11	89.18
3 & 4	106.01	102.81	100.49	97.35	95.24	92.05	90.21	88.06	86.78	85.29	84.44
4, Low	99.34	96.35	94.20	91.24	89.28	86.27	84.51	82.53	81.34	79.97	79.15

Masonry or Concrete—Interior Suite Entrances, Length More Than 4 Times Width

First Story—Square Foot Area

Quality Class	2,000	2,500	3,000	4,000	5,000	7,500	10,000	15,000	20,000	30,000	40,000
Exceptional	166.42	160.13	155.63	149.51	145.48	139.43	135.93	131.90	129.56	126.87	125.30
1, Best	158.62	152.62	148.35	142.51	138.65	132.87	129.55	125.72	123.48	120.93	119.38
1 & 2	149.36	143.74	139.69	134.19	130.57	125.14	122.02	118.41	116.32	113.87	112.44
2, Good	142.72	137.34	133.48	128.23	124.76	119.55	116.57	113.11	111.13	108.78	107.43
2 & 3	132.03	127.03	123.48	118.62	115.42	110.60	107.84	104.64	102.80	100.68	99.38
3, Average	124.13	119.46	116.10	111.53	108.49	104.00	101.38	98.39	96.65	94.61	93.45
3 & 4	117.44	113.01	109.81	105.54	102.67	98.37	95.93	93.09	91.45	89.51	88.43
4, Low	109.99	105.82	102.87	98.83	96.16	92.15	89.82	87.21	85.63	83.85	82.78

Second and Higher Stories—Square Foot Area

Quality Class	2,000	2,500	3,000	4,000	5,000	7,500	10,000	15,000	20,000	30,000	40,000
Exceptional	156.05	150.46	146.44	141.01	137.41	132.03	128.93	125.93	123.32	120.94	119.55
1, Best	148.82	143.47	139.64	134.45	131.05	125.89	122.94	119.57	117.58	115.30	113.95
1 & 2	141.11	136.04	132.43	127.51	124.26	119.38	116.59	113.37	111.52	109.34	108.07
2, Good	135.93	131.06	127.56	122.84	119.71	115.02	112.31	109.22	107.42	105.32	104.11
2 & 3	125.37	120.90	117.65	113.30	110.41	106.11	103.61	100.76	99.09	97.15	96.03
3, Average	117.76	113.54	110.53	106.42	103.71	99.66	97.33	94.61	93.06	91.26	90.19
3 & 4	111.49	107.48	104.60	100.74	98.15	94.34	92.11	89.57	88.10	86.37	85.38
4, Low	104.47	100.75	98.02	94.38	91.98	88.42	86.32	83.96	82.55	80.94	80.00

Wall Height Adjustment

The square foot costs for medical-dental buildings are based on the wall heights of 10 feet for first floors and 9 feet for higher floors. The main or first floor height is the distance from the bottom of the floor slab or joists to the top of the roof slab or ceiling joists. Second and higher floors are measured from the top of the floor slab or floor joists to the top of the roof slab or ceiling joists. Add or subtract the amount listed in this table to the square foot of floor cost for each foot of wall height more or less than 10 feet, if adjusting for a first floor, and 9 feet, if adjusting for upper floors.

Perimeter Wall Adjustment

A common wall exists when two buildings share one wall. Adjust for common walls by deducting the linear foot costs below from the total structure cost. In some structures, one or more walls are not owned at all. In this case, deduct the "No Ownership" cost per linear foot of wall not owned. If a wall has no exterior finish, deduct the "Lack of Exterior Finish" cost.

Masonry or Concrete—First Story

Class	For a Common Wall, Deduct Per L.F.	For No Wall Ownership, Deduct Per L.F.	For Lack of Exterior Finish, Deduct Per L.F.
1	$257.00	$521.00	$196.00
2	202.00	353.00	129.00
3	146.00	291.00	68.00
4	109.00	224.00	44.00

Masonry or Concrete—Second and Higher Stories

Class	For a Common Wall, Deduct Per L.F.	For No Wall Ownership, Deduct Per L.F.	For Lack of Exterior Finish, Deduct Per L.F.
1	$241.00	$471.00	$196.00
2	196.00	381.00	129.00
3	146.00	291.00	68.00
4	129.00	257.00	44.00

Masonry or Concrete—Wall Height Adjustment, Square Foot Area

Quality Class	1,000	1,500	2,000	3,000	4,000	5,000	7,500	10,000	15,000	20,000	40,000
1, Best	4.50	3.51	2.96	2.32	1.96	1.75	1.38	1.19	.97	.80	.58
2, Good	3.88	3.05	2.55	2.03	1.72	1.54	1.21	1.03	.82	.72	.48
3, Average	3.39	2.65	2.21	1.78	1.51	1.33	1.09	.89	.74	.65	.43
4, Low	2.98	2.37	1.97	1.55	1.32	1.16	.92	.81	.66	.51	.38

Medical-Dental Buildings—Wood Frame

	Class 1 Best Quality	Class 2 Good Quality	Class 3 Average Quality	Class 4 Low Quality
Foundation (9% of total cost)	Reinforced concrete.	Reinforced concrete.	Reinforced concrete.	Reinforced concrete.
First Floor Structure (4% of total cost)	Reinforced concrete slab on grade or standard wood frame.	Reinforced concrete slab on grade or standard wood frame.	Reinforced concrete slab on grade or 4″ x 6″ girders with 2″ T & G subfloor.	Reinforced concrete slab on grade.
Upper Floor Structure (6% of total cost)	Standard wood frame, plywood and 1-1/2″ lightweight concrete subfloor.	Standard wood frame, plywood and 1-1/2″ lightweight concrete subfloor.	Standard wood frame, 5/8″ plywood subfloor.	Standard wood frame, 5/8″ plywood subfloor.
Walls (9% of total cost)	Standard wood frame.	Standard wood frame.	Standard wood frame.	Standard wood frame.
Roof Structure (6% of total cost)	Standard wood frame, flat or low pitch.	Standard wood frame, flat or low pitch.	Standard wood frame, flat or low pitch.	Standard wood frame, flat or low pitch.
Exterior Finishes: **Walls** (8% of total cost)	Good wood siding with 10 to 20% brick or stone veneer.	Average wood siding or stucco and 10 to 20% brick or stone veneer.	Stucco with some wood trim or cheap wood siding.	Stucco.
Windows (5% of total cost)	Average number in good aluminum frame. Fixed float glass in good frame on front.	Average number in good aluminum frame. Some fixed float glass in front.	Average amount of average aluminum sliding type.	Average number of low cost aluminum sliding type.
Roof Cover (5% of total cost)	5 ply built-up roofing on flat roofs. Heavy shake or tile on sloping roofs.	5 ply built-up roofing on flat roofs. Avg. shake or composition, tar and large rock on sloping roofs.	4 ply built-up roofing on flat roofs. Wood shingle or composition, tar and pea gravel on sloping roofs.	3 ply built-up roofing on flat roofs. Composition shingle on sloping roofs.

(continued)

Medical-Dental Buildings—Wood Frame (*continued*)

	Class 1 Best Quality	Class 2 Good Quality	Class 3 Average Quality	Class 4 Low Quality
Overhang (3% of total cost)	3″ sealed overhang, fully guttered.	2″ sealed overhang, fully guttered.	None on flat roofs. 18″ unsealed on sloping roofs, fully guttered.	None on flat roofs. 12″ to 16″ unsealed on sloping roofs, gutters over entrances.
Floor Finishes: **Business Offices** (3% of total cost)	Solid vinyl tile or carpet.	Resilient tile or carpet.	Composition tile.	Minimum grade tile.
Corridors (2% of total cost)	Solid vinyl tile or carpet.	Resilient tile or carpet.	Composition tile.	Minimum grade tile.
Waiting Rooms (1% of total cost)	Carpet.	Carpet.	Composition tile or carpet.	Minimum grade tile.
Private Offices (2% of total cost)	Carpet.	Carpet.	Composition tile or carpet.	Minimum grade tile.
Treatment Room (2% of total cost)	Sheet vinyl or carpet.	Sheet vinyl.	Composition tile.	Minimum grade tile.
Bathrooms (1% of total cost)	Sheet vinyl or ceramic tile.	Sheet vinyl or ceramic tile.	Composition tile.	Minimum grade tile.
Interior Wall Finishes: **Business Offices** (3% of total cost)	Good hardwood veneer paneling.	Hardwood paneling or vinyl wall cover.	Gypsum wall board, texture and paint.	Gypsum wallboard, texture and paint.
Corridors (2% of total cost)	Good hardwood veneer paneling.	Gypsum wallboard and vinyl wall cover.	Gypsum wallboard, texture and paint.	Gypsum wallboard, texture and paint.
Waiting Room (1% of total cost)	Good hardwood veneer paneling.	Hardwood paneling.	Gypsum wallboard and paper, some wood paneling.	Gypsum wallboard, texture and paint.

234

Medical-Dental Buildings—Wood Frame (*continued*)

	Class 1 Best Quality	Class 2 Good Quality	Class 3 Average Quality	Class 4 Low Quality
Treatment Room (3% of total cost)	Gypsum wallboard and vinyl wall covering.	Gypsum wallboard and enamel.	Gypsum wallboard and enamel.	Gypsum wallboard, texture and paint.
Bathrooms (2% of total cost)	Gypsum wallboard and enamel with ceramic tile wainscot.	Gypsum wallboard and enamel or vinyl wall covering.	Gypsum wallboard and enamel.	Gypsum wallboard, texture and paint.
Ceiling Finish (4% of total cost)	Suspended "T" bar and acoustical tile.	Gypsum wallboard and acoustical tile.	Gypsum wallboard and acoustical tile.	Gypsum wallboard and paint.
Plumbing (6% of total cost)	Copper tubing, good fixtures.	Copper tubing, good fixtures.	Copper tubing, average fixtures.	Copper tubing, economy fixtures.
Lighting (6% of total cost)	Conduit wiring, good fixtures.	Conduit wiring, good fixtures.	Romex or conduit wiring, average fixtures.	Romex wiring, economy fixtures.
Cabinets (7% of total cost)	Formica faced with formica tops.	Good grade of hardwood with formica tops.	Average amount of painted wood or low grade hardwood with formica top.	Minimum amount of painted wood with formica top.

Note: Use the percent of total cost to help identify the correct quality classification.

Square foot costs include the following components: Foundations as required for normal soil conditions. Floor, wall and roof structures. Interior floor, wall and ceiling finishes. Exterior wall finish and roof cover. Interior partitions. Cabinets, doors and windows. Basic electrical systems and lighting fixtures. Rough plumbing and fixtures. Permits and fees. Contractors' mark-up. In addition to the above components, costs for building with more than 10,000 feet include the cost of lead shielding for typical X-ray rooms.

Medical-Dental Buildings—Wood Frame—Exterior Suite Entrances,
Length Less Than 2 Times Width

Estimating Procedure

1. Use these figures to estimate medical, dental, surgical, and similar professional buildings in which access to each office suite is through an exterior
entrance. Buildings in this section have more plumbing fixtures per square
foot of floor and smaller room sizes than general office buildings. Note also
that buildings with more than 10,000 square feet are assumed to have lead
shielded X-ray rooms.
2. Establish the building-quality class by applying the information on pages 233–235.
3. Compute the first floor area. This should include everything within the exterior walls and all insets outside the main walls but under the main roof.
4. If the first floor wall height is more or less than 10 feet, add to or subtract
from the first floor square foot cost below the appropriate amount from the
wall height adjustment table on page 248.
5. Multiply the adjusted square foot cost by the first floor area.
6. Deduct, if appropriate, for common walls or no wall finish. Use the figures
on page 246.
7. If there are second or higher floors, compute the square foot area on each
floor. Locate the appropriate square foot cost from the table on page 237.
Adjust this figure for a wall height more or less than 9 feet, using the figures
on page 248. Multiply the adjusted cost by the square foot area on each
floor. Use the figures on page 246 to deduct for common walls or no wall
finish. Add the result to the cost from step 6 above.
8. Multiply the total cost by the location factor listed on pages 207–215.
9. Add the cost of heating and air conditioning systems, elevators, fire sprinklers, exterior signs, paving and curbing, miscellaneous yard improvements,
covered porches and garages.

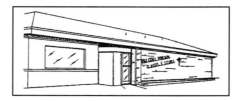

Medical–Dental building, Classes 2 and 3

Medical-Dental Buildings—Wood Frame—Exterior Suite Entrances,
Length Between 2 and 4 Times Width

Estimating Procedure

1. Use these figures to estimate medical, dental, surgical, and similar professional buildings in which access to each office suite is through an exterior
entrance. Buildings in this section have more plumbing fixtures per square
foot of floor and smaller room sizes than general office buildings. Note also
that buildings with more than 10,000 square feet are assumed to have lead
shielded X-ray rooms.

Wood Frame—Exterior Suite Entrances, Length Less Than 2 Times Width

First Story—Square Foot Area

Quality Class	1,000	1,500	2,000	2,500	3,000	4,000	5,000	7,500	10,000	15,000	20,000
Exceptional	158.00	151.87	148.36	146.00	144.32	142.01	140.47	138.13	136.77	135.16	134.24
1, Best	145.05	139.39	136.21	134.05	132.53	130.39	128.99	126.83	125.55	124.11	123.24
1 & 2	136.75	131.44	128.42	126.39	124.95	122.94	121.59	119.56	118.35	116.98	116.16
2, Good	129.37	124.33	121.46	119.55	118.20	116.28	115.02	113.09	111.99	110.67	109.89
2 & 3	120.13	115.44	112.77	111.02	109.74	107.95	106.81	104.99	103.99	102.74	102.04
3, Average	112.44	108.08	105.56	103.89	102.73	101.07	99.97	98.31	97.33	96.20	95.52
3 & 4	105.10	101.02	98.66	97.12	96.01	94.44	93.47	91.89	90.97	89.91	89.27
4, Low	98.13	94.32	92.17	90.71	89.67	88.25	87.27	85.83	84.98	83.97	83.37

Second and Higher Stories—Square Foot Area

Quality Class	1,000	1,500	2,000	2,500	3,000	4,000	5,000	7,500	10,000	15,000	20,000
Exceptional	140.85	137.29	135.21	133.79	132.76	131.31	130.34	128.82	127.92	126.87	126.25
1, Best	129.49	126.20	124.29	123.01	122.06	120.74	119.84	118.43	117.62	116.63	116.06
1 & 2	121.11	118.07	116.28	115.07	114.17	112.92	112.08	110.80	110.01	109.09	108.56
2, Good	117.97	115.01	113.29	112.09	111.22	110.02	109.21	107.93	107.12	106.28	105.75
2 & 3	109.02	106.25	104.65	103.57	102.74	101.62	100.87	99.71	99.00	98.21	97.71
3, Average	101.45	99.25	97.38	96.34	95.61	94.58	93.87	92.77	92.13	91.40	90.93
3 & 4	94.81	92.41	91.02	90.06	89.37	88.39	87.73	86.73	86.12	85.39	85.00
4, Low	88.68	86.45	85.15	84.25	83.60	82.70	82.05	81.12	80.57	79.90	79.48

2. Establish the building-quality class by applying the information on pages 233–235.
3. Compute the first floor area. This should include everything within the exterior walls and all insets outside the main walls but under the main roof.
4. If the first floor wall height is more or less than 10 feet, add to or subtract from the first floor square foot cost below the appropriate amount from the wall height adjustment table on page 248.
5. Multiply the adjusted square foot cost by the first floor area.
6. Deduct, if appropriate, for common walls or no wall finish. Use the figures on page 246.
7. If there are second or higher floors, compute the square foot area on each floor. Locate the appropriate square foot cost from the table on page 239. Adjust this figure for a wall height more or less than 9 feet, using the figures on page 248. Multiply the adjusted cost by the square foot area on each floor. Use the figures on page 246 to deduct for common walls or no wall finish. Add the result to the cost from step 6 above.
8. Multiply the total cost by the location factor listed on pages 207–215.
9. Add the cost of heating and air conditioning systems, elevators, fire sprinklers, exterior signs, paving and curbing, miscellaneous yard improvements, covered porches and garages.

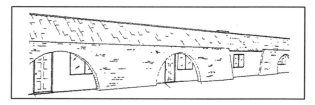

Medical–Dental building, Classes 1 and 2

Medical-Dental Buildings—Wood Frame—Exterior Suite Entrances, Length More Than 4 Times Width

Estimating Procedure

1. Use these figures to estimate medical, dental, surgical, and similar professional buildings in which access to each office suite is through an exterior entrance. Buildings in this section have more plumbing fixtures per square foot of floor and smaller room sizes than general office buildings. Note also that buildings with more than 10,000 square feet are assumed to have lead shielded X-ray rooms.
2. Establish the building-quality class by applying the information on pages 233–235.
3. Compute the first floor area. This should include everything within the exterior walls and all insets outside the main walls but under the main roof.
4. If the first floor wall height is more or less than 10 feet, add to or subtract from the first floor square foot cost below the appropriate amount from the wall height adjustment table on page 248.
5. Multiply the adjusted square foot cost by the first floor area.

Wood Frame—Exterior or Suite Entrances, Length Between 2 and 4 Times Width

First Story—Square Foot Area

Quality Class	1,000	1,500	2,000	2,500	3,000	4,000	5,000	7,500	10,000	15,000	20,000
Exceptional	161.34	153.71	149.43	146.61	144.62	141.81	140.00	137.21	135.61	133.74	132.65
1, Best	148.09	141.11	137.18	134.59	132.73	130.19	128.53	125.97	124.51	122.79	121.80
1 & 2	139.42	132.87	129.16	126.71	124.99	122.58	120.99	118.62	117.20	115.64	115.29
2, Good	131.68	125.63	122.09	119.80	118.17	115.88	114.40	112.12	110.82	109.29	108.43
2 & 3	122.35	116.61	113.32	111.20	109.65	107.54	106.17	104.08	102.84	101.46	100.63
3, Average	114.46	109.10	106.06	104.07	102.60	100.63	99.34	97.38	96.24	94.88	94.16
3 & 4	106.92	101.90	99.06	97.20	95.87	94.02	92.79	90.96	89.91	88.68	87.96
4, Low	99.86	95.16	92.49	90.75	89.48	87.80	86.65	84.92	83.94	82.78	82.10

Second and Higher Stories—Square Foot Area

Quality Class	1,000	1,500	2,000	2,500	3,000	4,000	5,000	7,500	10,000	15,000	20,000
Exceptional	142.50	137.97	135.37	133.64	132.38	130.65	129.49	127.70	126.68	125.48	124.78
1, Best	130.84	126.65	124.27	122.67	121.54	119.93	118.87	117.24	116.31	115.20	114.56
1 & 2	124.31	120.37	118.10	116.57	115.49	113.99	112.98	111.41	110.53	109.49	108.85
2, Good	119.32	115.52	113.35	111.91	110.84	109.38	108.44	106.96	106.09	105.05	104.48
2 & 3	110.35	106.83	104.85	103.48	102.49	101.15	100.28	98.88	98.09	97.14	96.60
3, Average	102.23	99.00	97.12	95.89	94.99	93.74	92.93	91.63	90.88	90.04	89.52
3 & 4	96.10	93.08	91.28	90.09	89.25	88.10	87.30	86.12	85.45	84.63	84.15
4, Low	89.19	86.36	84.75	83.64	82.86	81.77	81.04	79.95	79.32	78.54	78.09

6. Deduct, if appropriate, for common walls or no wall finish. Use the figures on page 246.

7. If there are second or higher floors, compute the square foot area on each floor. Locate the appropriate square foot cost from the table on page 241. Adjust this figure for a wall height more or less than 9 feet, using the figures on page 248. Multiply the adjusted cost by the square foot area on each floor. Use the figures on page 246 to deduct for common walls or no wall finish. Add the result to the cost from step 6 above.

8. Multiply the total cost by the location factor listed on pages 207–215.

9. Add the cost of heating and air conditioning systems, elevators, fire sprinklers, exterior signs, paving and curbing, miscellaneous yard improvements, covered porches and garages.

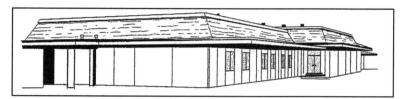

Medical–Dental building, Class 1

Medical-Dental Buildings—Wood Frame—Interior Suite Entrances, Length Less Than 2 Times Width

Estimating Procedure

1. Use these figures to estimate medical, dental, surgical, and similar professional buildings in which access to each office suite is through an interior entrance. Buildings in this section have more plumbing fixtures per square foot of floor and smaller room sizes than general office buildings. Note also that buildings with more than 10,000 square feet are assumed to have lead shielded X-ray rooms.

2. Establish the building-quality class by applying the information on pages 233–235.

3. Compute the first floor area. This should include everything within the exterior walls and all insets outside the main walls but under the main roof.

4. If the first floor wall height is more or less than 10 feet, add to or subtract from the first floor square foot cost below the appropriate amount from the wall height adjustment table on page 248.

5. Multiply the adjusted square foot cost by the first floor area.

6. Deduct, if appropriate, for common walls or no wall finish. Use the figures on page 246.

7. If there are second or higher floors, compute the square foot area on each floor. Locate the appropriate square foot cost from the table on page 243. Adjust this figure for a wall height more or less than 9 feet, using the figures on page 248. Multiply the adjusted cost by the square foot area on each floor. Use the figures on page 246 to deduct for common walls or no wall finish. Add the result to the cost from step 6 above.

Wood Frame—Exterior Suite Entrances, Length More Than 4 Times Width

First Story—Square Foot Area

Quality Class	1,000	1,500	2,000	2,500	3,000	4,000	5,000	7,500	10,000	15,000	20,000
Exceptional	168.66	159.31	154.08	150.64	148.19	144.83	142.65	139.29	137.38	135.16	133.89
1, Best	155.18	146.58	141.78	138.62	136.35	133.26	131.25	128.19	126.42	124.35	123.18
1 & 2	145.93	137.85	133.30	130.34	128.20	125.33	123.41	120.53	118.85	116.95	115.84
2, Good	137.77	130.16	125.88	123.08	121.05	118.32	116.54	113.80	112.21	110.43	109.37
2 & 3	127.85	120.74	116.79	114.18	112.34	109.78	108.12	105.57	104.11	102.45	101.48
3, Average	119.54	112.97	109.20	106.78	105.04	102.67	101.08	98.73	97.38	95.80	94.88
3 & 4	111.60	105.44	101.98	99.71	98.05	95.85	94.37	92.19	90.89	89.45	88.62
4, Low	104.17	98.40	95.18	93.05	91.52	89.44	88.09	86.02	84.83	83.51	82.70

Second and Higher Stories—Square Foot Area

Quality Class	1,000	1,500	2,000	2,500	3,000	4,000	5,000	7,500	10,000	15,000	20,000
Exceptional	147.32	141.49	138.20	136.07	134.55	132.46	131.05	128.99	127.78	126.40	125.57
1, Best	135.30	129.96	126.97	125.00	123.59	121.67	120.40	118.48	117.38	116.09	115.36
1 & 2	128.42	123.33	120.49	118.64	117.31	115.45	114.25	112.44	111.38	110.18	109.50
2, Good	122.84	117.97	115.27	113.45	112.17	110.44	109.28	107.54	106.54	105.41	104.70
2 & 3	113.53	109.04	106.51	104.88	103.67	102.08	101.02	99.40	98.44	97.42	96.78
3, Average	105.53	101.39	99.05	97.51	96.41	94.91	93.91	92.41	91.55	90.58	89.98
3 & 4	98.74	94.83	92.68	91.23	90.20	88.79	87.85	86.47	85.66	84.75	84.19
4, Low	92.20	88.59	86.49	85.19	84.23	82.91	82.03	80.75	79.97	79.11	78.61

8. Multiply the total cost by the location factor listed on pages 207–215.
9. Add the cost of heating and air conditioning systems, elevators, fire sprinklers, exterior signs, paving and curbing, miscellaneous yard improvements, covered porches and garages.

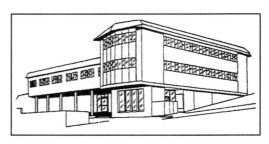

Medical–Dental building, Class 3

Medical-Dental Buildings—Wood Frame—Interior Suite Entrances, Length Between 2 and 4 Times Width

Estimating Procedure

1. Use these figures to estimate medical, dental, surgical, and similar professional buildings in which access to each office suite is through an interior entrance. Buildings in this section have more plumbing fixtures per square foot of floor and smaller room sizes than general office buildings. Note also that buildings with more than 10,000 square feet are assumed to have lead shielded X-ray rooms.
2. Establish the building-quality class by applying the information on pages 233–235.
3. Compute the first floor area. This should include everything within the exterior walls and all insets outside the main walls but under the main roof.
4. If the first floor wall height is more or less than 10 feet, add to or subtract from the first floor square foot cost below the appropriate amount from the wall height adjustment table on page 248.
5. Multiply the adjusted square foot cost by the first floor area.
6. Deduct, if appropriate, for common walls or no wall finish. Use the figures on page 246.
7. If there are second or higher floors, compute the square foot area on each floor. Locate the appropriate square foot cost from the table on page 245. Adjust this figure for a wall height more or less than 9 feet, using the figures on page 248. Multiply the adjusted cost by the square foot area on each floor. Use the figures on page 246 to deduct for common walls or no wall finish. Add the result to the cost from step 6 above.
8. Multiply the total cost by the location factor listed on pages 207–215.
9. Add the cost of heating and air conditioning systems, elevators, fire sprinklers, exterior signs, paving and curbing, miscellaneous yard improvements, covered porches and garages.

Wood Frame—Interior Suite Entrances, Length Less Than 2 Times Width

First Story—Square Foot Area

Quality Class	2,000	2,500	3,000	4,000	5,000	7,500	10,000	15,000	20,000	30,000	40,000
Exceptional	133.76	131.58	129.99	127.80	126.36	124.14	122.84	121.31	120.41	119.34	118.76
1, Best	126.65	124.58	123.06	121.01	119.61	117.51	116.29	114.86	114.01	113.01	112.43
1 & 2	119.62	117.68	116.25	114.31	113.00	110.99	109.86	108.48	107.66	106.71	106.20
2, Good	113.48	111.64	110.29	108.44	107.18	105.30	104.19	102.94	102.15	101.29	100.75
2 & 3	105.41	103.67	102.44	100.73	99.55	97.80	96.77	95.52	94.88	94.05	93.59
3, Average	98.85	97.25	96.05	94.43	93.36	91.72	90.76	89.64	88.98	88.24	87.77
3 & 4	92.97	91.44	90.35	88.81	87.82	86.27	85.34	84.31	83.67	82.95	82.52
4, Low	87.44	86.01	84.98	83.55	82.58	81.13	80.29	79.32	78.68	78.04	77.63

Second and Higher Stories—Square Foot Area

Quality Class	2,000	2,500	3,000	4,000	5,000	7,500	10,000	15,000	20,000	30,000	40,000
Exceptional	122.64	121.31	120.35	118.99	118.09	116.68	115.86	114.92	114.35	113.71	113.32
1, Best	116.30	115.02	114.12	112.81	111.97	110.66	109.87	108.98	108.45	107.81	107.43
1 & 2	110.42	109.21	108.31	107.11	106.29	105.03	104.32	103.47	102.95	102.37	101.65
2, Good	105.45	104.28	103.45	102.29	101.50	100.31	99.64	98.79	98.32	97.75	97.41
2 & 3	97.43	96.34	95.58	94.51	93.77	92.70	92.04	91.29	90.84	90.32	90.00
3, Average	90.63	89.64	88.90	87.90	87.24	86.23	85.61	84.92	84.50	84.00	83.73
3 & 4	85.19	84.27	83.60	82.75	82.02	81.07	80.49	79.83	79.43	78.98	78.71
4, Low	80.02	79.14	78.51	77.63	77.04	76.13	75.61	74.99	74.60	74.19	73.93

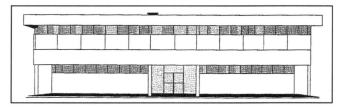

Medical–Dental building, Classes 1 and 2

Medical-Dental Buildings—Wood Frame—Interior Suite Entrances, Length More Than 4 Times Width

Estimating Procedure

1. Use these figures to estimate medical, dental, surgical, and similar professional buildings in which access to each office suite is through an interior entrance. Buildings in this section have more plumbing fixtures per square foot of floor and smaller room sizes than general office buildings. Note also that buildings with more than 10,000 square feet are assumed to have lead shielded X-ray rooms.
2. Establish the building-quality class by applying the information on pages 233–235.
3. Compute the first floor area. This should include everything within the exterior walls and all insets outside the main walls but under the main roof.
4. If the first floor wall height is more or less than 10 feet, add to or subtract from the first floor square foot cost below the appropriate amount from the wall height adjustment table on page 248.
5. Multiply the adjusted square foot cost by the first floor area.
6. Deduct, if appropriate, for common walls or no wall finish. Use the figures on page 246.
7. If there are second or higher floors, compute the square foot area on each floor. Locate the appropriate square foot cost from the table on page 247. Adjust this figure for a wall height more or less than 9 feet, using the figures on page 248. Multiply the adjusted cost by the square foot area on each floor. Use the figures on page 246 to deduct for common walls or no wall finish. Add the result to the cost from step 6 above.
8. Multiply the total cost by the location factor listed on pages 207–215.
9. Add the cost of heating and air conditioning systems, elevators, fire sprinklers, exterior signs, paving and curbing, miscellaneous yard improvements, covered porches and garages.

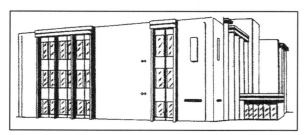

Medical–Dental building, Class 2

Wood Frame—Interior Suite Entrances, Length Between 2 and 4 Times Width

First Story—Square Foot Area

Quality Class	2,000	2,500	3,000	4,000	5,000	7,500	10,000	15,000	20,000	30,000	40,000
Exceptional	137.11	134.46	132.54	129.92	128.19	125.52	124.00	122.18	121.18	119.92	119.23
1, Best	130.28	127.73	125.92	123.44	121.77	119.26	117.77	116.08	115.11	113.92	113.25
1 & 2	122.86	120.46	118.75	116.40	114.83	112.48	111.08	109.49	108.55	107.47	106.78
2, Good	116.43	114.19	112.56	110.34	108.83	106.59	105.29	103.77	102.90	101.85	101.25
2 & 3	108.19	106.09	104.58	102.50	101.12	99.03	97.83	96.41	95.58	94.62	94.07
3, Average	101.37	99.39	97.97	96.02	94.76	92.77	91.63	90.31	89.56	88.65	88.11
3 & 4	95.65	93.80	92.45	90.62	89.42	87.56	86.48	85.24	84.49	83.65	83.16
4, Low	89.62	87.86	86.63	84.87	83.74	82.02	81.01	79.86	79.16	78.38	77.89

Second and Higher Stories—Square Foot Area

Quality Class	2,000	2,500	3,000	4,000	5,000	7,500	10,000	15,000	20,000	30,000	40,000
Exceptional	125.31	123.47	122.15	120.40	119.25	117.52	116.57	115.45	114.83	114.09	113.64
1, Best	119.41	117.66	116.42	114.73	113.63	112.02	111.08	110.01	109.41	108.69	108.30
1 & 2	112.79	111.13	109.95	108.36	107.34	105.80	104.92	103.93	103.34	102.69	102.32
2, Good	107.66	106.09	104.96	103.46	102.46	101.00	100.14	99.20	98.66	98.03	97.67
2 & 3	99.85	98.38	97.36	95.94	95.02	93.67	92.87	91.99	91.49	90.89	90.57
3, Average	92.57	91.19	90.25	88.93	88.09	86.82	86.10	85.29	84.81	84.27	83.96
3 & 4	87.44	86.14	85.23	84.00	83.20	82.01	81.32	80.57	80.10	79.59	79.28
4, Low	81.74	80.55	79.69	78.54	77.80	76.65	76.05	75.31	74.93	74.45	74.14

Wall Height Adjustment

The square foot costs for medical and dental buildings are based on the wall heights of 10 feet for first floors and 9 feet for higher floors. The first floor height is the distance from the bottom of the floor slab or floor joists to the top of the roof slab or ceiling joists. Second and higher floors are measured from the top of the floor slab or floor joists to the top of the roof slab or ceiling joists. Add or subtract the amount listed in this table to the square foot of floor cost for each foot of wall height more or less than 10 feet, if adjusting for first floor, and 9 feet, if adjusting for upper floors.

Perimeter Wall Adjustment

A common wall exists when two buildings share one wall. Adjust for common walls by deducting the linear foot costs below from the total structure cost. In some structures, one or more walls are not owned at all. In this case, deduct the "No Ownership" cost per linear foot of wall not owned. If a wall has no exterior finish, deduct the "Lack of Exterior Finish" cost.

Wood Frame—First Story

Class	For a Common Wall, Deduct Per L.F.	For No Wall Ownership, Deduct Per L.F.	For Lack of Exterior Finish, Deduct Per L.F.
1	$190.00	$369.00	$162.00
2	152.00	295.00	128.00
3	123.00	240.00	89.00
4	95.00	196.00	67.00

Wood Frame—Second and Higher Stories

Class	For a Common Wall, Deduct Per L.F.	For No Wall Ownership, Deduct Per L.F.	For Lack of Exterior Finish, Deduct Per L.F.
1	$128.00	$245.00	$162.00
2	95.00	190.00	128.00
3	89.00	184.00	89.00
4	84.00	172.00	67.00

Wood Frame—Interior Suite Entrances, Length More Than 4 Times Width

First Story—Square Foot Area

Quality Class	2,000	2,500	3,000	4,000	5,000	7,500	10,000	15,000	20,000	30,000	40,000
Exceptional	142.44	139.27	136.97	133.71	131.50	128.09	126.07	123.71	122.25	120.58	119.60
1, Best	135.06	132.07	129.87	126.80	124.70	121.45	119.54	117.26	115.92	114.33	113.38
1 & 2	127.28	124.47	122.39	119.49	117.50	114.47	112.63	110.53	109.25	107.76	106.88
2, Good	120.50	117.85	115.87	113.13	111.26	108.39	106.66	104.65	103.45	102.02	101.17
2 & 3	112.47	109.97	108.16	105.55	103.84	101.15	99.52	97.67	96.54	95.20	94.44
3, Average	104.83	102.51	100.80	98.41	96.80	94.29	92.78	91.06	89.96	88.74	88.02
3 & 4	101.63	99.41	97.72	95.44	93.84	91.42	89.97	88.27	87.25	86.07	85.33
4, Low	92.52	90.48	88.98	86.87	85.46	83.22	81.93	80.38	79.43	78.35	77.69

Second and Higher Stories—Square Foot Area

Quality Class	2,000	2,500	3,000	4,000	5,000	7,500	10,000	15,000	20,000	30,000	40,000
Exceptional	127.89	125.82	124.33	122.30	120.96	118.91	117.78	116.43	115.68	114.73	114.23
1, Best	121.27	119.31	117.90	115.97	114.69	112.79	111.67	110.42	109.65	108.81	108.28
1 & 2	115.09	113.20	111.87	110.04	108.82	107.02	105.96	104.76	104.06	103.22	102.75
2, Good	109.83	108.07	106.78	105.03	103.87	102.15	101.14	99.99	99.31	98.55	98.09
2 & 3	102.01	100.35	99.16	97.54	96.48	94.87	93.91	92.86	92.23	91.53	91.11
3, Average	94.43	92.93	91.82	90.30	89.32	87.82	86.99	85.99	85.40	84.74	84.33
3 & 4	89.18	87.72	86.69	85.27	84.34	82.94	82.10	81.19	80.51	80.01	79.63
4, Low	83.32	81.99	81.04	79.69	78.82	77.52	76.77	75.87	75.36	74.78	74.44

Wood Frame—Wall Height Adjustment, Square Foot Area

Quality Class	1,000	1,500	2,000	3,000	4,000	5,000	7,500	10,000	15,000	20,000	40,000
1, Best	1.49	1.18	1.01	.80	.70	.60	.48	.43	.36	.33	.22
2, Good	1.31	1.00	.87	.71	.58	.52	.43	.38	.32	.29	.21
3, Average	1.15	.88	.75	.61	.51	.46	.39	.34	.30	.24	.12
4, Low	1.02	.79	.67	.52	.46	.43	.34	.31	.24	.21	.12

248

Appendix D

Patient Care Considerations in the Construction Process

Steve Amsberry, DVM

THE FOCUS OF THIS appendix is to encourage you to view your construction project through the eyes of your patients. My assumption is that you are a patient advocate and want the best care provided for your patients.

Just as our patients cannot be treated for an anterior uveitis without considering the health of the rest of their body, we cannot view the construction process from only one perspective. When we consider what is best for the owner, staff, clients, and patients we will note many construction choices that will benefit all concerned. One example of this might be having the proper mechanical systems for heating, cooling, and odor control of all hospital zones. Occupying comfortable and odor-free spaces benefits all concerned. As an owner I enjoy my work and perform better if the air I breathe and smell is fresh and I'm not shivering or wiping sweat from my brow. The hospital staff responds in a like manner. Pet owners smell a clean hospital, see the pride we take in keeping the hospital comfortable, and equate that to quality care for their pets, therefore increasing their peace of mind. The pets arriving at a clean comfortable hospital appreciate their owners (i.e., stewards) being less stressed and the fact that their superior senses are not assaulted by the unchecked scents and odors from the previous hundreds of pets. Patient care considerations in the construction process cannot be compartmentalized from the considerations of the owner, staff, and clients. With this understanding in mind let's proceed.

I encourage you to rewind your thought processes to predesign time. As the title of this book alludes to, things are created twice, once in our minds and once in reality. We need to have the ability to articulate our dream before the building (form) will "follow function." As Dan Chapel mentions in chapter 8, this is the time to decide how you *want* to practice veterinary medicine in the future, not a recounting of how you *have* practiced in the past. Before any of the actual building process begins you need to honestly and thoroughly answer the question, Why am I undertaking this project? If your *entire* answer is to "increase your fame and fortune"—you may choose not to read the rest of this appendix. If your answer includes the desire to improve the level of care you deliver, please keep reading.

If your practice team has shared, strong core values that include excellent patient care, your foundation is set. As a leader you have "painted a picture" for the team of where your practice is heading. The team is excited about what will be and synergistically aids in the process. Change becomes exciting rather than threatening. The team support will be invaluable during the process and transition into the new "form." As a leader you have the responsibility to live your dream through your actions. If you talk about delivering the best pet care, yet have your flea-infested family dog on a chain in the backyard, your actions speak so loudly they can't hear a word you're saying. So if you haven't already done so, invest the time and energy to clarify your motives for taking on this building project. If you are reading this part way into the actual building process it is certainly not too late to benefit from "rewinding" the process and "dubbing in" missing parts.

Embracing a core value of patient advocacy is very important for you and your team. As this foundation is laid it can then be shared with clients, architects, bankers, interior designers, contractors, subcontractors, and so on. Let them all know of the benefits you want your patients to enjoy. I suspect that in general, humans want to be part of a project that benefits so many living beings.

If you review the literature related to construction of a veterinary hospital, most of it relates to the actual process. Topics include demographics, finances, building team, codes, variances, change orders, cost overruns, inspections, and so forth. Recently we are starting to see more consideration given to staff and client needs. Larry Gates includes in chapter 3 some thoughts on determining what your clients want. We are starting to see more information published regarding ergonomics in the workplace. There is a growing science of psychoneuroimmunology (the study of creating environments that prevent illness, speed healing, and promote well-being). My literature searches provided little information specifically regarding patient care considerations in the veterinary construction process. Keeping in mind the anecdotal flavor to this information, I am really encouraging you to use the creative portion of your brain to think about what our patients would view as benefits. For most of us this creative thought exercise is very awkward and long ago suppressed. We come from educational training backgrounds that emphasize there is only one right answer for every problem.

Mind mapping is not a technique commonly taught in veterinary school. Mind mapping is a tool used to unleash the creative right brain we all possess. We put a little damper on our yes/no, right/wrong, black/white thinking patterns. The individual or group goal of this technique is to focus on a topic we want ideas about (e.g., patient advocacy) and then get as many crazy, wild, doable, or undoable ideas as possible on the board in the shortest period of time. The quantity of ideas is more important than the quality. Initially no value judgments, criticisms, or even constructive critiques are offered.

I am going to list some logical and not-so-logical ideas for patient care to get you started with the process. This will be followed by some anecdotal suspected patient conversations. Get your creative juices turned on.

- No toxic plants in landscaping.
- Relieving "station" for dogs prior to entering the hospital.
- Glass front door so pets can see what they're getting into.
- Living-room-like atmosphere (pets have moved from barnyard to bedroom).
- Separate canine, feline, avian, and exotic reception and lodging areas.
- Fish tanks for feline consult/exam/lodging areas.
- Aroma therapy, soothing music.
- Glass doors in holding kennels instead of jaillike gates.
- Lots of glass block in lodging areas to allow natural light and a nonconfinement feeling for the pets.
- Floors with traction for dogs (i.e., tile, textured concrete, some newer sheet vinyl, etc.).
- Carpeted areas in feline-only spaces/rooms.
- No phones ringing/distracting in reception or consult/exam rooms.
- Videos/DVDs, etc., for the pets, fish aquarium screen savers if computers in consultation rooms.
- Quiet lift tables—nonstainless steel surfaces for pets.
- Soothing colors for humans and pets.
- Full-spectrum natural lighting.
- Glass in most doors to decrease anxiety of unknowns for pets and people.
- Video monitoring of post op/ICU/lodging areas (in-house and off-premise monitoring).
- Sound control throughout hospital (insulation, double layers of sheet rock, sound-absorbing panels and wall hangings, walls extending up through attic spaces as needed, proper placing of canine lodging).
- Odor control throughout hospital. Individually operated fans in rooms needing quick relief.
- Proper zones for exchange and filtration (odor, contamination, and sound control).
- Canine lodging ideas—executive suites (TV, chair, rug, more room), heated floors, day care activities, bathing/spa services, treadmills, outdoor exercise

areas, agility course, swimming pond, behavior training on site, volunteers who come in to just play with the boarding pets, courtyards to view with live animals, glass block partitions, natural light, puppy day care options, etc.
- Feline lodging ideas—cat condos, exercise arboretum, viewing pleasure (fish tanks, outside bird feeders, TVs, etc.), no dog odors or sounds.
- Consultation/visiting room with mobile kennel to allow owner visitations in calm, quiet environment.
- Owner seating in consult/exam room near exam table to decrease separation stresses.
- Enough exam consultation rooms to negate need for two cats or dogs to be in reception at one time.
- Comfortable space for family gathering for patient euthanasia—homelike atmosphere.

As mentioned earlier, we can't really separate patient consideration from client, staff, and owner perspectives. Generally speaking if we can earn the trust of the client and patient—providing peace of mind for both—all of us benefit. The human-animal bond is powerful and as recent surveys indicate— pets are becoming very important family members.

As an anthropomorphic lighthearted exercise, let's try to imagine a conversation between two dogs comparing their trips to the veterinarian.

Vignette #1

Rocky (three-year-old neutered black lab) talking with Byron (five-year-old neutered golden retriever).

Rocky: Hey Byron, didn't you go to the doctor for your checkup and vaccinations last month?

Byron: Yes, it was a long time ago, during the last full moon.

Rocky: Well, I just went yesterday and I'm here to tell ya I'm not looking forward to the next time and I don't think they are either. You should have seen them back off when I showed 'em my teeth and red gums!

Byron: I really like to go for my checkup—what's so bad about your trip?

Rocky: Well, here's the way my day went! Judy tricked me to get into the car with some sardines. I should have remembered she did the same thing last year. The car ride makes me feel sick to my stomach, so Judy gets ticked off because I drooled on her new skirt. We get to the hospital and the parking lot is so small just the workers use it—we have to walk two blocks in the pouring rain and I get to hurry because we're late for the appointment. We walk in and there are three immigrant dogs and a freaked-out cat in the tiny waiting area. I got a whiff of Jack's signature on the corner of the desk and having a full bladder I had plenty of "ink" to cover his up. For some reason my signing objects stresses Judy out and she's scolding me, tugging on my leash,

I back up, sit on the cat, and she nails me in my tail foundation, then climbs her human's back. That human starts yelling at Judy and everyone retreats to their corner. The floor is so slick I panicked and ice skated into the food display, knocking a few bags off.

We calmed down a little, but the phone kept ringing and I got a whiff of the new gang from 32nd Street—had to bite my tongue to keep from signing a few more places.

We finally had our names called and went into the exam room. The walls were so thin I could hear the cat next door hissing and the dog on the other side screaming about some shot. Judy was really anxious and I fed off her stress. I don't think either of us heard anything the doctor said. The nurse body-slammed me against the wall and I got two shots and then the nurse and veterinarian put on their big smiles and asked us if we had any questions. We were anxious to leave. Judy answered "no" and we went back to the dark waiting room. Judy nearly choked me standing on my leash while she wrote out the check. Then in her sweet voice she says, "You were so good Rocky, I'm so proud of you!" We walked through the pouring rain—I had to ride in the back so I could drool properly—then home we came. I think I'm going to pull the snarl technique next time Judy tries to get me in the car.

Byron: Man, that sounds awful. Let me tell you what my visit was like. Maybe I can drop a hospital brochure at your door for Judy. I'll have Kristi bump into Judy on our walks and I'll bet they tell their vet stories to each other. Maybe you'll get to go to my hospital next time.

Rocky: Well I'd appreciate any help I can get. I really don't want to resort to force to prevent this from happening again.

Byron: Since I was a young puppy about thirty some years ago I've been pretty used to my visits there. Our whole pack family went to some really fun puppy parties. We played games, got to meet other puppies' packs, got lots of treats from everyone, and got comfortable with the building.

It isn't uncommon for Stephanie to be driving by the place, pull in for a treat stop and I get to sniff all the treat givers that work in the building and then off we go to do the rest of our errands. So every time we go for a checkup I'm actually looking forward to the experience!!

My routine is to get out of the car, go over to the fire hydrant in the garden and see if my signature is bold enough to cover up everyone else's. If it's raining, I make this quick so I can get under the big roof next to the garden. As we are walking in I check everything out through the windows. The most dogs I've met in a visit is two, and I rarely see or hear any other people partners. After I get my treat and get loved up I usually go over and lay down by the fireplace and listen to the music and watch the waterfalls while Stephanie gabs with the treat givers. Pretty soon they call us in to the smaller room where the doctor checks me over. It's kind of like a chair massage with a few strobe light distractions. I never have heard all the commotion or been manhandled like you described. The only weird smells I notice are the treat givers often have chocolate smells on their hands, but I never have seen a chocolate. I vaguely feel the needle pokes, but I'm usually too distracted snarfing some of their bakery food to notice much. After the exam we say our good-byes to the doctor and then Stephanie gets her homework, pays the lady, and we go right through the fireplace room and back to the car. The whole visit seems pretty sedate compared to your experience. I don't even mind going in for my teeth cleaning every ten to twelve moons and that visit is for a whole daylight visit. Everyone treats me so well and I really like the new nap gas they have. When I'm waking up after they cleaned my teeth they have me in this warm tunnel and one of the treat givers holds my head in her lap. I don't think Stephanie even gets jealous of all the special treatment because she is always so appreciative when she picks me up.

So Rocky, I guess the simplest way for me to describe my visits to the doctor is—I look forward to them and so does Stephanie. We just don't experience the stress you described. In a different way being there is more comfortable than being at home.

Rocky: As a fellow canine good citizen, all I can say is please hurry up and get Judy to talk with Stephanie!!!!

Vignette #2

Seal (five-year-old spayed female Russian Blue) sharing information with her cousin Louie (four-year-old neutered male Sphynx).

Louie: Hey Seal, got some time before your nap to lend an ear?

Seal: For you I'd even delay my nap!

Louie: Sally cornered me yesterday, rolled me in a towel, and took me in for my checkup. I'm so stressed out I'm going to make her pay for a few days. I know she loves me, but every time she does this to me I get more and more ticked off.

Seal: What could be so bad, besides the needles they stick in you?

Louie: Well, one of the worst things for me is the anticipation. I get so worked up, Sally starts to tense up and give off bad vibes. We just have this pattern and neither of us can stop it. When we get there she acts like everything is cool and then tells me not to embarrass her! Yesterday, the two beagle twins were in the waiting room and they acted like I was a rabbit. There was so much noise and commotion I wet my blankie—I just started screaming for help. Finally they came to get us and I thought things might improve.

Seal: Did it get any better in the next room?

Louie: Instead of letting me walk out of the carrier on my own free will, the nurse grabbed both of my back legs and yarded me out breech. I escaped and jumped through a big round hole in the cupboard door—right into the trash can. I smelled at least six other cats—one was an untutored male—so I just barely had enough urine to cover up all their scents. The nurse caught me with a head noose and flung me onto the cold slippery stainless steel table and then threw a towel over me. As they talked about how they would handle me from there, I listened to Sally's anxious voice, two beagles howling, and another cat screaming next door.

Another nurse burst into the room from I don't know where and grabbed my scruff—pressing me against the cold metal. The doctor talked to Sally for a few minutes, stuck me with two needles, and the nurses released me back into my wet jail box. We went back to the noisy, busy waiting area—Sally apologized for my behavior and they said I was pretty normal! I think they said I have to go back in a year. I'm so worn out! And on top of that I'm feeling bad about myself because I'm giving Sally the cold shoulder.

Seal: I'm getting pretty upset just listening to you describe your visit.

Louie: I don't think it's fair you come back from the doctor's office in such a good mood. Why is it so different for you?

Seal: From what you've described I have an entirely different experience. I've been going multiple times a year and when I was in my teens I got to go to youth parties. I started to enjoy my visits to the hospital. The reception area is calm, quiet, and they play relaxing music. I've never had a dog approach me. I don't even hear any phones ringing. We are greeted when we arrive and go right into the exam room. The only odd smell I get a whiff of is some disinfectant. When I get there, Christian and the nurse start talking and I get out of my carrier to go look at the fish in the tank. Then we play a few games before they lift me up to the padded table. The doctor gives me a good nose to tail exam that I put up with because she is so kind and gentle—plus she calls me by my name and tells me I'm a "queen on high." I'm not tempted to hide anywhere because there are no small open spaces. When I get poked with the needles I'm usually distracted by food or the cool mobile they have above the exam table. After my checkup and shots the nurse talks to Christian about something, he pays, and we just leave without stopping in the reception space.

Louie: Well I can tell I've been living on the wrong side of the tracks. When do you think we can orchestrate getting Christian together with Sally to talk about my disaster visit. I want to go to your hospital next time!!

These two vignettes may be a little too cutesy for you, but the outcome I'm after is to get you to view this building project from the patient's point of view. Using this primer information will hopefully stimulate your creative right brain to come up with some excellent ideas to benefit your patients. Enjoy!!! (Please keep in mind—buildings come and go, families are forever!!)

Patient Care Considerations in the Construction Process Review Issues

- Clarify your core values before starting the process—what do you want in your building and why?
- Attempt to see the construction outcome through the eyes of your patients—shift your paradigm.
- Pay close attention to sight, sound, touch, and smell issues.
- Decrease the stress for the pet owner to decrease the stress for the patients.
- Your team includes not only your banker, accountant, contractor, consultant, and attorney but also your staff, clients, family, and patients. The project is an extension of you and those you care about.
- Enjoy the ride!!!!

Appendix E

Outpatient and Inpatient Flow and Other Fine Details

Thom A. Haig, DVM

THIS APPENDIX IS MEANT to follow the title in stimulating the practitioner's thoughts outside his or her current box. The following programs and ideas are meant to start a discussion with your architect and management team. What new programs or ideas can we implement in our new hospital that we can't do in the current physical plant? How much can we afford to plan for future growth? Not all of these ideas are for every hospital, but one or two may strike your fancy! Let's take a tour through our dream hospital.

Let's start in the front and work our way through the dream. What does your waiting room say to your client? Warm and fuzzy is an option. Sterile and high tech could be the opposite extreme. Windows to view the treatment and surgery areas or solid barriers in between are two more options. Whether you do exotics or cats, separate entrances or "safe" dividers may be appropriate. Those dividers don't have to be walls. They can be fish tanks or planters. Consider planning an interactive computer center. You can have educational games for children. Human-companion animal bond (HCAB) education like Delta Society web site and pet selection programs are other options. Guiding your clients to good on-line education such as Veterinary Information Network's Pet Care forum; the Missouri, OSU, or Don Levesque's seizure web sites; Y2Spay; AOL's pet selection; or Jan Bellow's dental web site are all suggestions. Retail sales have come and gone a couple of times. Do you want a retail area in your waiting room? Do you want display shelves for dog food, behavior toys, or training aids? It's easier to leave some wall space now for the next fad than to add it later.

What about the reception area? Plan for enough computer workstations to allow for growth. Look at a floor plan and traffic flow that separates the client relations area into its various functions. A place to greet clients and welcome them to the practice is your first requirement. Next you need a place for the telephone receptionist. Hopefully you have an on-line real-time appointment book that places this person someplace else! There is nothing worse than having a receptionist on the phone ignoring the client in front of her. Unless of course it is that poor receptionist with the same client breathing down her neck while trying to quietly placate the irate client on the phone! Another option is cordless phones that allow the receptionist to wander freely while still maintaining control of the phones. Then you need a place for checkout. Two options here are a back counter or window near the exam rooms or enough computers and workstations to do in-room checkout. With exam room checkout a back hallway and exit allows for efficient traffic flow. The client from the exam room never has to go back up to the waiting room or front reception areas. Don't forget the files. Whether you've switched to paperless or still use conventional medical records, you need to plan adequate and convenient storage space. Plan space either here or in the pharmacy for prescriptions to go home and for large bags of special order diets. Is the fax machine going to be up front or in the business office?

A side issue may apply to hospitals with large boarding and grooming facilities. The real income source for veterinary hospitals is the additional medicine brought in by these frequent visitors. All boarders and groomers in a veterinary-associated establishment should be screened as patients for wellness items as well as recommended procedures. Some state boards hold veterinarians to a higher standard of care than a nonveterinary boarding establishment. Using the recall-remind function of your computer, a pet partner can screen the pet's record for any missed care suggested by the doctor and deferred by the client. These items include therapeutic drug screening for chronic medications, past due wellness items like vaccinations, heartworm tests or fecals, medical progress checks (rechecks), and of course surgical and dental procedures. Consider a separate check-in area off the waiting room for these clients. All boarders should be screened prior to the owners leaving to allow for approval of these procedures prior to departure. Successful completion of these missed items is much more likely to be accomplished while the client is still present rather than later. Many clients prefer the convenience of having these procedures done while they are away rather than during a second trip later.

The next idea concerns number of exam rooms. High-density scheduling is a Tom Cat program covered in detail in *Building the Successful Veterinary Practice: Volume 2: Programs and Procedures*. In a nutshell: It requires staff utilization and allows you to see up to 40 percent more clients in the same period of time. This is accomplished with an outpatient nurse-doctor team seeing patients in two rooms with staggered appointments. I have had architects tell clients they never need more than four exam rooms. *Wrong!* Not if you want to do high-density scheduling. You need a minimum of two exam rooms per outpatient doctor. I say per outpatient doctor because with this type of scheduling you can have a doctor doing surgery part or all of the day in back. You may even have an inpatient doctor working up one doctor's cases while he or she is still seeing patients. This requires good interdoctor cooperation and is the subject of several other publications including *Veterinary Healthcare Services: Options in Delivery*. So how many doctors will be seeing patients at one time? You will need twice that many exam rooms plus the number discussed below!

There are other uses for exam rooms. Our generic recommendation is to build an odd number of exam rooms. The even number is for the docs seeing outpatients as just discussed. The odd exam room can have so many uses you may want two! The first is technician appointments. If tech appointments are legal in your state, these may be blood draws for therapeutic monitoring. They may be rabies-only clients. They may be preferred clients that have had a recent doctor exam and are back for routine vaccinations. You may want to have a tech take out drains or sutures in front of the client. If the client doesn't object, these animals may also be taken directly to the inpatient team. This "extra exam room tech" is not your outpatient nurse or doctor's assistant. This is an additional staff member with his or her own appointments.

This room may be used in the morning for the surgeon or surgical nurse to admit the day's surgery patients. This room may be used for discharge appointments after a surgery or hospital stay. By booking this room for surgical or medical discharge you can virtually eliminate—okay, minimize—the 5 o'clock rush. If you have an inpatient doctor, one of his or her functions can be to see walk-ins and emergencies. This is a real practice builder that many hospitals avoid. Now you can see why you may need more than one extra exam room. You can use the room for surgery check-ins in the morning and alternate walk-ins with tech appointments and releases during the day, then use it for discharges at night. I think you can now see where investing in one or two extra exam rooms may be beneficial. Don't forget to allow for practice growth in this final decision.

Certainly a discussion about your computer and records system deserves some thought pertaining to exam rooms. Even if you *never* want to go paperless, expanding technology will probably require a computer in every exam room at some point in time. Placing a piece of PVC pipe in the wall and an empty junction box in every room is far cheaper now than later. Then cable can be easily pulled at a later date for computers or video cameras or some new toy that hasn't been invented yet! Another consideration is the new telemedicine and otoscopy machines. Are you going to need to wheel carts through the door and up to the exam table or are you going to take every infected ear to the special procedures room?

Finally, think about the type of tables you want in the exam room. Many practices have several exam rooms with lift tables for big dogs. Then you have the scheduling problem of big dog and little dog rooms. Do you want a lift table in every room? This not only impacts the plumbing and cabinetry requirements but also the actual size of the room. Besides the lift tables there are wall-mounted tables, pedestal tables, and many unique custom-built tables to choose from. Discuss function and personal preference with your architect, but look "outside the box" before you decide!

The last use for this room overlaps with the "conference room" discussed below. If you build a "special purpose room" as your odd exam room, it may be larger and furnished differently than the other exam rooms. Then it can be used for euthanasia and grief counseling. It may be used for client conferences to discuss findings, treatment options, review radiographs, and so on. Additionally this room may be used as an alternative medicine room. If you have the need to keep a client in the room longer than normal for an Eastern history taking, acupuncture appointment with the client present, or chemotherapy discussion, you may want to use the odd room as a backup exam room. This way the regular exam rooms are not removed from the high-density rotation.

The next dream is a conference room. In this day and age it is a luxury that the new veterinary hospital cannot afford to forget. This room can double as the library, Veterinary Information Network (VIN)/Internet access room, interview room, doctor's meeting room, management team meeting room, employee counseling room, grief counseling room, acupuncture room, and general all-purpose place to get some privacy! A modern veterinary practice *is* a small business and needs meeting space and a place outside some doctor's office to find some privacy. Staff interviews for new staff or performance planning of existing staff are less threatening on neutral territory. Maybe you want to design a room big enough to hold a staff meeting or all-staff training session without dragging all the chairs out to the waiting room!

Speaking of office space, I hope you're not planning the group office for the docs and practice manager and everybody else! Docs can certainly share office space, maybe two per office. If you're building a new hospital, you need a practice manager and that job requires privacy. You probably have a bookkeeper and an inventory clerk. They require office space and privacy. Even though it's "wasted space" and "nonproductive," you must plan for it or you will be remodeling soon. His or her own office is a real perk for that employee who is often not appreciated for the work he or she does.

Now let's get back to our front-to-back tour. The pharmacy is next in line. What is in your pharmacy? Is it combined with your lab or do you do enough in-house lab work to make that a separate area? Depending on your medical records, checkout procedures, and use of outpatient nurses, you may need several computer workstations in this area. The amount of inventory and the way you fill prescriptions will determine the amount of storage necessary in the pharmacy. It may also dictate the need for a backup storage room. In a very big practice or one with multiple satellites and central purchasing, a locked central pharmacy may be advisable. If you plan a separate lab, it needs to be convenient to the treatment room but constructed in a way to minimize noise from both areas and with enough room to work comfortably. With all the in-house machines available today, you can't just put a microscope in a closet. Certainly odor and noxious fumes control is another consideration. Don't forget your OSHA eye wash station!

Now let's enter the treatment room. If you have never used a wet table, double the number you think you'll want. You need one for surgical prep for each surgeon. Another can be in the special procedures room for dentals and endoscopy. A third may be used for nonsterile procedures like abscesses and contaminated lacerations. This table could be in addition to the prep table if you have enough surgery to keep the surgeon busy all day. The outpatient and inpatient doctors may still be fighting over the third table for minor procedures. Some folks balk at doing blood draws and "nonwet" procedures on the grate. Depending on the grate's design, trapped toes can be a problem. Small spacing on the grate and/or throwing a towel on the grate easily prevent this problem. The flexibility of having multiple wet tables far outweighs its drawbacks. Obviously these functions can be combined depending on number of docs and caseload. Just like the exam rooms, you are far better planning the cabinetry and plumbing for one too many wet tables than too few! If the plumbing is in place, you can always add the table later. There are even inserts for wet and dental tables that can be added to existing cabinetry with just a cutout.

An average practice that is routinely grading teeth and has several levels of dental charges based on those grades can keep a technician-assistant team and a wet table busy all day. Dentistry is an enormous source of income that is mostly staff generated. Many people are annoyed by the whine of a high-speed hand piece, especially eight to ten hours a day. Design a dental alcove as an almost separate room off the main treatment room. Ensure adequate space to allow personnel to work all the way around the end of the table. I prefer a sit-down dental table with the end cut out to allow easy access by a technician or assistant who is sitting to do his or her work. This can be a commercial wet table from any of several manufacturers or a specially built custom cabinet with a dental insert. This room requires special thought given to plumbing, oxygen delivery, and possibly a wall-mounted anesthetic machine. Don't forget electrical and ceiling or wall mounting for a dental X-ray and counter space for a chair-side developer. If you are a really big practice, you may even consider a room big enough for two dental tables!

A special procedures room is another consideration that is very practice specific. It could include dental, but I would make special procedures separate. Different procedures require different design. Procedures that shouldn't be done in surgery or the spare exam room include endoscopy, ultrasound, echo, and telemedicine. The number of these procedures performed in your hospital and their frequency will obviously impact the design of this room. Related to special procedures in my mind is radiology. Do you still need a darkroom? With the new hospital you may be purchasing an entire new radiology suite with smart collimator and exposure settings or maybe the cassette-less system is now in veterinary price range. You certainly want to look at the space savings of a pass-through darkroom.

When you consider the design of the treatment room, remember that this is the center of your hospital. Room for records, white boards, doctor's workstations, computer terminals, and so on; all need to allow for future growth. Evaluate your use of technicians and assistants as you think through this plan. Are your docs still doing tech work? If the answer is yes, you will probably not plan enough tables for the teams to work. After you call a consultant to help you pay for this new building, you will need a place for the inpatient team to draw blood, place catheters, do initial and sequential TPRs, blood chemistries, and so forth. You will still need work space for the inpatient doctor to do medical progress exams, minor procedures, and emergencies. The goal of high-density scheduling is to do exams in exam rooms and everything else in back. This is an oversimplification, but you get the idea. You should not be drawing blood, placing IVs, and doing minor procedures in the exam room. If you are, consider how much work you could be sending to the back while you see the next client. If you switch to this system, consider how many tables you will need to support this effort.

In calculating the amount of cage space, several issues need to be considered. First is whether or not you are doing any boarding. VIP boarding and its possibilities and requirements need to be considered in the total numbers of runs, large cages, and wards. Review the overall plan and then determine the needs of just the hospital wards. It is always best to *not* comingle boarders and hospitalized animals whenever possible. Having said that, consider medicated boarding. There are two groups here. One is the perfectly healthy dog on a chronic medication like thyroid or Phenobarbital. Can this patient be part of the boarding population? The other is the ill dog on oral medication that would normally be treated at home. Is this animal a boarder or does it need to be hospitalized while Mom and Dad are on vacation? The next population is related to high-density scheduling and the day admit procedure for diagnostics. If you embrace this philosophy, how many patients will need a home for the day or a few hours? Finally, we have to consider the need for an isolation ward and special environmental conditions for an exotic ward or various types of exotics. Some clients tell me they see one case of parvo a year. Others see multiple cases at once several times a year. Obviously these two extremes would have significantly different requirements for isolation. The same applies to the numbers and types of exotics you may see. Sick birds and reptiles have vastly different humidity and temperature requirements than mammals. Do you see enough exotics to justify a separate ward or wards? Sometimes a closet with sliding glass doors, a humidifier, and separate temperature control is enough. If you do potbellied pigs, they might require some special soundproofing measures!

An area that has been touched on but requires thought to the overall plan is storage. I mentioned the pharmacy and possibility of a central pharmacy. Even a small practice needs some backup area for fluids, bulk shipments, diets, and other items too large to put in the hallway pharmacy. Don't forget X-rays, medical records, and other items required to be kept for several years past their active date. Do you need to finish the attic or basement or plan extra room in the business office for these items?

Outpatient and Inpatient Flow Review Issues

- Think outside the box.
- Tour this virtual hospital to get new ideas.
- Don't redesign what you've already got.
- Think teamwork and patient flow.

Appendix F

Emergency and Specialty Facility Concerns

Thomas E. Catanzaro, DVM, MHA, FACHE

Checklist for Facility Success

- Ensure you have a copy of the AAHA *Design Starter Kit for Veterinary Hospitals,* third edition, since building materials are building materials, and scale drawings of parts are parts (if I remember right, KFC was built on the "parts are parts" concept).
- Location visibility is not critical since most clients come from referral; you can put it at the back of an industrial park on *very* cheap dirt! The demographic information provided in the *Feasibility of the Veterinary Specialty Practice* Signature Series Monograph (www.v-p-c.com) may be of some assistance at this point.
- Storefronts in low-use shopping center areas work very well for low rent and happy landlords. Leasehold build-outs are cheaper than new construction, but if specialists are to be daytime users, a freestanding facility needs to be in the five-year plan.
- While landscaping is not usually important (except for zoning issues), the facility *requires* more outside lighting augmentation than any comparable veterinary facility; the parking lot must be flooded with light at night, and most all facets of the building should be accent lighted. A well-lit and obvious entry is a necessity.
- Brochures must have very clear strip maps, but those using night photos of the well-lit emergency practice have greater client appeal; day photos of a facility usually used at night is not good marketing.

- The entrance must be inviting, with wide sidewalks and wide doors so gurneys can move concurrent with staff and stressed clients. Curb cuts are for scissor gurneys as well as ADA, and smooth surface transitions are critical for patient movement.
- There *must* also be a security screening capability for potential incoming clients; a good-sized vestibule out of the elements, with remote camera imaging and a generous use of shatterproof glass equivalent to the interior, is more inviting than the brick airlock of the past.
- The use of remote imaging of all client areas is an important safety concern and includes the vestibule, reception, waiting, and even consultation rooms; this is not Big Brother, it is staff safety, so the more obvious, the better.
- Deposits for healthcare needs *must* be collected upon admission, but that does not require a cash drawer in front; all monies can be collected in the privacy of the consultation room, if there are adequate consultation rooms, and the cash drawer can be secured in the pharmacy area.
- The quality emergency practice most often becomes a twenty-four-hour critical-care and emergency healthcare facility, so the administrator's office (the person running the facility for the board) must be centrally located to the client access area, as well as for supporting the bookkeeper, central medical supply (CMS), and inventory management staff members.
- Medical records must be on paper for forensic liability, but since fax reports are usually needed in the morning transfer, electronic records are a great temptation for easier transmission. If this is the case, ensure hard copies are printed each morning and the attending doctor signs the paper record, which can then be archive-filed chronologically in a less central storage area than reception.
- Consultation rooms usually need to be larger than the standard eight-foot-by-ten-foot room in general practices. Lift tables and large, concerned, family groups are common for night emergencies, so there must be room for the people as well as the critical-care staff.
- Using white boards, augmented with corner scanning attachments that read the white board and computerize the marker writing/drawing, is a great time saver as well as liability protection; they should be in all consultation rooms as well as the conference room.
- The better emergency practices have a higher than usual admission for stabilization rate, and as such, a "stat" treatment area *behind* the consultation rooms is becoming common, with larger-than-normal sized cages for observation.
- The pharmacy and lab have a higher laboratory utilization, so about three linear feet of counter for each piece of apparatus must be in the plan, as well as a low wet sink area for the centrifuge, separated from the higher dry microscope counter to prevent vibration.
- Half refrigerators in multiple areas with supplies and drugs specific to the zone's needs are better than one large refrigerator centrally located.
- The treatment room needs multiple dry, single-use workstations, with computers closely located to the dry, lift, and wet tables, as well as four-foot-wide runs and oversized cage banks so providers can access patients needing care/monitoring more easily.

In a "stat" ICU/CCU setting, radiology, endoscopy, ultrasound, ECG, and
    other imaging capabilities must be readily available.

The imaging room should be directly off the central treatment area but should
    be large enough for all the imaging equipment as well as a darkroom with
    automatic processor.

- Most all cage banks need nasal oxygen and IV pump hookups and apparatus
space. Multiple concurrent cases mean that easy visibility from the treatment
area is an important time saver, so glass walls increase, providing noise control concurrent with visibility.

- The surgery suites need to be positive pressure (10 percent more air inflow
than exhaust out), single-use, impermeable surface, easy-to-clean rooms.
There should usually be two types in an emergency facility: a "stat" surgery
and a HEPA filter orthopedic suite, larger than the standard surgery suite.
Again, both should have predominantly glass walls.

If the daytime specialists include the board-certified surgeon, plan on two
    suites per surgeon.

With a surgery daytime specialty, a radiology film reading room (screen bank
    and/or computer screens) should be close to the surgery suites.

    - Surgery scrub can be in pack prep, with glass walls so cases in the sur-
gery suite can be observed, but it should be blocked from aerosol contamination from the prep area or treatment wet tables.

    - A good emergency facility has a staff lounge off treatment and lab, so
staff can react to either area quickly.

    - If the facility is to have a day specialist use, the radiology department
might become a central issue of concern. In these cases, we recommend
looking at elevators ($28,000–$40,000 each) to allow the vertical distance to become "zero" for lateral access.

When the footprint is tight, the primary aseptic surgery can be upstairs, with
    offices, conference rooms, and library.

In exceptionally large facilities, radiology is scattered to the needed work
    centers and connected via computerized X-ray records, so film files are not
    essential and hard copies can be sent to the referring practice(s).

In extremely diverse specialty practices, the MRI and CAT scan shielding
    suggests the radiology department becomes subsurface for best shielding
    (most cost effective).

- The isolation ward is seldom isolated, since emergency care is still a high visibility need, so again glass walls are important, as are remote monitoring
capabilities (sight and sound). When designing an emergency and specialty
center, many smaller ward units, each able to be sanitized and separated from
circulation contamination, are the rule.

- Doctor stations must be comfortable, centrally located (no bed), with Internet
access. They are separate from nursing stations or medical record stations and
are used to develop proper records of care as well as conduct case literature
reviews and case-centered research.

In the most progressive emergency practices, the slower dead-of-night hours
    are used to conduct literature reviews (e.g., VIN library, etc.), so the refer-

ring practice, as well as the emergency practice staff, has value-added supplemental information returned with the patient report in the morning.

In marketing-savvy specialty practices, the nonsignificant emergency patient causes the referring practice to get a researched "local or topical issue" (e.g., vaccination protocols, zoonosis emergence, CDC morbidity and mortality (M&M) release, etc.).

- Since the best advertisement for an emergency practice is referral from general practices, training of staff from the referring practice becomes a mission-essential element of facility planning. Observation space for small groups, as well as team-based healthcare delivery, requires a more spacious treatment and surgery floor plan. Mobile equipment allows easier reconfiguration, and in some cases, even walls are designed to be moveable (e.g., Hermann-Miller wall units).
- We are seeing some specialty centers colocate with upscale pet resorts that have respite care facilities (larger suites for the elderly animals needing higher levels of healthcare when their stewards are away). A VIP suite (eight foot by eight foot) can lease for about forty dollars-plus a night, and attracts the type of people that usually use emergency and specialty centers.
- Most boarding facilities have gone to centralized decontamination washing systems, and laundry facilities use only *industrial* machines; this is appropriate for a specialty/emergency practice due to staffing limitations.
- Most upscale boarding facilities have gone to self-watering runs, central food preparation, and dishwashers for animal bowls and trays; this is appropriate for a specialty/emergency practice due to staffing limitations.
- With an emergency practice, there is inadequate staff to appropriately clean a facility after a hard night or weekend, so morning janitorial services provided by a healthcare-skilled contractor become an essential line item. This includes medical waste removal on a daily basis.
- Snow removal (northern areas) cannot wait until morning in an emergency practice setting, so there must be a "first flake" contract, with an outside agent, for ensuring a cleared parking lot and safe facility access.

To put this all into perspective, a "renovation" floor plan has been included. This was an emergency practice with added specialists that was moving to an existing facility (an old dinner club), and we helped them "find a fit." The local architect had placed a staggered six exam room diagonal in the outpatient area where we now have nine consultation rooms, the endoscopy room, and the specialized treatment room for opthalmology and dermatology behind the special exam rooms (two part-time specialists share the space on alternating days). Like many neophyte architects who automatically pattern specialty hospital designs from the traditional veterinary teaching hospitals, he had overused hallway access; in the VTH, hallways (single-use circulation space) are needed for moving students, while in private veterinary facilities, they are usually just *very* expensive "turf" boundaries ($150 a square foot plus) and a waste of essential working space. The client room was added next to the elevator due to the long distances clients often travel for specialists and comes equipped with Internet access, telephone, and television; the client view into the lab was an added benefit for a high-tech environment. The stat surgery in the main treatment room allows the surgical specialists to have the second floor for their own domain, and the ultrasound room allows internal medicine to access it more readily than by crossing the treatment space. The center cages in treatment are for urgent care cases, common with emergency practices and ICU surveillance. The long counter on the diagonal wall (which was actually a high window wall) provides plenty of work space for medical records and nursing staff. Staff access was directly into the lounge area (with lockers) as well as the stairway up to the staff office cubicles. Office space was virtually eliminated from the main floor and moved to the second floor, while radioisotope areas were moved to the basement for safety reasons.

Glossary

Ad infinitum: The time when veterinarians wish to make changes to blueprints and construction documents, usually due to poor planning earlier.

Afterthought: An expensive change order when told to a contractor post-bid order.

Air conditioning: The process of treating air so as to control simultaneously its temperature, cleanliness, humidity, and distribution to meet the requirements of the conditioned space.

Air-handling unit: An assembly of components used to cool or heat, filter, humidify or dehumidify, and circulate air to occupied spaces to maintain a controlled environment.

American Institute of Architects: Professional society that does not license architects.

Anesthesiology: The suspending and restoring of consciousness, depending upon the patient's mental and physical status; it is used to maintain circulation, respiration, and vital signs during surgery.

Animal: Patient with fur, fins, feathers, or other living attributes.

Architectural registration: State licensing procedure based upon testing and application.

Average daily census: Patient days divided by 365.

Average length of stay: Number of days spent in hospital cage/run divided by number of patients.

Average patient days: Number of cages/runs divided by 365.

BTU monitoring: A system of instrumentation to determine the total amount of energy being used.

Cardiology: Diagnosis and treatment of heart, artery, and vein disease; it makes use of surgery, electrical heart monitoring, radioactive tracing, high-frequency sound study, and cardiac catheterization and angiography.

Central plant: A central grouping of mechanical, heating and ventilation, and electrical equipment designed to provide maximum flexibility, maintainability, and operating efficiency over the useful life of the facility.

Central-vac: An installed system of vacuum tubes to allow easy cleaning of hospital by staff.

Centrex: A type of central telephone system that permits direct dialing between telephones in that system.

Chiller: A mechanical device used to chill water that is circulated throughout a building to terminal cooling coils; it consists of a compressor to compress vapor refrigerant, a condenser to convert the pressurized refrigerant into a liquid, and an evaporator to chill the supply.

Circuit breaker: A device designed to automatically open an electrical circuit at a predetermined overload.

Condenser: A device in which refrigerant vapor is condensed in a closed shell with a cooling medium circulated through an assembly of tubes within the shell.

Constant volume system: An air-conditioning system designed to deliver air to occupied spaces at a fixed, predetermined flow rate.

Converter: A device designed to transfer heat from steam to water; used to generate hot water for heating with steam from a steam boiler.

Cooling tower: An enclosed device for cooling water by contact with air that is moved through the unit by one or more fans.

Critical path method: Type of scheduling using a computer input that maps various desirable inputs to time.

Cystoscopy: A procedure in which the doctor looks into the bladder through a lighted tube.

Dentistry: A program of oral health promoted for better breath and long life of companion animals and horses.

Dermatology: The treatment of skin disorders; it uses various treatments and procedures such as cryotherapy (freezing cancerous tissues) and photochemotherapy (a combination of light and drugs).

Domestic water heater: A piece of mechanical equipment used to heat potable water for delivery to plumbing fixtures such as sinks, showers, or laundry equipment.

Ductwork: A system of sheet metal conduits used to convey conditioned air to and from occupied spaces.

Electric distribution: A general term used to describe the building's electrical system from the main building electrical service to the loads that it serves, including wiring, controls, and protective devices.

Electric resistance heating: A radiation heating unit in which the heat is generated by passing an electrical current through a resistance-type wire.

Emergency generator: An engine-driven device that generates electrical power to serve essential needs when the normal power supply is out of service.

Endocrinology: The study of tiny endocrine glands that control growth, maturation, and reproduction, including the pituitary, thyroid, adrenals, parathyroids, ovaries, and testes glands; hormonal disorders such as hyper- and hypothyroidism, diabetes mellitus, and severe hypoglycemia are treated, and patient education and counsel are given.

Endoscopy: The internal examination of hollow areas of the body using a long, flexible periscope-type instrument.

Energy audit: Breaking down total energy consumption so it can be analyzed.

Fan coil unit: A prefabricated assembly including heat transfer coils, a fan driven by an electric motor, air filter, controls, and air outlet; it is located in occupied spaces to provide a controlled environment within that space.

Fast-tracking: Advanced construction phases (such as building utilities and foundation) before construction drawings have been completed.

Feeders: Sets of electrical conductors extending from the main service to the panelboard.

Fire alarm system: A system designed to detect the presence of fire or smoke in a building and to automatically transmit signals that are used to initiate certain automatic and manual procedures in a fire emergency.

Fire detection system: A system of devices within occupied and unoccupied spaces and within the air-conditioning system to provide an early warning that fire is present.

Fire protection: A term loosely used to describe a system of sprinklers, hose outlets, fire extinguishers, fire and smoke detectors, and alarms designed to detect smoke or fire, extinguish a fire, and warn personnel.

Fire zone: An area separated from other areas by walls and doors having a high resistance to fire, designed to prevent the spread of fire to or from adjacent fire zones.

Four-pipe system: A system that utilizes two heat transfer coils, one for heating and one for cooling. Heating or cooling is available at any time.

Full-spectrum lighting: Specially designed bulbs that provide the entire visual light spectrum; essential for effective tissue evaluation.

Gastroenterology: Problems affecting the organs of the digestive tract—esophagus, stomach, intestines, liver, pancreas, and biliary duct system.

General surgery: The beginning of all surgical subspecialties and still the most extensive range of procedures.

Ground fault: A type of short circuit caused by an electrical contact between an energized electrical conductor and any part of the grounding system that results in a flow of currents in grounding conductors.

Health maintenance organization: Group formed to supply healthcare insurance services on a prepaid plan, not yet available in veterinary medicine.

Hematology: The study of blood, including nutrients, proteins, hormones, white blood cells, platelets, and bone marrow, to aid in diagnosing a medical condition or disease.

Hot water coils: A component of an air-handling unit consisting of pipe with metal fins on the outside; designed to transfer heat from hot water within the pipe to the air contacting the fins.

Incremental units: A prefabricated assembly that includes a refrigeration system, steam, or air filters, electric motor-driven fan, heater, and controls. The heater can be hot water, steam, or electric resistance. The unit is located on an exterior wall within the occupied space.

Indemnity insurance: Similar to car insurance, where there is risk sharing (not transfer) between insurance company and property owner. Reputable pet insurance falls into this category.

Induction unit: A prefabricated assembly, including heat transfer coils, air filters, controls, and a connection to a central, conditioned, primary air supply; room air is induced into the unit by primary air, they mix, and the mixture is delivered to the room to provide a controlled environment.

Interstitial space: Unoccupied space between floors, approximately six to ten feet high, enabling mechanics to work on air conditioning and equipment without disturbing the occupied floors.

Laboratory and pathology: The performing of tests to confirm (or not) diagnoses, tracing and identifying microbes that cause infectious diseases, running the blood bank and hematology test section, and studying chromosomal abnormalities (cytogenics), tropical diseases, and parasites (parasitology).

Life-cycle costs: Process by which total costs are determined over a selected period of years; included are yearly maintenance costs, yearly energy costs, and the initial purchase price, including installation costs. The process is effective in determining the most economical system by comparing life-cycle costs over the normal life expectancy.

Lightning protection: A special wiring system designed to intercept atmospheric lightning and cause it to flow to the ground, thereby preventing damage to structure or building.

Load shedding: A process of shutting down electrically operated equipment in a predetermined sequence to limit the maximum demand and thereby reduce electrical costs.

Medical gases: Gases used in medical treatment and laboratory procedures; they include air, gas, oxygen, nitrous oxide, and vacuum.

Medicine: The general category of subspecialties includes cardiac, endoscope, pulmonary, and internal medicine.

Nephrology: Study of the kidneys; kidney dialysis (artificial kidney machine) and kidney transplant depend on this service.

Neurology and neurosurgery: The study and treatment of brain, spinal cord, and nervous system disorders or injuries, including seizures, tumors, multiple sclerosis, and headache; stroke, vision, cancer complications, and blood pressure are all related to neurology.

Nuclear medicine: The application of internally administered radiopharmaceuticals to diagnose or treat conditions.

Obstetrics: Obstetrics is the specialty dealing with pregnancy, labor, delivery, and postpartum care. Patients with high-risk pregnancies are now referred to specialists in perinatal-neonatal services.

Ophthalmology: Treatment of diseases of the eye; programs with special diagnostic aids and specialized surgical equipment.

Oral surgery: Correction of facial deformities and joint dysfunction and removal of cysts and tumors from the jaws.

Orthopedics: Surgical and nonsurgical care of patients with problems of the musculoskeletal system, such as back problems, fractures, torn ligaments, and torn tendons.

Otorhinolaryngology: Specialty dealing with the ear (otology), nose (rhinology), and throat (laryngology).

Oxygen system: A large central supply and piping to locations where oxygen is used in treatment.

Panelboard: A unit designed for control of a number of individual lighting and other electrical loads, including automatic overload protection devices.

Passive solar energy: The use of a building's exposures to the sun to absorb heat.

Patient days: Admissions multiplied by length of stay; average daily census divided by target occupancy.

Perinatal and neonatal pediatrics: Intensive care nurseries, constant care, and transitional nurseries for twins, jaundiced infants, breech birth or cesarean section infants, and infants who are underweight or overweight at birth; neonatologists become involved in high-risk pregnancies long before delivery.

Physical medicine and rehabilitation: Treating disabled patients; a rehabilitation team involves physical and occupational therapists, rehabilitation nurses, and animal caretakers.

Pneumatic controls: A system of controls for regulating system functions, operated by air pressure from a central air system.

Power factor: The ratio of the true power, or watts, to the product of the current and voltage in an alternating current electrical circuit.

Pressure differential: The difference in pressure across a device, expressed in pounds per square inch or inches of water.

Primary care: Deals with minor illnesses or injuries and includes general practitioners, outpatient facility, or primary care center.

Pulmonary medicine and respiratory therapy: The treatment of lung and breathing disorders, including chronic bronchitis, emphysema, asthma, sarcoidosis, and lung cancer, as well as respiratory failure accompanying shock, trauma, burns, surgery, and various medical diseases.

Radiant heat: A heating unit located in occupied spaces; heating is provided by a combination of radiation to objects within the space and conduction to surrounding air, which is circulated by natural convection.

Radiation therapy: A tissue-destroying procedure primarily directed toward diseases characterized by tumor or new growth, using cobalt gamma rays and radiation of varying intensities.

Radiology: The use of radiant energy in treatment; also brain scanning by computerized tomography (CAT scan and MRI).

Reheat: A process related to control of space humidity during the cooling season. Air is cooled to the dew point to remove excess humidity and then reheated to the temperature that, when delivered to the space, will provide the proper space temperature.

Retrofit: Existing building space remodeled for a different function.

Secondary care: More specialized services such as metabolic diseases, general surgery, and diagnostics; usually involves hospitalization in quality health-care 24-hour environment.

Shock and trauma: Subspecialty of emergency with advanced diagnostic, resuscitative, and monitoring techniques.

Short list: Reducing the number of professional or contracting firms down from many to a few for final selection.

Smoke damper: An automatic damper in an air duct system designed to close and prevent the spread of smoke to occupied spaces.

Smoke-purging mode: A particular arrangement of equipment components and controls that causes smoke removal from within a space or spaces without circulating it to other spaces.

Smoke zone: An area separated from other areas by walls and doors to prevent the spread of smoke to or from adjacent smoke zones.

Sprinklers: A system of piping containing water under pressure and sprinkler heads designed to automatically trip at the presence of heat, thus spraying water on a fire.

Standpipes: Vertical piping containing water under pressure with valved hose outlets at strategic locations for use by personnel in fighting fires.

Step-down: Care for patients who need monitoring but not intensive, direct viewing; return to ward patients from ICU/CCU.

Tertiary care: Most specialized medical care available, including advanced surgery, neurology, internal medicine, ophthalmology, radiologists, and similar "board-certified" specialist care; receives referred patients from primary and secondary care facilities and includes a teaching program or major affiliation; examples are university medical school hospitals and large private institutions.

Thoracic and vascular surgery: Surgery on vital organs of the chest and vascular system.

Two-pipe system: A system that utilizes one heat transfer coil for both heating and cooling. Chilled water is supplied to the coil during hot weather, and hot water is supplied during cold weather. The water is changed from cold to hot in the fall and from hot to cold in late spring. The disadvantage is that one cannot switch back and forth between heating and cooling; only one is available at any time.

Unit heater: A direct heating, prefabricated assembly including a heating element, a fan driven by an electric motor, and an air outlet.

Urology: Diagnosis and treatment of the urinary system and the male reproductive system; subspecialties include fertility, sterility, reconstructive surgery, oncology, infectious disease, and renal (kidney) surgery.

Utility services: A term used to describe the main utility services to a building from a larger system owned by a municipality or utility company. These services include electrical power, water, sanitary sewer, storm drainage, natural gas, and telephone.

Water treatment: Chemical treatment of water to prevent corrosion or the growth of bacteria and algae in mechanical equipment and piping.

Bibliography

AAHA Chart of Accounts. Lakewood, CO: American Animal Hospital Association Press, 2002.

AAHA Standards for Veterinary Hospitals, www.aahanet.org/web/practice_accred.html.

Architectural Graphic Standards. Washington, DC: American Institute of Architects.

Beyond the Successful Veterinary Practice: Succession Planning and Other Legal Issues, by Thomas E. Catanzaro, Robert W. Deegan, and Edward J. Guiducci. Ames: Iowa State Press, 2000.

Building the Successful Veterinary Practice: Volume 1: Leadership Tools, by Thomas E. Catanzaro. Ames: Iowa State Press, 1997.

Building the Successful Veterinary Practice: Volume 2: Programs and Procedures, by Thomas E. Catanzaro. Ames: Iowa State Press, 1998.

Building the Successful Veterinary Practice: Volume 3: Innovation and Creativity, by Thomas E. Catanzaro. Ames: Iowa State Press, 1998.

Design Starter Kit for Veterinary Hospitals, 3rd ed., by Thomas E. Catanzaro. Lakewood, CO: American Animal Hospital Association Press, 1996.

General Standards of Construction and Equipment for Hospital and Medical Facilities. Oakbrook Terrace, IL: Joint Commission on Accreditation of Healthcare Organizations.

Healthcare of the Well Pet, by Thomas E. Catanzaro and Caroline Jevring. New York: Saunders Company, 1999.

Life Safety Code. Quincy, MA: National Fire Protection Association, 2000.

Minimum Requirements of Construction and Equipment for Hospital and Medical Facilities. Hyattsville, MD: U.S. Department of Health, Education, and Welfare, Public Health Service, Health Resources Administration, DHEW (HRA) Publication No. 79-14500, 1979.

National Building Cost Manual. Carlsbad, CA: Craftsman Book Company, 2002.

Promoting the Human-Animal Bond in Veterinary Practice, by Thomas E. Catanzaro. Ames: Iowa State Press, 2001.

Veterinary Healthcare Services: Options in Delivery, by Thomas E. Catanzaro, Thom Haig, Peter Weinstein, Judi Leake, and Heather Howell. Ames: Iowa State Press, 2000.

Veterinary Management in Transition: Preparing for the Twenty-First Century, by Thomas E. Catanzaro. Ames: Iowa State Press, 2000.

Veterinary Medicine & Practice: 25 Years in the Future and the Economic Steps to Get There, by Thomas E. Catanzaro and Terry H. Hall. Ames: Iowa State Press, 2002.

Veterinary Practice Management Secrets, by Thomas E. Catanzaro and Philip Seibert, Jr. Philadelphia: Hanley & Belfus, Inc., 2000.

Veterinary Practice Consultants® Signature Series® Monographs (www.v-p-c.com)

Client Relations Zone Operations (encompasses former Monograph, Recovered Pet Recovered Client, and has medical record audit forms on disk).

Compensation Strategies for a Client-Centered Quality Healthcare Delivery Team (with sample contracts; Doctor & Manager, Assessment tests, benefit & survey tables, and more on diskette).

Feasibility of the Veterinary Specialty Practice (includes sample business plan on disk).

Fundamental Money Management for the Veterinary Practice (with QuickBooks® Chart of Accounts diskette and sample budgets).

Fundamental Operations of a Critical Care Practice (includes diskette with basic operating plan & QuickBooks® file).

High Tech Needs High Touch in Program Delivery (includes feasibility and planning forms for realistic assessment of investment on disk).

Internal Promotion Tips & Tricks for QUALITY Veterinary Practices (includes diskette with customizable client communication tools).

Keeping Controlled Drugs Under Control (self-inspection checklist, sample forms, disk).

Leadership Action Planner (includes action planning forms on disk).

Profit Center Management (2nd Edition, w/ budget planning template and 10 essential charts to track critical information, diskette).

Recovered Pet and Recovered Client Programs (includes Preferred Client Program, disk).

Staff Performance Planning and Goal Setting (includes sample performance plans, disk).

Staff Training and Orientation (w/orientation checklists, sample job descriptions, plus disk).

Strategic Response & Practice Positioning (includes Mission Focus worksheets on disk).

Veterinary Medical Records for Continuity of Care & Profit (includes sample forms on disk for customization)

Your Personal Veterinary Practice Marketing Review (includes marketing checklists, disk).

Zoned Systems & Schedules for Multi-Doctor Practices (includes high density, plus sample schedules on disk).

Index